AIDS
Today, Tomorrow

D1506967

AIDS
Today, Tomorrow

An Introduction to the
HIV Epidemic in America

Second Edition

ROBERT SEARLES WALKER

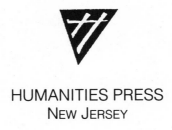

HUMANITIES PRESS
NEW JERSEY

First published in 1991 by Humanities Press International, Inc.,
Atlantic Highlands, New Jersey, 07716

Second edition published 1994, reprinted 1995

© Robert S. Walker, 1991, 1994

Library of Congress Cataloging-in-Publication Data
Walker, Robert Searles, 1930–
    AIDS — today, tomorrow : an introduction to the HIV epidemic in America /
Robert Searles Walker.—2nd ed.
       p.   cm.
    Previously published: 1991.
    This is an updated and revised ed.
    Includes bibliographical references and index.
    ISBN 0-391-03859-1
    1. AIDS (Disease)—United States. I. Title.
RC607.A26W35   1994
362.1'969792'00973— dc20

                               94-17975
                                CIP

A catalog record for this book is available from the British Library.

Printed in the United States of America

Contents

List of Illustrations

List of Tables

Preface

In 1985 I lost the first of many friends to AIDS. During the hours of visiting at the hospital, I tried to understand what was happening, to make some sense of it. Why should he have been so afflicted at so young an age, only twenty-seven? How was it that in medically advanced America, there was no effective treatment, much less a cure? Like most Americans, I grew up believing that we could deal effectively with all but the rarest ailments. But AIDS was becoming increasingly common, and it targeted youth—the age group that enrolled in my classes. By 1986 the Human Immunodeficiency Virus had already infected one out of every thirty American men between the ages of twenty and fifty. My friend's death led to a personal research effort as I sought answers.

In 1987 I was obliged to organize my general understandings of the epidemic. Biology Professor Richard Siegel (University of California at Los Angeles) invited me to give some lectures on the political and social aspects of the epidemic. Dr. Siegel was a pioneer in the development of general education, sexually transmitted diseases courses. His efforts in this field were, like mine, a personal response, but of a different sort. His children asked him why his college was not offering any general courses on a topic of increasing interest to those in their sexually active age group. They definitely wanted to know about AIDS—not as a problem of retrovirology—but as a problem confronting their lives. Dr. Siegel responded with an excellent and successful course at UCLA. In the process of preparing my lectures for that course, the themes of this book began to emerge. Overall, this book is the product of trying to make sense out of the tidal wave of death that was beginning to break over the nation—threatening my children, my students, and my friends.

The spread of the virus is uneven, both globally and within the United States. However, it will gradually spread everywhere. Although the focus of this book is on the national picture, I have used data from Texas, including my home city of San Antonio. I hope thereby to encourage readers *to look to their own areas*, their state and city health agencies and their communities for parallels and comparisons. The data can easily be obtained from state and local health departments. There is a strong tendency to shrug off the agonies and lessons of New York City and San

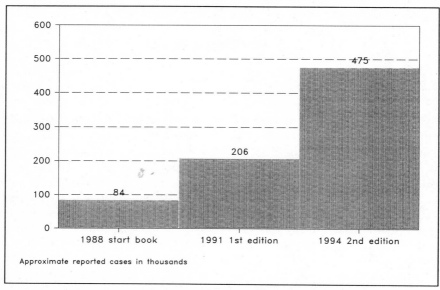

FIGURE P.1 Reported AIDS Cases and *AIDS: Today, Tomorrow*

Francisco as irrelevant to "our town." But they definitely are relevant! It is just a matter of time. The mid-1993 statistics indicated that the rate of AIDS cases increased in sixty-two cities by 10 or more per 100,000, while six cities posted gains of fifty to one hundred. Further, data from 1990 onwards indicate that the virus had begun to spread into our smaller cities and rural areas.

Since the first printing of this book in 1991, there have been significant increases in the reporting of AIDS cases both here and abroad. Under the 1993 revised definition of AIDS issued by the Federal Centers for Disease Control, the end of the 1993 recorded about 350,000 cases—a number that was originally projected for mid-1994. Thirteen states have registered a gain in their AIDS rate of five cases or more per 100,000, while San Francisco leads the nation with a rate of 280 per 100,000. The nation posted a gain in the overall rate from 17.6 cases to 32.4* and is currently recording about eight thousand new AIDS cases each month. AIDS has become the leading cause of death in men aged twenty-five to forty-four and one of the top five causes among women of the same age group.

With the dissolution of the Soviet empire and the establishment of more

---

* See Figures 3.7, 3.8, and Appendix 2. Part of the extraordinary increases registered in the 1993 data resulted from the use of a new and more inclusive definition of AIDS that commenced in January 1993.

open and honest governments, we are finally getting a peek at previously denied problems. Extraordinary increases in cases are being reported to the World Health Organization: Russia 271 percent, Bulgaria 133 percent, Poland 338 percent, and Romania 4,680 percent! Epidemiologists are recording an explosion of case reports from India, East Asia, and Latin America. In 1991, for example, Asian/Pacific infections were estimated at five hundred thousand; by 1994 that estimate had quadrupled. Similar figures are emerging in Latin America. The World Health Organization estimates conservatively that there are 14 million HIV infections globally, 3 million of which have progressed to the still-fatal AIDS.

As the AIDS epidemic grows, it will capture an increasing share of the nation's attention and resources. More people will be compelled to confront it intellectually and emotionally. If you assume that each Person with AIDS (PWA) relates to just five other people—family and friends—then the total intimately affected by the epidemic equals a substantial portion of our population. Even those not directly and personally affected will feel the impact as taxes, lost productivity, and other costs begin to mount. As President Clinton put it in his 1993 World AIDS Day Address, "For nearly every American with eyes and ears open, the face of AIDS is no longer the face of a stranger."

Willingly or otherwise, millions of people will be thinking about AIDS. The range of issues raised by the epidemic is extraordinary—from simple problems (avoiding infection), through tangled ones (the political difficulties of ensuring catastrophic health care), to the downright baffling (the complexities of vaccine development). It is my hope that this study, by viewing the epidemic from many different perspectives, will help concerned individuals to think about the problems raised by AIDS for themselves, their communities, their nation, and their world. Think about AIDS we must, for it is idle fantasy to imagine that any of us will be left untouched by the greatest biologic scourge of our time.

This is a brief introductory work. Like all of its kind, it must oversimplify—sometimes embarrassingly so. The epidemic is an exceptionally complex phenomenon in all its manifestations, from the nature of the virus itself to the epidemic's impact on our culture. In all cases I have tried to point the reader to more extensive treatments of whatever topic the text takes up. For example, chapter 2 renders a very generalized, elementary account of the life cycle of the virus, but the reader will find reference to more complex and comprehensive descriptions up to and including those from molecular biology and virology. I would have my readers regard each of the chapters as a door through which they can pass in order to view in greater detail, if they wish, some aspect of this far-reaching event.

I would like to thank my friend Esta Wolfram for her generous and significant assistance both in collecting data and in editing the text. Major Robert Munson, M.D. (USAF) enriched my data and journal files with a steady stream of medical bulletins and journals. Finally, my wife, Joyce, was always present with encouragement and constructive comments as *AIDS: Today, Tomorrow* progressed through its various incarnations.

San Antonio, Texas

1

AIDS: Plague or Epidemic? What's in a Word?

In 1976 Professor William McNeill published a challenging and provocative book, *Plagues and Peoples*, that explored the impact of epidemics in history. In his conclusion, he noted the progress made in containing such historic killers as the bubonic plague, smallpox, and cholera, but he cautioned his readers to remember that the biologic agents of epidemics are always with us; they never just go away. Medicines and public health measures may keep them at bay, but none have been eradicated. Further, he reminded:

> it is always possible that some hitherto obscure parasitic organism may escape its accustomed ecological niche and expose the dense human populations that have become so conspicuous a feature of earth to some fresh and perchance devastating mortality.[1]

You and I are living out the scholar's careful reservation. Events force us to face the truth that we are in the beginning throes of a major world epidemic attributable to an "hitherto obscure parasitic organism," the Human Immunodeficiency Virus (HIV). We must recapture a knowledge our ancestors knew well, namely, that epidemics are natural, recurring events, that we can seldom do more than guess at their duration or impact, and that we have very limited ability to contain them. The Acquired Immunodeficiency Syndrome (AIDS) precipitated by HIV is not the first, nor will it be the last, epidemic illness to afflict humanity. It is but one of the inescapable hazards that are part of life on Earth.*

The AIDS epidemic illness is the "devastating mortality" that Professor McNeill's words foreshadowed. It is sometimes referred to as a "plague" and sometimes as an "epidemic" in sermons, media accounts, and general

---

*This chapter is based on a series of lectures delivered in January 1988 to the sexually transmitted diseases class at the University of California at Los Angeles.

1

conversation. Should the semantics make a difference; are the terms synonymous? What's in a word?

Words, our choice of words, matter enormously. Words denote the objects or ideas that we are trying to convey. They also carry a hidden baggage of emotion and prejudice that quietly but decisively direct action. A word can be like the proverbial iceberg, nine-tenths underwater, unseen, and ten times more deadly for that![2] So many illustrations of this come to mind that it is hard to choose. Consider the words that we have stricken from the acceptable public vocabulary in only the last twenty-five years— "nigger," "kike," "wop," "broad," "spic," and (almost, but not quite) "queer or faggot." We are in the process of excising these words from our public speech because they co-opt thinking rather than promote it, they cloud rather than clarify debate, and they inflame emotions rather then engage the mind.[3]

An example of change in word-usage directly attributable to AIDS is the current trend to replace the word "sex" with the word "gender," even though this usage constitutes a malapropism. AIDS, a fatal sexually transmitted disease, has made probing discussion of sexual behavior, male-female sexual differences, and sexual risks—indeed, the whole world of sex—not only commonplace, but necessary. This is in a society with a historic, religious-based aversion to direct portrayals or discussion of sex! Increasingly the response is to cushion the impact on our internal guilt-centers by using what is perceived to be a "softer," less direct, less threatening word, a polite word usable in the drawing room. So now we speak of gender differences, gender risks, gender behaviors. I suppose that eventually the classic "War between the Sexes" will become the "War of the Genders" and sexual intercourse will become "physically intimate gender-relating."

To be sure, there is a wryly amusing aspect to this as we reflect on the fads and foibles of our culture. On the other hand, it is wise to keep in mind that laughter alone may be a rather superficial reaction; behind the semantic usages and issues are deeper ones relating to our perception of society, deity, and of ourselves as members of a sexual species, issues about which we have always fought with both ballots and bullets.

How do such considerations apply to choosing a designation for AIDS— "plague" or "epidemic?" All the great mortalities of the past were known by one or the other term. For example, the devastation caused by *Yersinia pestis* has always been called the bubonic plague, and the havoc wrought by the *Vibrio Cholerae* is referred to as a cholera epidemic. We speak of a "plague" of locusts but of an "epidemic" of measles. The ancient curse is "A plague on both your houses!"—never "an epidemic." For AIDS, the emphatic choice must be "epidemic." AIDS is an *epidemic*, not a plague.

Why? What's in a word? Is it much ado about nothing? AIDS was quickly labeled a plague, although previous twentieth-century visitations (cholera in 1900, Spanish flu in 1918, and infantile paralysis) were all called epidemics. Is it just a matter of contemporary versus traditional usage? No, not really. The truly classic words used to name these terrible events were "pestilence" or "mortality." Perhaps we distinguish between "plagues" and "epidemics" based on their relative prowess as killers. There is, after all, a sense hovering around the word "plague" that suggests something extraordinarily deadly and fearsome. But truthfully, it requires a worst-case, long-term scenario for AIDS to match past mortalities. Cholera killed seven million people in the first twenty years of this century and struck again in 1960; there are current serious outbreaks in Africa, Asia, and South America, some of which involve new and deadly cholera strains. Complications from the Spanish flu killed approximately 20 million people in a mere two years after its outbreak in 1918. Smallpox, measles, typhus, and flu, which were introduced into the New World by the Spanish Conquistadores, killed 90 percent of the native population. Entire Indian civilizations simply disappeared, and the population dropped from 100 million to 10 million in just one hundred fifty years. Bugs conquered the New World for Spain; they changed the course of history, just as HIV promises to do today. Still, it is most unlikely that AIDS will match these historic mortality figures.[4]

So what *is* the difference between "plague" and "epidemic"? Clearly we do discriminate in our language. I would like to suggest that the discriminating criterion is subjective, not objective. Plague is a theological idea; it refers to an event that is imputed to God. In our emotional memory, plagues are terrifying, devastating, inescapable expressions of God's wrath and judgment. Those who die in them are targets, not victims; they are "Sinners in the Hands of an Angry God," to borrow Jonathan Edward's eighteenth-century sermon title. Epidemics, no matter how serious, pale into insignificance before direct manifestations of divine anger. The word "epidemic" is a term associated with the science of public health. Epidemics are understandable aspects of nature and are manageable with modern skills. People who die in them are unfortunate victims, not sinners. Epidemics come from a nonjudgmental "Nature," they arise from the lives of the people. Plagues come from God.[5]

The American media resurrected the fearsome label "plague" and applied it to AIDS. It is strange when you think of it—our encounters with the Spanish flu of 1918, polio, and more recently Legionaires Disease were never accorded that dread title. Why? If one keeps in mind the theological-political matrix, the answer seems obvious. A just and compassionate God would never strike a Christian nation fighting Barbarian Huns. He would never target children to suffer crippling paralysis and the embrace of an Iron Lung. Nor would he attack solid mainstream Americans meeting in patriotic convention. Thus those groups were visited by "epidemics."

AIDS was an entirely different matter. In the epidemic's opening years in America, its *visible* victims were male homosexuals living in New York City and San Francisco, "sinners" living in urban dens of iniquity.[6] The Western biblical heritage linked with the American agrarian tradition to generate a powerful ideology of condemnation and avoidance.[7] In 1986 the president of the Southern Baptist Association, clearly representing both traditions, proclaimed, "God created AIDS to show his displeasure into [sic] America's acceptance of the homosexual lifestyle." Baptist and Vatican orthodoxy met when Cardinal Kroll of Philadelphia pronounced the same judgment in 1987. Then American right-wing orthodoxy spoke through Patrick Buchanan, President Reagan's director of Media and Communication and later a major speaker at the 1992 GOP Convention, who told us that ". . . nature was finally exacting her price on homosexuals for having spilled their seed against her."[8] From the White House to millions of private houses, from thousands of pulpits, talk shows, news broadcasts, and editorials, AIDS was seen as God's punishment, a divine curse. It was semiofficially called the "Gay Related Immune Deficiency (GRID), or more bluntly, "The Gay Plague."[9]

Calling the AIDS epidemic a plague has the effect of indicting the ill, for in a plague the sick are not just sick, they are sinners. Illness itself is a mark of God's anger and is borne as a sign, a stigma, of that anger. The various signs, symptoms, or stigmata of affliction warn the righteous-well to shun the sick-sinner lest the contagion spread to them.[10] The plague mindset binds with tight theological knots the physical affliction and the putative moral failure. In biblical and medieval times lepers were made to bear signs, wear bells, and live in quarantined leprosaria. During plague times the Pope authorized special ceremonies of penance to cleanse the spiritual atmosphere of the sin that God was presumably attacking; victims of the bubonic plague desperately tried to conceal their affliction to avoid condemnation.[11] Today proposals are heard to quarantine and even brand HIV infected individuals with some public mark of their physical and moral affliction, their crime against nature.

However, as the theologian Alan Watts once pointed out, the only crime against nature is stupidity. People can and do get away with murder, but no person, no nation can escape the consequences of personal or public stupidity. A penalty is always assessed, and with little regard for constitutional notions of fair punishment. Early commentators on the epidemic ignored the fact that there is no such thing as a "gay" virus, one that targets people in terms of lifestyle or sexual preference. They ignored the clear international evidence that HIV kills men, women, and children of all ages and attacks all races, nationalities, religions, and lifestyles. Their stupidity helped pave the way for the spread of the Human Immunodeficiency Virus, the deadliest and most "equal opportunity" enemy we have ever faced.

The harm done by this revival of the plague mentality is incalculable. What's in a word? Words can heal; words can kill. In the AIDS epidemic, "plague" is a lethal, killer word. The mindset expressed by the word excused the slowness and weakness of governmental action at the national, state, and local levels. Because of it, churches failed to provide the leadership that we rightfully expect of them—namely compassionate understanding and voluntary community care. I was amazed to read in the *San Francisco Chronicle* a headline stating, "Some churches *begin* counseling on AIDS" (my emphasis). This article appeared in December 1987, four years after the problem was manifest in the Bay area. In that same period, San Antonio's Northside Christian Church asked a long-standing, active member of the congregation "to voluntarily refrain from attending our gatherings" when it was discovered that he was suffering from AIDS. He died without the support of the church he had long supported. Even ministers were not immune to the stigma and shunning. The Rev. Jimmy Allen, former pastor of San Antonio's large First Baptist Church and son of a former president of the 17 million-member Southern Baptist Convention, was discouraged from even attending church with his family when it was discovered that HIV was in the family. His wife had received an HIV contaminated blood transfusion in 1982 and later gave birth to two infected sons. After 1985, when the infection was discovered, none of them were welcome at church.[12] Interfaith efforts to address the epidemic in a helpful and compassionate way are still hamstrung by the notable absence of Catholic and Southern Baptist leaders.[13] As Rev. Allen put it, "Jesus was the first one to reach out and touch the lepers. Our churches haven't followed in the spirit of Christ." In times of crisis it becomes an obligation of the church and synagogue to lead, not run. Ignorance, fear, and the ancient doctrinal hatred of homosexuals flowed together to transform a deadly viral epidemic into an even deadlier "Gay Plague."

How downright stupid this can get was revealed, I think, after the post office issued the AIDS awareness stamp in December 1993. A San Antonio philatelic clerk, Randy Chittick, revealed that many collectors refused to buy the stamp even though it meant a break in their collection, saying, "They associate it with homosexuality and dirtiness." The owner of a stamp collector's shop commented, "people just don't want to see the AIDS stamp on their mail. They think people might get the wrong idea." One letter to a philatelic magazine lambasted the post office for issuing an immoral stamp and concluded, "I definitely will never purchase these stamps . . . let alone lick one."[14]

There was also a touch of wishful thinking on the part of mainstream Americans. After all, if AIDS was a judgment of God, then presumably the fate of the victims was deserved, and no extraordinary effort was called for to divert the calamity. President Reagan's budget officials resisted pressure to increase expenditures for AIDS-related programs, candidates in the 1984 elections totally ignored the developing crisis, and churches contented themselves with traditional moralizing. Average Americans went about their daily business encouraged in the false belief that, while AIDS was a sad affair, it was something that affected "them" not "us," and "they" (being undesirables anyway) were dispensable. In this heterosexual fantasy-world, thinking about AIDS as a plague to punish homosexuals seemed to divert the Grim Reaper from the front doors of most Americans.[15]

Finally, in the darkest recess of the mind, in Dante's deepest level of Hell (reserved for leaders found unworthy of his mandate to rule justly), another and most ugly thought keeps breaking through the eternal lake of ice. With fervor and consistency, Americans have been taught that homosexuality is a perverse disposition, demonic or psychiatric in origin, to challenge nature and offend the godly. If AIDS was commonly seen as divine retribution, then how many of our leaders believed that doing nothing was the appropriate response? What to do? Do nothing! Let God work his will; let the Reaper mow! For some, such an outcome might be seen as a way to help resolve the conundrums posed by homosexuality, drug abuse, and crime-ridden slums swarming with people of dubious pedigree and worth—an adaptation of Adolph Hitler's "Final Solution."[16]

But then the children began to die. The nation was compelled to face a thorny problem of the plague mentality—the problem of the "innocent victim."[17] How does a reasonable person explain away the fact that God's aim seemed a trifle imprecise? Why would sexually innocent children, non-IDU heterosexuals, women, hemophiliacs, health care workers, accident victims, and those who simply sought needed surgery get caught in the fire and brimstone of divine retribution?

Cyprian, Bishop of Carthage, commenting on the Great Plague that was devastating his Mediterranean world of the third century A.D., gave the classic answer:

> Many of us are dying in this mortality, that is many of us are being freed from the world. This mortality is a bane to the Jews and pagans and enemies of Christ; to the servants of God it is a salutary departure. As to the fact that without any discrimination in the human race, the just are dying with the unjust, it is not for you to think that the destruction is a common one for both the evil and the good. The just are called to refreshment, the unjust are carried off to torture; protection is more quickly given to the faithful, punishment to the faithless.[18]

Bishop Cyprian's position has a childlike simplicity. The rational mind cannot easily address it; it is a statement of faith. If you get sick and die, then it must be part of God's plan. Either you will be sent to hell for your transgressions, or called to heaven for your goodness. Since the human mind cannot know which will happen or why, it is best not to ask questions.

This "explanation" will hardly satisfy the modern mind. If we applied it consistently, then we should allow all who sicken from cholera, measles, flu, cancer, or the bubonic plague, to die and be done with it. All these afflictions and more were at one time viewed as expressions of God's judgment. Nonetheless, echoes of Cyprian's position, usually presented as objective analysis, appear frequently in the press. For example, here is the commentary of nationally syndicated columnist John J. Kilpatrick:

> I would treat AIDS for what it is: a disease that mortally afflicts a tiny fraction of the population whose willful behavior results in the infection. The fellow who dies of sodomy is no more special than the fellow who dies of two packs of cigarettes a day.[19]

Kilpatrick's position has a superficial appeal. He states that "This disease overwhelmingly is a disease that afflicts two classes—drug addicts and homosexual men." Both contract the disease through voluntary, dangerous behavior, and, consequently, there is no moral compulsion for society to exert itself unduly or feel much compassion.

Kilpatrick implies that his views are the result of objective analysis. Thus we can subject them to critical analysis. He is correct in stating that the spread of AIDS is partly traceable to the practice of sodomy, a word which today broadly denotes illegal oral or anal sex. There is little evidence that oral sex presents a major risk for the transmission of HIV; however, anal intercourse is another matter (see chapter 5). In the United States, anal intercourse has been a major mode of sexual expression in the homosexual community and a secondary mode in the heterosexual community. Historically anal intercourse has been a widespread technique of birth control, and today it is practiced, for example, in nations where for various reasons condoms are not readily available. There is absolutely no question that anal intercourse, without condom protection, is exceedingly dangerous in this age of AIDS. Kilpatrick is also correct in pointing to the use of unsterile needles among drug addicts as a significant path of transmission both here and in Europe. However, he is wrong to suggest that by eliminating these practices (or the people who practice them), the epidemic will be contained. It might be slowed, it will not be contained.

An enormous, frightening reservoir of possibly 14 million individuals around the globe are already HIV infected. The overwhelming majority of these were not infected through the behavior that offends Kilpatrick (see Figure 1.1).[20] Further, most of the infected are unaware of the danger to

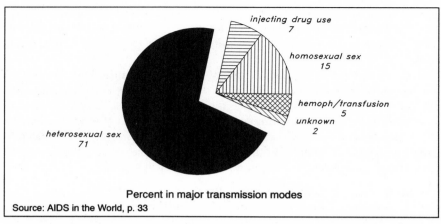

FIGURE 1.1 Global Adult AIDS (cumulative to 1992)

themselves or the danger they pose to others. These people undoubtedly will act as the source from which HIV can flow to the uninfected population. This is a fact of international life with AIDS. No one has formulated an acceptable policy to deal with it.

Another problem with the Kilpatrick analysis is the analogy drawn between smoking and lung cancer on the one hand and sodomy and AIDS on the other. He argues that both involve voluntary behaviors which, if stopped, would eliminate most of the problem. However, *the analogy is false.* AIDS is a communicable disease that can spread along several transmission routes; lung cancer is not. If all smoking stopped tomorrow, lung cancer would gradually become a rare ailment instead of the multibillion dollar medical problem it is today. If all heterosexual and homosexual anal intercourse ceased tomorrow, and if all addicts began using sterile equipment, the Human Immunodeficiency Virus would nonetheless continue its deadly way, multiplying and spreading. To be sure, its spread would be slowed and fewer people would be infected for a while, but the virus would remain undiminished in its virulence.

Finally we should never discount the capacity of HIV to mutate variants with more efficient modes of transmission. The flexibility in transmission enjoyed by *Yersinia pestis*, the agent of bubonic plague, should give us pause for thought in this regard. It was transmitted in three different ways. First, there was the standard form by which disease was carried to the human host by fleas from infected rats. This form had an incubation period of from two to seven days and a mortality rate of about 60 to 75 percent. Second, the rare septicemic system infection killed in a few hours, with 100 percent certainty—a person could go to bed healthy and die before waking.

Finally, there was the rarest and most dangerous mode from the standpoint of transmission and the only one that passed from human to human, that is, the pneumonic or airborne mode. This form, which could be transmitted in the droplets of a sneeze, was 100 percent fatal in less than 48 hours; pneumonic bubonic plague is considered the most dangerous of all bacteria-based human infections. The analogy between bacterium and virus cannot be carried too far, but my nightmare is that HIV will mutate the superbly efficient pneumonic form and become transmissible in the droplets of a cough or sneeze, like a flu virus or tuberculosis. The odds against such an event are great, and there is absolutely no evidence, I repeat, *absolutely no evidence*, that HIV has done so. On the other hand, there is absolutely no reason why it cannot. Luc Montagnier of France's Pasteur Institute and the discoverer of HIV and Robert Gallo of the National Institutes of Health, two of the world's leading virus researchers, disagree on the possibility that HIV might mutate a variant transmissible through casual behaviors like coughing or kissing. Montagnier thought it possible; Gallo thought it impossible. They agreed on "highly improbable" as a joint response to inquiries.[21] I think it would be criminally stupid to play the odds! The smart money is on research and more research. A genetic first cousin of HIV, the Simian Immunodeficiency Virus (SIV) has evolved an as yet rare variant that kills its monkey host in a mere six days, as compared with the many years it takes HIV to kill humans. Virologists have already identified seven strains or variants of HIV—all of which have different transmissibility characteristics as well as striking variations in virulence.[22]

Only at our peril dare we forget that the virus is a living entity. It will seek, like all living things, to assure its survival by evolving biomolecular strategies to nullify, compensate for, or circumvent the drugs or behavioral changes we use to thwart it.[23] If the Human Immunodeficiency Virus should mutate a casual or pneumonic form before we have completed our basic research into the virus and developed some effective countermeasures, then every human being on this planet will be staring down the throat of a biologic black hole.

It is at this point the true danger of such a view as Mr. Kilpatrick's become clear. If it prevails sufficiently to slow progress in research and treatment, we may all pay a dear price. However, notwithstanding its deficiencies and dangers, it is a position with great public appeal. This is not because of the facts or logic of it, but because it ties into our ancient plague mindset. The key phrase in the editorial is the phrase "a tiny fraction of the population." The fraction referred to is, of course, the "queers and junkies"—the undesirable and dispensable fraction of the population. Gallup polls show that about one half of the adult population is sympathetic to this position, and I suspect the number is actually much higher.

The poll results are undoubtedly affected by the fact that it is no longer considered good manners publicly to express one's prejudices. White prejudice against Blacks, Gentile prejudice against Jews, and heterosexual prejudice against homosexuals are all deeply rooted in Western culture; it is unlikely that they have been eradicated, though they may be concealed by current forms of polite discourse.[24]

Kilpatrick reveals the real origins of his position by invoking the ancient category of the innocent victim. He advises us to take care of the kids and leave the rest of those sinners to God, a position that at the end of the 1980s emerged as one of the most influential views effecting the AIDS funding policy of the national and state governments. If by "innocent" victim he means to indicate those who did not by knowing, voluntary action bring the affliction upon themselves, then we must care as much for the homosexual and the drug user as for infected wives, infants, hemophiliacs, and heterosexuals. The truth of the matter is that most of those who are sick and dying now were infected as long as a decade or more ago, when few were aware of the nature and danger of the Human Immunodeficiency Virus.[25] No one can be said to have voluntarily exposed themselves to AIDS at that time; it was unknown. Even by the plague mentality's own terms, most of those currently ill are "innocent victims."

The real mainspring of the plague position is revealed as old-fashioned hatred of homosexuals, a hatred that has been a festering boil on Western culture for millennia. This is supplemented by a disdain for those who use drugs other than those approved by the majority. For those with a more open and compassionate sensibility, it should be evident that a plague is a church event, not unlike a heresy trial. A plague is not the work of God; it is a negative and self-destructive interpretation of the work of God. This interpretation has spread its poison into all aspects of our national response to the appearance of HIV in America.

In November 1991 basketball superstar Magic Johnson revealed his infection and in doing so provided a striking illustration of the plague stigma's power. In an effort to minimize the damage that he would incur by going public, he and his publicists made a great point of stating that his infection was heterosexually acquired. Since, as they insisted, he was a straight, non-injecting drug user, his infection proved that "anyone" could get it. There was an outpouring of sympathy, and President Bush appointed him to the National AIDS Commission. Nonetheless, within three months he had lost all but one of his commercial sponsorships while fans, sports writers, and others in basketball were saying that he should stay off the courts—the course he chose after some hesitation.

One consequence of these stupidities has been that private and public funding for the care of those who are sick, except infants, has been hopelessly inadequate and slow to appear; the leadership of American society has simply dismissed the sick as dead and "deservedly" so. Government money is overwhelmingly funneled into research and hopefully preventive education. In Texas fully one third of the State House of Representatives refused to sign a resolution offered in memory of the thirty-five hundred Texans who have died of AIDS and in appreciation of the private community groups that had provided the care that the state withheld. The same legislature has also severely cut state grant funds supporting hospice and home day care for fear the money might fall into the hands of homosexual caregivers;[26] the result has been to force AIDS patients into the much more expensive, and less appropriate, hospital environment, or to deny terminal care altogether.[27] There is no question that our cultural prejudices, our homophobia in particular, have contributed to a slow and stupid response to the epidemic, a response that can be measured in deaths—a sad commentary upon a people who profess to honor Christ.[28]

Clearly, America desperately needs presidential leadership in order to effectively address the HIV epidemic. Only the White House pulpit has the power to neutralize the plague pulpits and give us the confidence to assay, fund, and fight the battle against AIDS. Given the strength of our cultural bigotries, the president must constantly remind the nation that it faces a public health emergency, an epidemic, not a religious crisis. The only moral dimension involved in this epidemic relates to the adequacy and compassion of our national response. For reasons time will sort out, President Ronald Reagan was unwilling to exert this kind of leadership; Congress forced his reluctant administration to develop the programs of the early years. Someone must have asked him, or perhaps he asked himself, "What should I do?" History records the answer, "Do nothing."

President George Bush was offered the challenge and opportunity to set an appropriate national tone and build a constructive government agenda to confront HIV. At a conference of the National Leadership Coalition on AIDS in March 1990, he did call for compassionate and nondiscriminatory care for the sick, but he stopped short of concrete proposals. It was a step, but just a step, in the right direction.[29] As the National Commission on AIDS pointed out, rhetoric had to be matched with funded programs.[30] However, even while the president spoke, the funds available from both private foundations and his administration to meet the various costs of providing care were, in fact, diminishing.[31] President Bush's proposed budget for fiscal 1993, when amounts are corrected for inflation, incorporate still further cutbacks in research funding. In fact, he never did seize the many opportunities to move beyond rhetoric. His words remained just that, words; policy remained in the Reagan mold. It was left to his successor in office, President

Clinton, to lead as presidents should.

Properly considered, I am not talking about presidential inclinations, preferences, or policy choices, but rather the most important of presidential responsibilities. Decisions on the budget, the make-up of the weapons system, the funding of Medicare, and the like, can be and are made by many competent people in authority. However, only the president of the United States, who is our Head of State, can lead the entire nation down constructive paths. We distinguish our great leaders from the merely competent ones by their willingness and ability to educate the public in attitudes and policies that, in the long term, will benefit the commonwealth—not Republicans or Democrats—but the whole people. George Washington set the precedent for this overriding presidential responsibility in his "Farewell Address to the Nation," and we have measured our leaders by their success in building upon this foundation. President Roosevelt, in his "Quarantine Speech" of 1937, warned Americans that, whether they liked it or not, they could not isolate themselves from the affairs of the world. It was an unpopular message, one that a large segment of the nation did not want to hear. By leading the way, he inspired a massive public educational effort, joined by ministers, journalists, educators, and all ranks of public officials, to wean the public away from its foolish and self-destructive isolationist position. He began preparing the public mind for the events that would tragically unfold in the Japanese bombardment of Pearl Harbor. After the battlefield conclusion of World War II, Winston Churchill set the tone for Western public attitudes toward Stalin's Soviet Union with his famous "Iron Curtain" speech. John Kennedy in his Inaugural and "Berlin Wall" addresses defined fundamental American domestic and international positions in an increasingly dangerous world—a world that held its breath during the Cuban missile crisis. Now it is Bill Clinton's turn to lead the way; his opportunity to move beyond competence to greatness (see chapter 6).

Of course, the deadly virus will not be contained by words alone, even healing presidential words. People, facilities, and money must all be mobilized and targeted, and we all must do what we can to create and administer enlightened national, state, and local policy. But as the chairman of Levi Strauss & Co. so rightly observed, our best efforts will be of little avail "if there is darkness in the White House."[32] President Clinton must do the job that only a president can do; he must help the nation see the "Demon Plague" for what it is—a dangerous religious throw-back to our past, which serves only to confuse and frustrate the present.

Notes

1. Professor William H. McNeill, an eminent historian at the University of Chicago, is the author of many noted books among which is *Plagues and Peoples* (New York: Anchor, 1976), 289. At the point of my quotation from Professor McNeill's book, he refers to Richard Fiennes, *Man, Nature and Disease* (London, 1964), 124, which projects possible population die-offs in case of the spread of new agents.
2. S. I. Hayakawa, Language in Action (New York: Harcourt, Brace & Co., 1941).
3. One of the more interesting rhetorical-political developments in this area has been the deliberate and provocative use of the term "queer" by one of the major confrontational gay lobbying groups, Queer Nation. By this device they call attention to their outcast status and pointedly reject the negative connotations of the term as used by the straight community.
4. McNeill, *Plagues and Peoples*, chap. V.
5. Consider the structure of the word epidemic. Epi, from, prefixed to Demos, people. An epidemic is of and from the people.
6. By the early 1980s HIV had made major inroads into the injecting drug user population in New York City, but the members of this group were, and largely still are, "invisible" to middle-class America, including its epidemiological and journalistic investigators. Social workers whose work took them into the slums, the crack houses, and so on, were aware of serious illnesses but attributed them to drug effects.
7. An ideological tradition deeply imbedded in the American mind, which goes back through Jefferson to Rousseau, asserts that virtue resides in the plain country folk who make their living by honestly tilling the good earth. The city is viewed with suspicion as a place of corruption, venality, and sin. In the fight over repeal of prohibition in Oklahoma, for example, the "dry" ministers warned their parishioners that Oklahoma would become "like New York City" if prohibition were repealed. See: Robert S. Walker and Samuel C. Patterson, *Oklahoma Goes Wet: The Repeal of Prohibition in Oklahoma* (Eagleton Institute, Cases in Practical Politics, Rutgers, The State University; New York: McGraw Hill, 1960). For a good discussion of the interrelationship of the AIDS epidemic and American church establishments see Albert R. Jonsen and Jeff Stryker (eds.), *The Social Impact of AIDS in the United States* (Washington, D.C.: National Academy Press, 1993), chap. 5.
8. See: Paul Monette, *Borrowed Time: An AIDS Memoir* (New York: Harcourt, Brace, Johanovich, 1988).
9. The Centers for Disease Control, early in the epidemic, used the term Gay-Related Immunodeficiency Disease, or "GRID." The media shortened it to the more dramatic "Gay Plague." The English experience was remarkably parallel to the American. Peter Aggleton and Hilary Thomas, *Social Aspects of AIDS* (London: Falmer Press, 1988).
10. Susan Sontag, *AIDS and Its Metaphors* (New York: Farrar, Straus & Geroux, 1988).
11. The old nursery rhyme we all learned as children, "Ring around the Rosy, / Pockets full of posies / Ashes, ashes, / All fall down," is a grim expression of this. "Ring around the rosy" refers to the physical appearance of the pustules that erupted on the skin of the infected. "Posies" were the aromatic herbs the

infected carried in an attempt to disguise the sick smell emitted by the boils. "Ashes" refers to the practice of burning clothing, bedding, and sometimes the victim. Finally, "All fall down"—in the end, death conquered.

12. *San Antonio Express-News*, September 13, 1992, "Minister vs. AIDS Prejudice," p. 1, 13a.

13. "Religious Leaders Exhorted to Press U.S. on AIDS Crisis," *New York Times*, December 5, 1989, A14. This article is a report on a large interfaith meeting in Atlanta at the Carter Presidential Center.

14. Mary Sabota, "AIDS Awareness Stamp Getting Mixed Reviews from Philatelists," *San Antonio Express-News*, February 6, 1994, 1B.

15. The fundamentalist American Council of Christian Churches, which claims to speak for 2 million people, asserts the plague mentality forcefully and without qualification. However, many churches find themselves caught between the pull of classic plague doctrine and a more contemporary view. The Bishops of the Catholic Church, meeting at their national conference in Baltimore, November 1989, issued ambiguous statements reflecting the apprehension that, if they flatly denied divine authorship of the epidemic, they might thereby open the door to more basic questions as to God's intervention in mundane affairs. Doctrinal conservatives of all faiths generally shied away from any statement that could be construed as a departure from the traditional position of "homosexuality as sin," even if it produced the logical, if questionably Christian, result that they approved the epidemic as an instance of divine retribution. After all, how can one not approve of divine action of any kind? Heresy lurks in such questioning. Various polls indicate that at least 25 percent of the population will admit to the "divine retribution" view. See the *New York Times* Service report which appeared in various newspapers on November 19, 1989 relating some of these conflicts of conscience. Also see J. Gordon Melton's, *The Churches Speak on AIDS* (Santa Barbara, Calif.: Institute for the Study of American Religion, 1989). Melton is the director of the Institute.

16. For those whose first reaction to this conjecture is to dismiss it out-of-hand, I would suggest several works: James H. Jones, *Bad Blood: The Tuskogee Syphilis Experiment* (New York: Free Press, 1981), 17–48. Jones examines the theories of racial inferiority that were used to justify the use of Blacks in syphilis medical experimentation. For example, nineteenth-century White physicians explained the high rate of syphilis in the Black population on the ground that Blacks were immoral and promiscuous (exactly the perception of gays today). Black vice, in turn, reflected the fact that "personal restraints on self-indulgence did not exist because the smaller brain of the Negro had failed to develop a center for inhibiting sexual behavior." On the AIDS epidemic as seen by one of the most important gay activists in the nation, see Larry Kramer, *Reports from the Holocaust: The Making of an AIDS Activist* (New York: St Martin's Press 1989). And finally, Evelynn Hammond's provocative article, "Race, Sex, AIDS, the Construction of the 'Other,'" *Radical America* 20, no. 6 (November/December 1986): 28–38.

There is a strong feeling within the more activist AIDS groups that a political-biomedical decision was made early in the epidemic to dedicate most federal research money to basic research and the discovery of a "complete cure"—thus the emphasis on the development of nucleoside analogues (like AZT) which disrupted the replication of the virus. This decision was made even though biomedical science has never produced a "complete cure" for an infection wherein the virus is able to integrate its genetic materials into the human cellular genome. Infection in such cases—HIV, herpes, and hepatitis—is chronic and permanent. The "find-a-cure" strategy (which clearly has failed, at least as of 1994) shortchanged and slowed the development of palliative/management treatments for the bacterial and fungal diseases which develop in late-stage HIV infection, and thus condemned hundreds of thousands (of mostly "dispensable" gay men and IDUs) to a difficult and foreshortened life.

17. For example, the story of little Celeste Garrian, who died at the age of twelve in 1989, after having been born with AIDS in 1977 and having suffered the affliction her entire life. She survived longer than any other child born with AIDS. Bruce Lambert, *New York Times*, November 7, 1989, 1.

18. Cyprian, *De Mortalitate* (Hannon translation) as quoted in McNeill, *Plagues and Peoples*, 122.

19. *San Antonio Express-News*, June 1988.

20. Dieter Koch Weser and Hannelore Vanderschmidt, eds., *The Heterosexual Transmission of AIDS in Africa* (Cambridge, Mass.: ABT Books, 1988).

21. Robert Gallo, *Virus Hunting—AIDS, Cancer, and the Human Retrovirus: A Story of Scientific Discovery* (New York: Basic Books 1991), 232–33.

22. For example, Dr. David Ho, a leading HIV researcher, has found that only one class of virus could transmit by sexual contact, but once inside the body quickly mutated into noninfectious but more deadly forms. *San Antonio Express-News*, August 28, 1993, 18a. For a discussion of variations in the lethal characteristics of various HIV strains, see the article "HIV Tropism," by John Moore and David Ho, in *Nature*, January 28, 1993.

23. HIV has already developed an effective resistance to the drug AZT, which has been the "first-line of defense" to the progression of infection to AIDS. Another disturbing development is the resurgence of old diseases, like syphilis and measles, in new resistant forms. Brian Goldman, "'Old' Diseases Stage a Comeback—And Its Not Child's Play This Time," *Observer* (American College of Physicians) 9, no. 10, (November 1989): 1.

24. R. J. Blendon, et al. (Harvard AIDS Institute, Harvard School of Public Health) "Discrimination Against People with AIDS: A Public's Perspective," *New England Journal of Medicine* 319 (October 13, 1988): 1022–26. A. Comfort, "AIDS: Public Panic," *Journal of the Royal Society of Medicine* 81, no. 10 (October 1988): 618. This destructive mentality is clearly fostered in the nation's influential evangelical ministry. TV preachers such as Jimmy Swaggart, Oral Roberts, Jerry Falwell, and Pat Robertson earnestly preach the plague-mindset position, and their followers dutifully reflect their position. See the August 31, 1987 Gallup Report on public attitudes toward AIDS sufferers which pinpoints "Evangelicals and those who have not completed high school as the groups most likely to see AIDS as a punishment from God."

25. D. Huminer, J. B. Rosenfeld, "AIDS in the Pre-AIDS Era," *Review of Infectious Diseases* 9 (1987): 1102-1108.

26. As an example, The Texas Department of Health refused to renew the funding for the Dallas AIDS Resource Center's free food bank because the center is operated by the Dallas Gay Alliance. *Austin American-Statesman*, January 4, 1990, A1.

27. *San Antonio Express-News*, Kay Northcott's Comment, "AIDS Bill Emphasizes Criminality," May 19, 1989.

28. John Davide Dupree, and Glen Margo, "Homophobia, AIDS and the Health Care

Professional," *FOCUS: A Guide to AIDS Research* (San Francisco, Calif.: The AIDS Health Project of the University of California San Francisco, 1988).

29. *New York Times*, March 30, 1990, A1. The membership of the National Leadership Coalition on AIDS consists of the executives of large businesses.

30. See the *Report of the National AIDS Commission*, December 1989, which challenges the president to "match rhetoric with action."

31. Marisa Venegas and Tom Watkins, "AIDS Funders of Last Resort Cutting Community Services," *Medical Tribune, International Medical News Weekly*, January 11, 1990, 1. See *New York Times*, "AIDS Groups Are Worried by Looming Fiscal Crisis," May 6, 1990, 19.

32. *New York Times*, March 30, 1990, A1. Remarks of Robert D. Haas, Chairman of Levi Strauss & Co., at the meeting of March 29, 1990, sponsored by the National Leadership Coalition on AIDS.

2

Parasites and People: Cohabitors of Earth

THE HUMAN IMMUNODEFICIENCY VIRUS

Webster's Collegiate Dictionary defines a parasite as "a plant or animal living in, on, or with, some other living organism at whose expense it obtains food, shelter, or the like." We all "live in, off, or with" some other organism—the parent and child relationship, for example. The key element of the definition is the phrase "at whose expense." There is the feeling that parasites somehow take without giving and that the relationship between host and parasite is unilateral and possibly destructive. If the parasite has made any positive contribution, it must be on the very broad level of evolutionary development. Parasites come in all shapes and sizes—mistletoe, ticks, mosquitoes, *Y. pestis*, and our own human immunodeficiency virus. The character of the parasitism also varies. Some use the host for support and shelter, others for food, others for some phase of their life cycle, and for still others the host is their total environment. HIV-1 and HIV-2 are retroviral intracellular microparasites that spend their entire life cycle in the human host. Their classification as parasites stems from the fact that they use their genetic templates to convert the cellular activity of key human cells into a process that replicates viral cells. In effect, they are able to convert our cells into surrogate mothers giving birth to an ever increasing quantity of HIV cells; in approximately thirty viral generations (about four to six weeks) following infection, HIV will replicate about 1 billion copies of itself. It is worth emphasizing that our virus is *our* virus, it is the *Human Immunodeficiency Virus*. Even the virus' genetic structure overlaps ours.[1] HIV does not naturally occur in any other animal.[2]

When HIV came to the notice of the Western world, it inspired the usual cold war, conspiracy, and extraterrestrial theories of origin. Soviet KGB agents spread rumors in Africa that it was a genetically engineered product of American biological warfare distributed by the CIA as part of a racist war

17

against Black Africans. The theme has been picked up by several American groups, one of which, for a $29.95 video, will "document" the whole conspiracy and tell you how you can escape impending doom by following its advice. One of the more intriguing theories was that HIV made its earthly debut riding on a comet from outer space.[3] Dr. Robert C. Gallo of the National Cancer Institute suggested in 1987 that it might have been a mutation, several times removed, of a similar virus infecting the African Green Monkey, *Cercopithecus aethiops*, which may have cross-infected a human at some time. The green monkey is hunted for food in Central Africa, so a cross-infection was possible.[4] Research following up Gallo's suggestion indicated that the etiology of HIV was more complex. Although HIV and SIV (Simian Immunodeficiency Virus) did have much in common, advancing research made it seem at least as likely that SIV was a mutation of the human virus or that both evolved from a preexisting virus.[5]

More recently, Dr. Charles Gilks of Oxford proposed that people inoculated with fresh monkey blood in a series of malaria control experiments in the period from 1920 to 1950 might have received the progenitor of today's HIV.[6] There has also been speculation that HIV could have been a byproduct of testing oral polio vaccine in Africa during the late 1950s. Indicating, I suppose, that everyone can get into the act of theorizing about HIV's origins, a major article in this debate appeared in *Rolling Stone*, a magazine not usually considered as being on the cutting edge of biological science.[7] When discussions of the origin of HIV arise, the air is generally full of "could have beens" and "might have beens"—sometimes I am reminded of the endless "explanations" of President Kennedy's assassination.

It is probable that HIV appeared as a human pathogen sometime in the last one hundred years.[8] However, it may well be that scientists will never pin down the precise time, area, and mode of its appearance. This should not be surprising; we cannot produce birth certificates for the polio virus, the malaria plasmodium, the blastomycosis fungi, or most of the other nasty organisms that prey upon us. Scientists have been debating the origin of the syphilis spirochete for over fifty years without resolution. Disease agents have been around at least as long as we have. In any case, although the mad scientist manufacturing death for the planet, like Dr. Doom of the Spiderman comic strip, is part of our fantasy world, he is not part of our scientific and rational world. A nature capable of evolving an organism as complex as each of us is quite capable of churning out viruses by the bucketful.

The beginning point for understanding the cataclysm we call an epidemic is the concession that, from the standpoint of the natural world, it is not cataclysm at all. It is just another event like an earthquake, a volcanic eruption, or the birth or death of a star or a species. Writers have awarded our species many designations, most of them complimentary (man the tool maker, the risen ape, and so on), conceding pride of place only to God. Whatever else we are, it is clear that we are the most egotistical species. Because we generally believe that the universe revolves around us, we often forget that the first law of organic nature is that there is no such thing as a free lunch. Even though we are evolution's most successful, top-of-the-line predator, still, we cannot eat without being eaten.

TABLE 2.1 Human Diseases

VIRAL DISEASES		BACTERIAL DISEASES	
DISEASE	USUAL MODE OF TRANSMISSION	DISEASE	USUAL MODE OF TRANSMISSION
Smallpox	Airborne	Pneumonias	Airborne
Measles	Airborne	Diphtheria	Airborne
Influenzas	Airborne	Tuberculoses	Airborne
Mononucleosis	Oral contact	Lyme disease	Ticks
Enteroviruses (65 types)	Stool/hand/mouth	*Salmonella*	Stool/hand/food
Hepatitis B NonA/nonB	Stool/hand/mouth Transfusion	Leprosy	Prolonged close contact
Warts	Skin to skin	*Staphylococci*	Open wounds
Arboviruses	Mosquitoes, ticks	Bubonic plague	Fleas, airborne
Herpes simplex	Sexual contact	Gonorrhoea	Sexual contact
Cytomegalovirus	Sexual contact	Syphilis	Sexual contact
HIV-associated diseases (including AIDS)	**Sexual contact, *in utero*, transfusion**	Cholera and typhus	Contaminated water

Masters of all we survey, we tend to ignore what we cannot see, a humble, infinitesimally small virus quite capable of destroying us in the process of reproducing itself. The virus stands at the beginning step of life while we stand at the complex end of it; it is humbling, or should be. We are in the initial stages of a world epidemic that has the potential of reversing past trends of global population growth and collapsing third-world

economies.[9] Balanced perspective begins with understanding that this epidemic is a natural event, with the concession that HIV is part of nature just
as we are, that it has a role in the unimaginably intricate chain of being just
as we do, and that it is very unlikely that either of us will eradicate the other.
Our problem is to find a way of living with the virus, instead of dying from
it. A good place to start is to see HIV as just one among many organisms
that live in, on, or with us. The illustrative list in Table 2.1 is meant merely
to display some of the popularly known microbes with a taste for you and
me and to place HIV in company with its companions. Table 2.1 contains
some of the common assaults upon our species. It ignores many rare, but
deadly "assaults" such as the Viral Hemorrhagic Fevers, or widespread debilitating ones like Schistosomiasis, endemic in the fresh water of many nations.
The point to be emphasized is that we are the preferred environment for a
long list of bugs. Like it or not we are *part of* the chain of existence. The HIV
is dramatically reminding us of that fact of life.

Although it is not unique in targeting a human host, HIV is certainly the
most dangerous and insidious viral enemy we have ever faced.[10] Prior to
1981 it was just a suspicion, an apprehension that there was "something out
there"; physicians and epidemiologists in Africa, Europe, and America were
recording a puzzling new collection of ailments that defied classification and
resisted all medical interventions. In 1981 five cases *Penumocystis carinii*
pneumonia (PCP) and twenty-six cases of Kaposi's sarcoma (KS) were
reported to the Centers for Disease Control; both afflictions were medically
known, but rare. All cases were in homosexual men from New York and
California; unnoticed in the early years of the epidemic (because of their
"social invisibility"), there were also many cases of HIV infection among East
Coast IV-drug users. In 1982 the CDC officially classified a new collection
of clinical conditions, as a syndrome, and began monitoring a now officially
recognized illness. Later a separate classification was established for children. The first cases of hemophiliac and transfusion infections were also
recorded in 1982. Still, no one knew what was causing the newly observed
health problems and deaths. Then in 1983 Luc Montagnier, leading a team
of scientists at France's Pasteur Institute, isolated a virus believed to be the
cause of the collection of illnesses observed, a virus eventually named the
Human Immunodeficiency Virus. The French discovery was supported by
findings from America's National Cancer Institute.[11] Finally, in 1983 the first
cases of heterosexual male to female cases were discovered. By this time,
HIV, spreading quietly for at least forty years, had infected as many as 10
million people worldwide, and at least one million Americans.[12]

HIV is an approximately round retrovirus of about one ten-thousandth of
a millimeter in diameter. The skin, envelope, or surface membrane has

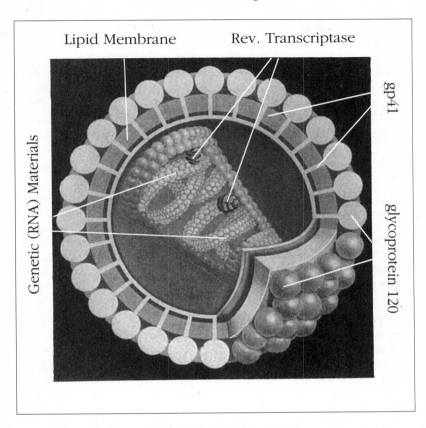

FIGURE 2.1 Structural Model of HIV

Source: Jose Esparza, "Prospects for a Vaccine," *World Health: The Magazine of the World Health Organization,* October 1989, p. 10.

molecular spikes (glycoproteins 120 and 41) that enable it to attach to and fuse with human cells having CD4 molecular receptors on their envelope surface (Figure 2.1).[13] HIV's membrane surrounds a dense inner core containing various protein molecules, enzymes, and amino acids. When the virus encounters a human cell with CD4 receptors, it attaches itself and then disgorges its genetic materials into the host cell. Upon infecting a cell, HIV commences a process that replicates the virus while eventually destroying or functionally disrupting the host cell. Over a period of time, the process of viral replication so seriously compromises the system that survival itself is threatened. AIDS is our first experience with a viral-based primary immune-regulating illness. HIV's life cycle directly assaults the very walls that nature has constructed over the aeons of hominid evolution to protect us against bacterial and viral invaders.[14]

The virus is sensitive to its environment. It thrives and is exceedingly tough in its natural environment—our circulatory system—but is fragile outside of it. Contact with air, for example, is fatal, though how rapidly depends upon environmental circumstances. Fortunately a wide range of common materials like household detergents, bleach, alcohol, iodine, hydrogen peroxide, and even human saliva are toxic to it.[15] A good deal of public misunderstanding relating to the probabilities of transmission and the possibilities of developing a vaccine stem from the virus' dual, "tough but fragile" character.[16]

HIV has a family and a life cycle. It is part of the lentivirus branch of a larger family group known as retroviruses; the prefix *lenti* expresses the fact that members of this branch produce an infection which develops very slowly—in the case of HIV, over many years. It is one of about fourteen genetically related microbes that trace their ancestry back over millions of years, perhaps to some common origin. Actually HIV is not one virus, but two: HIV-1—a species that has seven known subtypes (called A-F, and O) with hundreds of strains characterized by varying virulence and transmissibility characteristics[17]—and HIV-2. They are closely related and produce similar results, although it appears that HIV-2 (found mostly in West Africa) is somewhat less pathogenic and less likely to be transmitted mother to child. In this book, I will simplify the matter by simply referring to "HIV" and ask the reader to understand that I am mostly referring to HIV-1 (subtype B), which accounts for the overwhelming majority of American infections.[18] All members of the lentivirus family seem to have one common characteristic— they make whatever animal they inhabit very sick, whether it be cattle, horses, sheep, chickens, reptiles, mice, monkeys, or your pet cat. Many of them produce in animal hosts effects similar to those which HIV produces in us. For example, here is a description of Feline Immunodeficiency Virus (FIV) disease (infecting about 5 percent of the cat population) from the Bexar County Veterinary Medical Association:

> FIV infection occurs in two stages. During the initial stage, many FIV-infected cats appear healthy. Therefore, many cats go through Stage I with the disease unnoticed by their owners. Generally problems are not detected until Stage 2 when the immune system weakens and other infections occur. Common signs during Stage I are enlargement of lymph nodes, fever, poor coat condition, and lethargy. During Stage 2 there is often loss of appetite, weight loss, persistent diarrhea, oral lesions or sores, and skin, urinary and upper respiratory infections. Adult free-roaming male cats are at the highest risk for FIV because they tend to fight other cats. . . . There is no evidence to suggest that FIV can be transmitted from cats to humans.[19]

This could almost pass for a simplified version of Human Immunodeficiency Virus disease; for what its worth, we are not alone.

HIV'S LIFE CYCLE AND THE TACTICS OF COMBAT

Since its isolation in 1983, retrovirologists have traced the stages of HIV's life cycle in considerable detail. It is important to have some general understanding of the process because it is on the foundation of this knowledge that our strategies of prevention, cure, or treatment must rest. The technical language describing it is the arcane language of molecular biology; understanding that what follows is gross oversimplification, allow me to cast the process as occurring in four stages and in terms of familiar images (see Figure 2.2).[20]

Stage 1, Injection: Imagine that HIV is a small boat of guerrilla raiders launched sometimes by you, sometimes by others, into the river of your bloodstream. HIV circulates in the currents of the bloodstream until it encounters a likely docking site. It can only dock at wharves the configuration of which match that of the boat. Various cell-wharves offer such facilities.[21] Stage 2, Infection: When the virus boat docks at an appropriate wharf, the raiders take over and unload their cargo of replication materials. Stage 3, Replication: The patrol leader (an enzyme called *reverse transcriptase*) directs the host cell's residents in building and stocking new boats for further raiding. Stage 4, Recapitulation: Finally, they launch the new, freshly provisioned boats into your bloodstream to start the process over again but this time in greater numbers. As parting thanks, they always disrupt and sometimes destroy the host cell.[22] Within the framework of these four stages it is possible to gain some appreciation for the incredible complexity of fighting the HIV.

INJECTION

The first stage, of course, involves the introduction of the virus into the bloodstream. Technically it is not a stage of infection, but the necessary prelude to infection. If the virus never enters a human cell, even though it is within the blood stream, then no infection takes place. This may seem an empty distinction, but it is critical in Stage 2, as we shall see. Injection of the virus into the bloodstream can occur as a result of carelessness in the handling of infected materials, just plain rotten luck as in a hospital accident, or culpable industrial negligence in the transfusion of blood or blood products. It can also result from another kind of transfusion such as when contaminated syringes or needles are used by injecting drug users (IDUs) . It can result from being born to infected parents. Finally HIV injection can result from unprotected (condomless) sex with an infected partner, male or female. Various other means of transmission have been suggested (kissing, insect

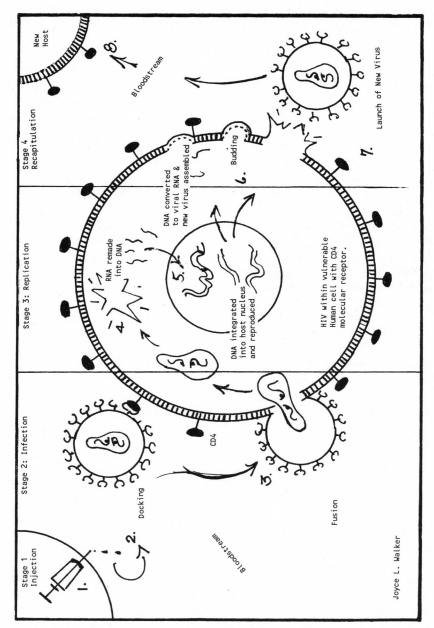

FIGURE 2.2   Life Cycle of HIV

bites, and toilet seats, for example). However, responsible research now resting upon literally hundreds of thousands of cases has failed to document these other routes. They are within the realm of theoretic possibility (see "The Hazards of Living," in chapter 5) but not life's real probabilities.[23]

Understanding there are occasional freak transmissions that cannot be anticipated, prevented, or classified, these various routes are the usual ones, and each requires different prevention strategies to prevent the initial infection. Minimization of blood transference in accident and health care situations can only be achieved through ongoing educational campaigns within the industry, and the provision of as much operational safety as is consistent with the job. Measures can range from hospital training seminars for paramedics, through the development of new protective materials, to rules requiring double-gloving in surgery. The health care industry is now acutely aware of the dangers, and new protocols and training programs are developing rapidly.[24] The general efficacy of protective procedures designed for health care workers is attested by the very small number worldwide who have been infected in the line of duty (see "The Hazards of Health Care," in chapter 4).[25] However, extra protection does not come free. Estimates in late 1990 put the additional health care costs at $337 million per year.[26]

Dr. Marcus Conant, a physician at the University of California, San Francisco School of Medicine, has published the recommendation that a physician suffering a needle stick injury immediately commence a self-prescribed AZT regimen as a way of decreasing risk of seroconversion.[27] However, no measures can eliminate risk, some is inevitable, and the possibilities are definitely not negligible. It is estimated that one in every two hundred and fifty accidental needle-sticks sustained by health workers caring for seropositive patients results in viral transmission and, further, that a surgeon, 10 percent of whose patients are HIV+, has a 1:200 chance of becoming infected within each working year.[28]

Attention to the possibility of injection during health care procedures has tended to focus on the dangers to the health care worker, but there are many more instances of patients being infected in what can only be called health care industry negligence. One of the most tragic cases developed in the Soviet Union in the period from 1981 through 1989. As reported at Montreal's International Conference on AIDS, a Russian male working in Guinea was infected, and then infected his wife upon returning to the Soviet Union. She became pregnant; the baby was born infected in 1984. The child sickened and was hospitalized in Elista, capital of the Kalmuk Republic on the Caspian Sea. The hospital was operating with an inadequate supply of hypodermic syringes due to a national shortage.[29] The nurses, departing from proper procedure, used the same needle for multiple patient injections and the original infection spread to fifty-one other children in the pediatric ward. Then one of the newly infected infants was transferred to a hospital in Volgorod where exactly the same thing happened, spreading the infection to twenty-two more. In addition, eight mothers were infected, possibly through breast feeding—their babies' mouths had bleeding sores, and the mothers were infected through minute cracks in their nipples. All told, eighty-one infections can be traced back to the original Guinea contact, seventy-eight of them attributable to health care negligence.[30] A popular Soviet weekly, *Ogonyok*, prophesied that, unless the scarcity of antiseptic hospital conditions is corrected, AIDS could spread to millions of Soviets by the year 2000.[31]

By far the largest number of individuals infected through industrial negligence were infected in the United States, France, and Germany as a result of the transfusion of contaminated blood and blood products. The story of the mulish reluctance of America's blood bank managers to begin screening procedures is one of the saddest chapters in the history of our early nonresponse to the threat of AIDS. As early as 1982, experts, studying patterns of infection in hemophiliac recipients of blood products, considered it highly probable that HIV could be transmitted by blood transfusion.[32] In late 1982 and early 1983 President Reagan's Food and Drug Administration (the agency charged with regulating the blood bank industry) issued recommendations to reduce the risk of possible transmission. In 1983–84 the virus was isolated, but not until 1985 did the FDA issue mandatory screening regulations.

The position of industry leaders was that no one had "proved conclusively" that AIDS could be transmitted through transfusion. Lacking such evidence, screening was too expensive. The industry position reminds me of the tobacco industry's persistent claim that "100% certain" scientific proof of a causal link between smoking and lung cancer has not been established, or of the explanation given by California Governor Wilson's for his 1994 veto of needle-exchange programs designed to slow the spread of HIV. By the time blood bank administrators bowed to the mounting evidence and implemented the FDA regulations, an estimated 70 to 90 percent of the population of severe hemophiliacs (8,000–11,000)[33] and approximately 12,000 surgical patients were added to the growing list of AIDS victims.[34] The Ryan White Comprehensive AIDS Act of 1990 (see chapter 6) requires the states to develop public information campaigns targeting people who received transfusions between January 1, 1978 and April 1, 1985 and inform them of the availability and need for health services.[35] As of 1994, two thousand hemophiliacs have died of AIDS, and there are now hundreds of individual lawsuits pending against various blood banks as well as a major national class action suit seeking hundreds of millions in damages.[36]

The 1993 scandals that unfolded in France and Germany, however, told a story that was worse, much worse. In both countries persons responsible for the quality and distribution of blood products acted in a manner that was unconscionable, impossible to justify. In both cases, blood and/or blood products that *were known to be HIV infected* were distributed. In France, the motive seems to have been a perverse combination of national pride and government budgeting,[37] while in Germany it was simply business profit. Old stupidities in the administration of the blood supply continue to surface (in Canada, for example), but today the problem of contaminated blood has been reasonably well addressed, at least in industrial Europe and North America. The supply has never been and never will be 100 percent free of possible disease contaminants, for nothing is absolutely safe. The Centers for Disease Control estimate that there currently are about five transfusion-related viral transmissions from a total 4 million transfusions annually and that approximately 4,619 persons have been infected through transfusion.[38] In the United States the supply is as clean as one can get anywhere in the world today.[39] However, I would not want to receive a transfusion in Mexico, Central or South America, the Caribbean, Africa, the Middle East, the Eastern Mediterranean, India, or Southeast Asia—a fair chunk of the world. U.S. government operations with contingents in these areas (such as the U.S. military, the Peace Corps, the State Department, the Central Intelligence Agency) fly their personnel to Europe or America or use previously banked blood when transfusions are needed. It is not a question of the nations involved being unwilling to screen; it is usually that they are unable to screen for economic or technological reasons.[40]

It is also possible to get infected in the health care setting itself, where one has gone to get solutions for health problems. The most publicized problem has been that of the infected physician. The cases of Dr. David J. Acer, dentist, and Dr. Rudolph Almaraz, surgeon, both of whom died of AIDS, are radically altering the rules covering sterilization procedures, protocols on invasive surgical procedures, and the practice of medicine and dentistry. Dr. Acer infected six of his patients (as of 1994 two have died). Dr. Almaraz infected no one. But other troubling cases involving either HIV+ doctors or dangerously inept medical administration keep cropping up—for example, the distribution from 1985 to 1990 of fifty infected segments of skin, bone, and tissue from one donor for use in surgical transplants[41]—to remind us of the surrounding dangers posed by HIV.

It is probable that the risk of doctor to patient transmission is low. However, given that the entire purpose of medical intervention is to improve the health of a patient, it seems clear that no avoidable adverse condition—be it a septic condition of the surgery or the health of workers—should be permitted. The number of health care providers with AIDS or HIV infections constitutes a very small fraction of the almost 4 million individuals comprising the health care workforce, but the problem has been sufficient to inspire the American Medical and the American Dental Associations to issue new guidelines (January 1991) stating that health care workers had an ethical obligation to inform patients of a seropositive status. It remains to be seen whether state health departments will accept and enforce these new guidelines (see "The Patient Perspective," in chapter 4).[42]

There are also instances of what can only be called accident-accidents— events of such unpredictable and bizarre a character that there is little or no conceivable protection. I have in mind, for example, the case of an American tourist in Rwanda who was seriously injured along with other passengers in a bus crash. His open wounds were splattered with the blood of other passengers piled on top of him; one of them was HIV+, and the infection was transmitted.[43] Millions of Americans travel each year in third world countries where the conditions of life in all respects are more hazardous, where HIV prevalence is higher, where the male-female seroprevalence ratio is close to even, and where medical facilities themselves may be a significant source of infection. In late 1993 there was an American transmission from one HIV+ hemophiliac brother to another—apparently they shared razors.

Then there are the children infected in the womb, the citadel of life itself, in the birthing process, or through breast feeding. A child born to an infected mother has about a 25 percent chance of infection. Eighty-one percent of the pediatric cases in the United States (although not elsewhere) can be linked to IV drug use.[44] By 1994 the United States had already recorded five thousand cases of pediatric AIDS. The World Health Organization estimates that by the year 2000 the number of HIV+ children in sub-Saharan Africa will number in the millions.

In America, most AIDS babies will be born in a hospital, and most will never leave it. It is sobering to realize that an entire group of infants will come into and go out of our world without experiencing the holding, the bonding, and the love that forges a human being from the raw material of our species. Statistical analyses indicate that about 20 percent of infected newborns will develop AIDS within the first year of life and die during the next; the rest will progress to AIDS at the rate of 8 percent per year.[45] A quick tour of an AIDS pediatric ward would probably stifle most of the moralistic posturing about God's wrath. The tour would also illustrate a facet of our response to the epidemic. The national government and various charitable groups are funding pediatric care lavishly (it is politically acceptable to help the innocent victims), but adult care parsimoniously. In 1992, pediatric AIDS accounted for about 40 percent of the national budget for testing new treatments, even though pediatric cases are less than 2 percent of the total.[46] Unfortunately, good support does not change the result. Children are sometimes born to drunken parents, cruel and sadistic parents, careless and improvident parents, and parents who abandon them. Most of them survive it all. None survive AIDS.[47]

Finally, there is transmission as a result of our own high-risk behavior, risky sex, or injecting drugs with contaminated syringes (the Soviet and Romanian pediatric tragedies are instructive here). Prior to 1985 no one could be held accountable for failing to avoid behaviors that were and are risky in terms of AIDS for the simple reason that there was too little information, too much confusion, and no really authoritative guidance. But nature does not require culpability or intentionality in any sense. It is enough that if you do something that, in fact, is dangerous, you pay—no "ifs, ands, or buts." Most of those who have died or are sick and dying currently are in this group. They were infected in the late 1970s or early 1980s before anyone was really informed as to the nature of the illness, its forms of transmission, or the possible scope of the epidemic.

Increasingly from 1985 to the current period, the possibility of being honestly ignorant is very slowly decreasing as government agencies, churches, and educational institutions gradually educate the public. At this juncture, about the only mass-preventive weapons we have to fight this epidemic are educational campaigns such as that commenced in 1988 by former U.S. Surgeon General Koop at the national level, local efforts sponsored by America's thousands of AIDS service organizations, and an increasing number of educational programs sponsored by schools, businesses, and churches.

In aggregate, our attempts at public sex reeducation have been simultaneously impressive and inadequate. We are rapidly learning how little we know about how to convince people to change their basic ways or, indeed, even how to reach them with a message they can assimilate. I have been involved in local phases of this effort and have been humbled by the discovery that I knew much less about teaching than I thought; the elaborate plans—posters, pamphlets, programs—always sound great to the middle-class, educated warriors around the conference table but absolutely bomb when put into effect. I suspect that one major reason for failures has been the unwillingness to show the true face of AIDS in presentations to the general public. Children with AIDS have been the traditional "March-of-Dimes" poster children, heterosexual couples have been attractive and healthy looking, though somber, while gay men, at the most, have been shown with a small facial lesion of Kaposi's sarcoma. The truth is messier and uglier, much uglier. Still, people are learning, and, in any event, national and local educational campaigns are all we really have to slow the epidemic on a population-wide basis.

In January 1944, the Department of Health and Human Services launched a major program to reach the eighteen to twenty-five-year-old age group,

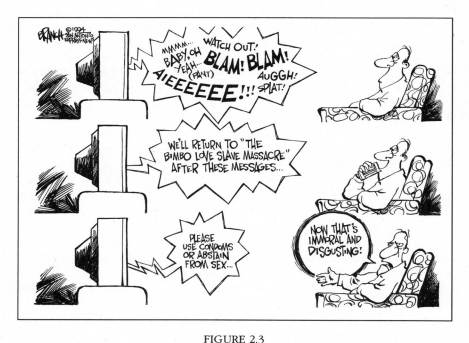

FIGURE 2.3

Source: Editorial Cartoon by John Branch, *San Antonio Express-News*, January 6, 1994

whose seroprevalence statistics are rising ominously. The Clinton administration clearly hopes that by using high-energy TV spots frankly promoting condom use, employing the talent of rock stars, and broadcasting on virtually all mass media channels it will be able to reach the sexually most active segment of the population. It was appropriate that the program was launched in Washington, D.C., a city with about thirty thousand seropositives.[48] There were the usual objections from the usual sources; my feeling is that anyone who, for reasons of sexual prudishness, religious doctrine, homophobic prejudice, or antipathy to drug use impedes these efforts, is, very simply and whether they intend to be or not, an ally of the epidemic.

INFECTION

If by one means or the other, the virus is injected into the human bloodstream, then conditions are set for stage 2, and the boat is launched. An entirely different set of problems arise. The newly seropositive person has lost control over the ultimate health of his or her body—a fact that makes it doubly important that he or she pay close attention to nutrition and other daily regimens of good health. For once the infection has passed, there is no known way of reversing it; there is nothing the individual can do other than live in such a way as to enhance general health, avoid contracting or transmitting further sexually transmitted diseases (STDs), and follow treatment protocols. Upon infection, at least for the person infected, the public health campaigns of Stage 1 have failed. Now matters are in the hands of research and clinical medicine. What happens, and what can be done?[49]

The virus will quickly encounter a human cell that it chemically recognizes as a potential host, and "dock." Docking involves the attachment of HIV's surface coat molecule gp120 to the CD4 molecule found on the surface of many human cells. Docking is followed by a fusion of HIV with the host cell through the action of another HIV surface molecule, gp41.[50] The vulnerable human cells are T and B lymphocytes, monocytes/macrophages, follicular dendritics, and Langerhams—all of which are essential to the effective functioning of our immune system and the glial cells of the brain and central nervous system.[51] Once it has transferred its materials into the host cell, HIV commences a process of replication which, within a few weeks, elevates the quantity of virus in the blood to very high levels and spreads it throughout the body. Within six weeks of infection, 50 to 70 percent of those infected will experience a temporary illness resembling flu or mononucleosis; standard blood tests given during this illness might not reveal the presence of HIV because the antibody response has not fully kicked in.[52]

In the meantime, an antibody response is mounted by normal, not-otherwise-compromised immune systems, and within three to six months it succeeds in greatly reducing the viral load in the peripheral blood system (see Figure 2.4, Walter Reed Model). The newly infected person resumes good health (assuming temporary illness) and may experience no further effects from the infection for many, many years. The immune response is very effective in eliminating HIV from the bloodstream. Indeed, it was long a puzzle to scientists how HIV could do so much damage with so few HIV infected cells detectable in the blood system.[53] The answer began to emerge in 1993. The virus is able to survive the immune system's counterattack by hiding in the lymph nodes, while being decimated in the peripheral blood system.[54] The nodes normally function to filter and hold alien invaders, presenting them for destruction. However in this case, they function like medieval fortresses for HIV, holding at least ten times more virus than the peripheral blood. Key cells of the lymphatic system are themselves infected and eventually, over the years, are so degraded by the presence of HIV that they can no longer filter. Then they release billions of virus into the bloodstream.

The virus adversely affects in some way the function of any cell it enters, and, in addition, it disrupts the exquisitely sensitive signaling system that the component parts of the immune system use to coordinate an attack on an alien intruder. Thus, the body's defense system is not only attacked directly but is also thrown into a state of confusion. The direct and measurable effects of HIV attack are seen in the gradual diminution of the T lymphocyte cells and the killer cells that are, together, responsible for the destruction of both invading and infected body cells.

Current research indicates that the gradually decreasing T cell counts typical of HIV disease progression may be partly a product of direct HIV killing action. However, more seriously, the decline may be the result of a triggering of T lymphocyte suicide. Cells are normally programmed to self-destruct when they can no longer function usefully or become a danger to the health of the overall system. This is a process known as apoptosis, and, among other things, it insures that our immune system's killer cells do not turn against us, destroying cells they are supposed to protect. When these internal programs go wrong, a person is faced with intractable autoimmune diseases, like multiple sclerosis—the body attacks itself. There is some evidence that HIV can trigger this kind of response in T lymphocytes. It disrupts the normal process of cell division in such a way that, apparently, the cell signals itself that it can no longer function which, in turn, precipitates a cellular suicide command.

Finally, the virus can confuse the basic intercellular communication system. The various cells of the immune system are bound together by an intricate system mediated by chemical signals. These signals tell a defending cell when to divide and multiply to meet an invader, what armor to put on, and where to go. The ability of HIV to sow confusion in this system must be one of the most successful forms of attack any pathogen has ever devised, and this confusion may, in the end, prove to be the most deadly effect of infection. There is nothing simple about this virus.

What can be done? There are two major strategies: (1) to prevent the docking and fusion of HIV to a host cell, or (2) to enhance the body's ability to destroy free virus or virus-infected cells. The first approach involves interfering with the process of docking so that the virus is left to drift, eventually to be destroyed by immune system defenders or by a specially targeted toxin.[55] There are many different drugs being tested to frustrate the process of docking and penetration. One approach has been to load the blood system with decoys in the form of recombinant soluble CD4 to which HIV could attach harmlessly, a floating cell receptor without a cell. Another approach seeks to attach additional molecules to the CD4 receptor. The wharf is thus structurally altered so that the boat will not fit, HIV's gp120 would be unable to attach.[56] In both cases, the virus would then be exposed to continual attack by the killer cells of the immune system. Although sound in theory, no effective means have been found to implement these initiatives.

The second strategy involves enhancing the body's natural immune response to the virus, and there are two approaches available. Either the system is enhanced after infection so as to more effectively fight an established infection, or a classic preventive vaccine is used to stop infection dead in its tracks, when and if it occurs.

With respect to the first approach, a number of therapies are being tried. Passive immunotherapy takes blood from a person with a high level of antibodies to the virus, kills the HIV in it, and then infuses it in another PWA. This gives the patient, in effect, a fresh supply of immunologically effective blood. Another is the use of DNCB, one of the current alternative and experimental approaches. DNCB's supporters state that it has the ability to boost the body's production of killer cells, which can then more effectively destroy HIV infected cells (see "Allopathic experiments," in chapter 4). Perhaps the greatest hopes for this approach have been placed upon the development of what is called a "therapeutic vaccine," that is, a vaccine administered *after* infection that is designed to challenge and boost the effectiveness of the natural system. Dr. Jonas Salk announced, in June 1989, that his research team had made some advances in producing such a vaccine. However, at the Berlin Conference in 1993 the optimistic tone gave way to a more somber mood as it became apparent that neither the Salk therapeutic vaccine, nor others like it, were producing significant benefit.[57]

The second approach involves the development of a classic preinfection vaccine, such as that used for polio, measles, some strains of flu, smallpox, and other diseases. Such a vaccine would not benefit infected individuals but would be the means to destroy HIV as a mother of epidemics. Developing such a vaccine involves the complicated business of producing a drug that would create a cellular "memory" of HIV before an individual is infected. Then, if and when a person is infected, the immune system would be able to mount an immediate and decisive defense. However, there is no expectation of an effective vaccine in this century. After ten years of intensive AIDS research, it is clear that science needs to know more both about the immune system and the virus before success is likely.[58]

The possibilities of a vaccine must be calculated within the context of the overall difficulties involved. One of the principals in a Simian AIDS vaccine research team cautioned that "the day when we come up with a human vaccine against AIDS is still far off."[59] A noted virologist stated, "The development of a vaccine against AIDS is hindered by the worst possible confluence of viral and pathogenic factors that seem to preclude any simple or easy resolution in the foreseeable future."[60] The press releases of the U.S. Surgeon-General, the National Institutes of Health, and various other groups have uniformly emphasized the difficulties and improbability of a human vaccine in less than a decade of research and testing![61] No one wants to say "never," but that is what it amounts to for the generation growing up today.

There are all sorts of problems that impede vaccine development.[62] One of the more ironic is that a vaccine that stimulates the production of necessary cells to defeat HIV might actually stimulate accelerated production of the HIV already there. Because HIV integrates its genetic material into the host cell's material, any division of the host cell in response to the injection of a foreign substance (the vaccine) automatically creates new viral materials. Seen from HIV's standpoint it is a brilliant strategy; seen from ours, it is a deadly and macabre minuet.

Another problem derives from the hypermutability of HIV. It is customary, especially in general literature such as this work, to speak of the HIV as though it was just one virus. Actually it is a complex family of rapidly mutating viruses, what virologists and molecular biologists are calling a "quasispecies." As mentioned earlier, there are seven known subtypes of HIV-1. They have varying characteristics and are found clustered in different parts of the world. For example, most North American infections are HIV-1(b), while most Central African and Asian are of HIV-1(f), a type that is transmitted more easily and produces a different pattern of opportunistic infections. However, each of the types shares the feature of being hypervariable. Findings from the Los Alamos National Laboratory indicate that HIV changes it genetic coding five times faster than the flu virus, which, until the appearance of HIV, was the most rapidly mutating virus known.[63] Flu vaccines must be developed or redeveloped every several years to keep abreast of viral changes (such as in the Hong Kong, the Spanish, and the Swine Flu). That level of "updating" would not be sufficient for HIV. Some researchers think that HIV may use its hypervariability as a tactic to "outflank the immune system"; its rate of change can outrun the capacity of the host immune system to generate responses.[64] HIV even mutates, over the decade of infection, within the individual, so that the same patient can harbor many variant strains of the original infecting virus.

The drug L661 developed by Merck & Co., a major pharmaceutical manufacturer, offers a sobering example of HIV's self-protective mutating ability. L661 held much promise as a means of inhibiting the ability of HIV to reproduce, and Merck spent millions bringing the drug to the trials stage. To everyone's dismay, it took the virus only a few weeks to mutate a form that completely nullified the drug's effects; Merck & Co. then turned to another drug.[65] Given such conditions, the production of a single, effective vaccine that will create the necessary "memory" upon which the immune system can act is improbable; if the vaccine approach is possible at all, HIV will require multiple vaccines that are continually updated. The rapidity of HIV mutation is not just a problem for vaccine development, it affects all drugs in a similar fashion. HIV has not only developed transmissible strains "born," as it were, resistant to drugs like AZT, but it can also develop a drug resistance at the time an individual is undergoing treatment with that drug.

A third problem stems from the fact, as noted above, that HIV is *our* virus. Few animals show any reaction at all, much less get sick, when inoculated with live virus. This means that we have no way to test (on other than human subjects) the toxicity and effectiveness of experimental vaccines.[66] In addition, the long time period involved in HIV infection makes it difficult to collect and maintain control data such that researchers can be sure that improvements are related to use of the vaccine. Finally, certain types of vaccines, such as inactivated whole virus vaccines, are hazardous because an imperfect manufacturing process might produce a vaccine that infected rather than conferred immunity.[67] Viral based infections have always proved difficult to counter—we have no vaccine or cure for the common cold, no universal vaccine for flu, none for any form of herpes, cytomegalovirus, Epstein-Barr, and so on through the viral pathogens that like us.[68]

REPLICATION

If cellular infection is not short-circuited, then HIV commences the intricate process of reproducing itself by using the facilities of the human cell. During this phase of its life cycle, the virus raider is skillfully camouflaged, invisible to immune system defenders because of its integration into a cell nucleus. However, it is vulnerable to intervention at some points, such as during the process of unloading its materials, and while building new boats (copies of the original) within the cell nucleus.

The business of replicating itself is a complex enzyme-directed process that may take place long after HIV has invaded the cell or very rapidly after infection. Upon entering the host cell, the raiders first unload their equipment. That is, HIV destroys its own nucleus membrane and frees its genetic materials within the cell. Then the enzyme reverses transcriptase directs a restructuring of the RNA strands containing HIV's genetic information into DNA strands matching those of the human cell. These newly constituted HIV-DNA strands are then inserted into the host cell DNA where they can be duplicated by that cell's normal division processes. In common with other members of its family, HIV cannot reproduce itself; it is at this point in its cycle that HIV's essential character as a parasite becomes clear.

The media has informed people on this aspect of HIV's life cycle more consistently than any other because, I suppose, everyone can identify with the process of reproduction and understand the significance of aborting it. Much scientific effort has gone into attempts to disrupt HIV's replication cycle. The most commonly known are those that inhibit the functioning of reverse transcriptase, the enzyme that directs replication on behalf of HIV. AZT (3'-azido-2',3'-dideoxythymidine) or Retrovir, the best known drug associated with HIV infection, is used for precisely this purpose. It works by fooling the enzyme (reverse transcriptase) that directs the process into incorporating a look-alike, but fake, molecular component into the viral make-up. This eventually disrupts the process and terminates replication—the molecular equivalent of throwing a monkey wrench into the works. AZT has been joined by other similarly operating drugs (ddI, ddC, d4t), and a good deal of research is directed to determining whether they will work in various combinations better than they work alone. There is considerable debate within the scientific and PWA community whether any of them work well enough, and last long enough (given HIV's mutation capacity), to be worth their toxic side-effects.[69] But it should be noted that no drug is trouble free; every one of them, even aspirin, can have serious side effects in some users.[70]

Disappointment with the results of replication inhibitors has led to a search for drugs which would attack the virus at an even more basic level, a level that would curtail all viral activity. These are drugs on the cutting edge of medicine, drugs that inhibit the action of specific genes within HIV's genome; they might be called gene inhibitors. The two approaches farthest along in drug development are Tat, Protease, and LTR (various segments of the HIV genome) inhibitors. They are in various stages of the clinical trial process, and it is unlikely that any answers as to their effectiveness will emerge until 1995.

HIV is, as one observer put it, "a replication machine," that is, it is a transmissible genetic program that commands host receivers: "Copy Me." As nearly as I can figure out, that is all it does. Why there should be such an organic program in the universe, I cannot fathom, but there it is. Efforts to disrupt such a highly specialized entity may well be very difficult. HIV *is* a replication machine, and a very good one.

RECAPITULATION

After its genetic materials are duplicated by human cell action, the materials are reorganized on RNA strands, as upon the original invading virus, and then reassembled as whole viruses in the outer portions of the host cell. If all else fails, attempts can be made to frustrate the final assembly and launch of the new viral boats (viral budding). There are several possible ways to go about this. There are at least two drugs in trial stage that, it is hoped, may confuse our raiders in the assembly and launch of their newly made boats. They are Castanospermine, which is derived from the Australian chestnut tree, and Hypericin derived from the common weed, Saint Johnswort.[71]

It is not certain, but it may be that the death and gradual depletion of essential human cells is partly a byproduct of the assembly and launching process. Although a slow production of individual HIV cells might not adversely affect the cell, it does appear that an accelerated production can disrupt its membrane as newly formed HIV cells swarm out. One of the goals of therapeutic medicine is to devise means of controlling, if not stopping, the production of HIV. A slow, controlled cycle would be tantamount to a chronic, but not necessarily fatal infection.

In any case, the raiders have achieved their goal, more boats and raiders. Biologically speaking, this is what both HIV and Homo sapiens behavior are all about, the survival of the species. Properly viewed, HIV's life cycle is seen as a continuous circle of events which, after initial injection, has neither beginning nor end. We can cut into it at various points to slow the deadly wheel, but so far, the only event that stops it is death of the host. Death results from one or more of the many afflictions enticed by HIV's impairment of our immune system. AIDS, the Acquired Immunodeficiency Syndrome, is the final, the terminal human response.

PROGRESSION TO AIDS

Each of the stages in the life cycle of HIV is repeated countless times, each time doing some additional minute damage. It is common, but a bit misleading, to speak of HIV's "latency or incubation" period as though this were a period of rest or inaction. What is usually being referred to is the long time lapse between infection and display of opportunistic disease symptoms.[72] The fact is, however, that by gradually depleting critical immune system cells and thereby compromising the system's effectiveness, the HIV infection (that is, the aggregate action of all the viruses) does damage throughout its tenure in the human body.[73] According to a model developed at Walter Reed Hospital (Figure 2.4), and based upon experience with military seropositives, HIV infection is seen as developing in six stages with identifiable diagnostic markers from (1) "asymptomatic seropositivity" through (6) "life-threatening opportunistic infections."[74] Initially the body's immune system does produce an effective response to the virus, but over the long run the response is inadequate. Viewing the same data in calendar stages (rather than diagnostic ones), the cross-over period during which the virus begins to gain the upper hand over the body's defense system, and symptoms begin to appear, seems to occur late in the seventh year after infection.[75] Prior to that, individuals can be quite unaware of their infection and may evidence no signs other than those which can be discerned only by lab testing (such as a gradually decreasing T4 cell count).

Another model, one that correlates the immune system's T4/CD4 cell counts with the appearance of disease symptoms, indicates that people will develop the indicator diseases necessary for an AIDS diagnosis from about the eighth year of infection. During the first six years no lasting symptoms

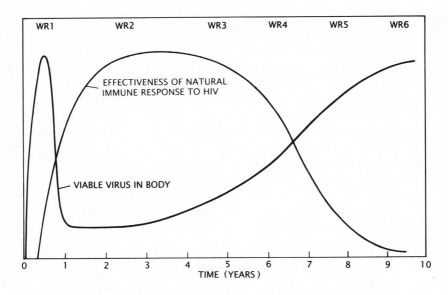

FIGURE 2.4 Walter Reed Progression-to-AIDS Model

ordinarily appear, but the cell counts drop from a healthy normal of 1000–1200 per cubic millimeter of blood to about 400. In the seventh year, blood cell counts drop further (200–400) and some relatively mild infections, such as oral thrush, bacterial skin infections, and shingles can appear. In the eighth year, with still lower cell counts (0–200), an HIV+ might experience serious fungal expressions (like severe athlete's foot), oral hairy leukoplakia, and tuberculosis. The ninth and subsequent years, when cell counts may drop to 50 or less, will present a variety of life-threatening infections which singly or in combination eventually produce a terminal prognosis.[76]

In individual cases the progress from infection to a display of the AIDS symptomology is extremely variable, and little is known about why these variations exist. Studies confirm that the older the individual is at the time of infection, the faster he or she progresses to AIDS, but what aspect of age affects the progression is unknown.[77] Various reports issued in 1993 indicate that drinking, smoking, and drug use speed progression, but, again, the exact mechanism involved for each remains unclear.[78] The virulence or quantity of the virus in a transmission may also influence speed of progression. Personal experience is no guide in this matter. As an AIDS foundation worker I have seen glowing specimens of health, people who are

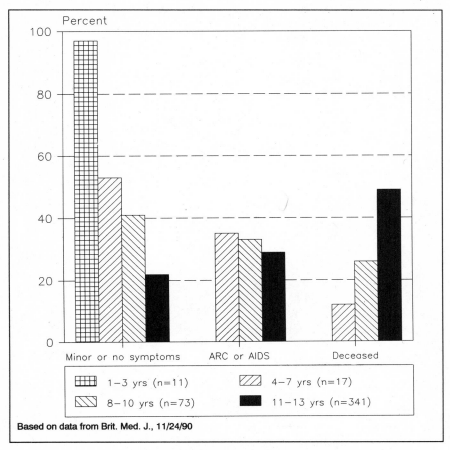

FIGURE 2.5 Clinical Symptons

careful with their diet and who exercise regularly, progress to AIDS faster than others who have clearly led a very unhealthy life. I have also seen the opposite. As in the case of cancer and other diseases, there may be genetic predispositions at work. Furthermore the reader should keep in mind that the "average" figures used in models are just that, averages of a large number of variable, unique cases. An individual history can depart strikingly from the statistical norms; for example, a counselee of mine watched his blood count drop from 900 to 526 in just two years, much faster than the average, but then the count remained at 526 for a year which, again, was not the average, expected reaction. Two other individuals enjoy good health with counts of 80 and 126 respectively, even though the standard charts and

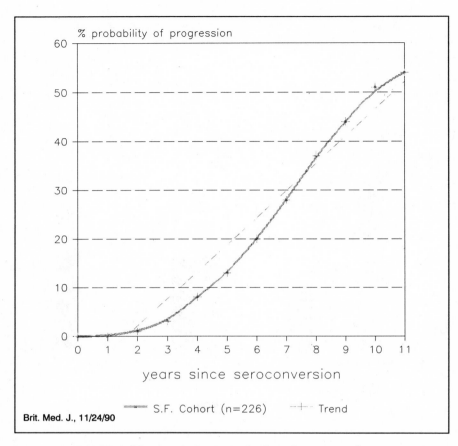

FIGURE 2.6 Progression to AIDS: Risk and Duration of HIV+

prognoses become very discouraging at these levels. As every physician with an AIDS practice can testify, the unusual is sometimes the usual in AIDS.

The average time from viral exposure to the onset of overt symptoms is seven to eight years. The median "incubation" time is thought to be from nine to eleven years, that is, half the subjects would develop clinical AIDS in less than that time, and half in more.[79] For individuals who have a documented seven-year clinical record, approximately 36 percent have progressed to AIDS, another 40 percent have measurable deterioration in clinical markers (such as decreasing T4 cell counts), and the remainder appear asymptomatic. These average figures, however, must be understood as very rough approximations for any individual case. For example, there is some evidence that

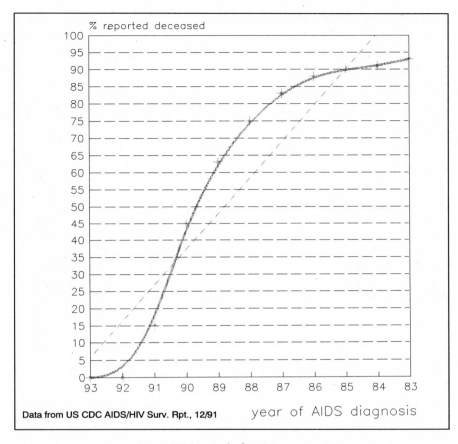

FIGURE 2.7 Survival after Diagnosis, U.S.

those who survive past six years may experience changes in their immune system that stabilize progression and produces a longer, slower infection— a plateau, as it were.[80] Assuming a normal immune system at the time of infection, the body is initially able to contain the damage of the invading virus, but over time the cumulative impact of HIV prevails.

It is not known whether everyone infected by HIV will develop AIDS, or how long the span of progression will ultimately prove to be. There are records now documenting a small number of long-term survivors, that is, individuals who have lived, in reasonable health, considerably beyond the usual projections. What the significant factors are that explain their longevity is unknown—perhaps genetic factors invest some people with unusual resistance or resilience, perhaps some were infected with a more benign strain of the virus, perhaps some have developed an especially effective, individually tailored treatment. Needless to say, all these variables and more are being examined. But it is likely that over a term of fifteen years or so, few will escape. The final stage involves an "irreversible decline . . . marked by successive, uncontrollable opportunistic infections, progressive general deterioration and debilitation, and often deteriorating mental capacity."[81] In the final stages all that anyone can do is help the PWA die with reasonable comfort and dignity.

HIV INFECTION AND AIDS

What is it that has developed? What is AIDS? What follows is a simple description of a complex phenomenon. However, it needs to be said up front that no set of descriptions can convey the reality of this disease. No one who has not heard the words, "I regret to say that your test results are positive for the human immunodeficiency virus" or who has not faced the final AIDS diagnosis, can possibly appreciate what it is like. The sinking feeling, the fear and then denial, the sense of separation from others, the final daily agony of watching your body sicken and age as though it had been suddenly switched to Fast Forward. Even those who have worked around AIDS patients cannot know. There is one book that does pierce the veil a bit—Emmanuel Dreuilhe's, *Mortal Embrace, Living with AIDS.*[82] It is a brief, beautiful, and anguished work that could only have been written by someone from within the agony.

HIV INFECTION

First, what is AIDS *not*? It is not equivalent to seropositivity, to infection with HIV. All people with AIDS will have been infected by the virus and generally will test positive, but only a minority of those who test positive at any given time will have AIDS. AIDS, as we shall see, is a defined collection of ailments, but HIV is a primary and initial infection. They are not the same. Like many other matters at this juncture, it is unclear just what HIV infection *by itself* entails beyond the observable damage to the immune system. No one knows what the physical consequences of just HIV infection would be without the later addition of opportunistic infections. Would HIV infection by itself be fatal? The problem arises from the fact that our morbidity and mortality data express people who have been infected and then have gone on to develop fatal infections of opportunistic pathogens. Finding the answer experimentally is difficult because there are no appropriate animal models. If there was an animal that reacted to HIV the way we do, then the animal could be inoculated and observed. If it died, then we could assert that HIV was fatal in and of itself. However, so far, the only animals that react to HIV are HIV-transgenic mice that are genetically engineered to

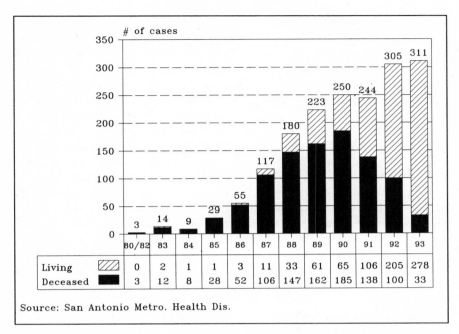

FIGURE 2.8 AIDS Cases and Survival after Diagnosis, Bexar County, Texas

express an HIV infection—the mice are born carrying portions of the HIV genome and then carefully insulated from exposure to other pathogens. The mice develop rather severe wartlike skin diseases from their "HIV infection" and die rather more quickly than otherwise they would.[83]

AIDS ETIOLOGY

What, then, is the relationship between HIV and AIDS? Does HIV "cause" AIDS? Western science has come a long way from the good old days of Newton and Hume when the notion of "cause and effect" seemed accessible and commonsensible. The old notion was neat—billiard ball "A" hits billiard ball "B," there is a transference of energy, and the second is impelled down the table, that is, "caused" to move in a certain direction. Then came the age of biology, evolution, relativity, and quantum mechanics, and everything got screwed up. Evolutionary and biological causation are clearly not of the billiard ball type, and now physicists can talk sensibly about "synchronicity," that is, paired events that occur separately in space, but occur synchronously in time—with no known connection between them.

Does HIV cause AIDS? The answer is yes and no. If one insists that a specific named disease be tied to a specific named pathogen, like bubonic plague is to *Yersinia pestis*, then "no," HIV does not "cause" AIDS. HIV "causes" HIV infection, which, as I have said, is not the same as AIDS. AIDS is, as we shall see, an official government definition. Let us say you are a PWA with a bad case of *Pneumocystis carinii* pneumonia. Did HIV "cause" it? The answer is "no"—it was caused by an agent common in our environment. Would you have reacted to that agent by developing PCP without having first suffered a significant depression of your immune system? The answer is "no"—approximately half the readers of this book have already encountered the pathogen and harbor it with no ill effects. Can such immune depression occur by various means? Yes—heavy use of antibiotics, administration of drugs designed to forestall organ transplant rejection, numerous forms of cancer therapy, being born with a defective immune system, and, of course, HIV infection. The dominant opinion today is that HIV infection is a necessary preliminary to the development of those further infections that will, cumulatively and inevitably, qualify as fitting the official government definition.

If this sounds to you a bit awkward and obtuse, you are right, it is. There are dissidents from the majority view that HIV causes AIDS, some of them members of an organization called the Group for the Scientific Re-Evaluation of HIV-AIDS Hypothesis. The range of positions in the dissident camp is broad. Some insist that the entire epidemic is some kind of manufactured fantasy composed of preexisting pockets of illness, environmental conditions, and media hype. Most of these folks also think that the moon landing was staged on a Nevada desert, that the Holocaust is a fiction developed to create sympathy for Jews, and that Elvis is still alive. Others admit the epidemic exists but insist that HIV has nothing to do with all the deaths. They are the result of lifestyle, drug use, and other factors.[84] Still others agree that HIV has a lot to do with AIDS but is not the whole story—HIV infection is perhaps a necessary but not a sufficient cause of AIDS. AIDS is conceptualized as a multistage, multifactorial disease of which HIV infection is just a part.[85] This is more than just a war of words. The distinctions are part of a significant debate the outcome of which could determine the flow of research funds and, therefore, research initiatives. If HIV has nothing to do with AIDS, then why are we spending billions studying the virus? If biologic, environmental, and behavioral co-factors are partly responsible for the epidemic, why not isolate and try to control them? Eventually these arguments will be settled by geneticists, virologists, microbiologists, epidemiologists, and others concerned with the characterization, evolution, control, and impact of disease pathogens. For now and for me, the evidence seem overwhelming that HIV infection leads inevitably to a bodily condition that meets the AIDS definition. In that sense, it "causes" AIDS. Much of the debate seems a bit like arguing whether the explosion that set off the avalanche that buried you was the proximate cause of death.

AIDS: THE ACQUIRED IMMUNE DEFICIENCY SYNDROME

AIDS was first defined in 1982 by the Centers for Disease Control of the Department of Health and Human Services. The CDC has the primary responsibility for defining, tracking, and containing epidemic diseases in the United States. The original and all subsequent definitions have been based on previous clinical and/or laboratory observations as to characteristics of HIV infection at various stages and in various populations studied, *as well as* the CDC's epidemiologic need to define it in such a way as to gather and collate needed data.[86] At any point then, AIDS equals a medical and scientific consensus as to the characteristics of a disease to be diagnosed, tracked, and recorded in accordance with an official government definition. The use of the word "consensus"—a very political word—should sound warning that there can well be political as well as scientific/medical aspects to disease definition. Indeed, politics plays a role. For example, women's groups rightly complained that there was no attention given in the CDC's 1982 and 1987 definitions to the unique expressions of HIV progression in women. In 1993 this defect was somewhat corrected with the result that the number of women reported with AIDS jumped sharply.

The 1982 definition has been changed twice, in 1987 and 1993, and on both occasions was expanded to include new conditions or characteristics. It is probable that it will be altered again in response to changing information, changing patterns of infection, and changing domestic and international politics. However, whether now or in the future, and in the CDC's words, "AIDS is the group of clinical conditions or laboratory markers that are indicative of severe immunosuppression due to HIV-infection."[87]

The current definition is found in the CDC's *Morbidity and Mortality Weekly Report,* "1993 Revised Classification System for HIV Infection and Expanded Surveillance Case Definition for AIDS Among Adolescents and Adults," December 18, 1992. It consists of two basic parts. First, is a list of twenty-five "indicator" diseases or symptomatic conditions (some of which have several parts); second, specifications of laboratory counts of CD4+ T lymphocyte cells that are considered "markers" or indicators of an underlying pathologic condition. Given an HIV infected person (not necessarily an HIV tested person), the cell counts and diagnoses of indicator conditions may be combined in various ways to meet the guidelines for a diagnosis of AIDS.

The indicator diseases on the list are what everyone else calls "opportunistic infections," infections that take advantage of the immune system's impairment to develop rapidly and severely.[88] Perhaps it would be more accurate to state that there are *groups* of opportunistic infections. For example, there are some twenty-four diseases associated with the central nervous system alone. The agents of some of these are common in our environment, such as that which causes *Pneumocystis carinii* pneumonia (PCP) or *toxoplasmosis*; a majority of the readers of this book have been exposed to the agents that causes them. However, the pathogens' damage potential is checked by a normal immune system.[89] On the other hand, Kaposi's sarcoma (KS) was an uncommon ailment largely confined to Mediterranean and African men prior to the HIV epidemic. It seems to be a separate epidemic STD with its own epidemiology, treatment, and impact, which somehow has become part of the HIV epidemic.[90] Other clinical indicators for AIDS are various cytomegaloviral infections[91] such as CMV retinitis, which blinds rapidly; cryptococcal meningitis, a dangerous yeast infection; oral candidiasis (thrush), which fills the mouth and esophagus with white choking fungus; severe herpes lesions; Mycobacterium Avium Complex (MAC) which produces many symptoms including high fevers, nausea, severe diarrhea and weight loss; a mycobacterial form of tuberculosis (that is becoming a major epidemic in itself); cryptosporidiosis (intestinal inflammations); acute renal failure[92] and on and on and on. The full clinical definition is distressingly long and complex.

The specific opportunistic infections that afflict any given individual will vary according to a number of variables. His or her previous health history and lifestyle will be obvious factors. Apparently unrelated matters can affect the health of a PWA. For example, bird droppings are a fertile source of *Toxoplasma gondii*, the agent of toxoplasmosis of the brain, and therefore immunocompromised people ought not to be around accumulations of, say, pigeon droppings. Similarly, *Mycobacteria avium* are commonly found in garden soil, poultry, dairy products, and red meats. Neither of these pathogens is dangerous to anyone with a normal immune system, but both can cause serious illness in a PWA. Even geographic locale can play a role. Different areas have varying concentrations of the pathogens involved. Thus in North America, the fungal agent responsible for histoplasmosis is found mainly in the Mississippi Valley. Current research indicates that few of the various opportunistic infections will take firm hold until an individual's immune cell counts fall below 200.

One problem that does not appear on the list, but perhaps should, is suicide. Although not an opportunistic infection in the ordinary sense, data nonetheless indicate an increased incidence of suicide for seropositives.[93] By the very fact of infection, the HIV+ is set aside, isolated from others. From biblical times into the twentieth century, lepers were quarantined for, as it turned out, no good reason. Happily we have learned, and no one in authority seriously proposes constructing HIV leprosaria. Nonetheless at the very time that a recent seroconverter most needs emotional support, he or she is least likely to get it. The fear of stigmatization is sufficient to prevent the new HIV+ from turning to those from whom he or she would normally seek help. Frequently there is a self-quarantine process, a distancing that results from fear of public exposure and a consequent loss of jobs, insurance, and friends. There is also the isolation that comes from the conviction that communication with "the others"—the uninfected—is futile since no one but another HIV+ can possibly understand about the shortened and difficult life ahead.[94] All this is exacerbated by feelings of disorientation, even madness, as all the fixed points of one's life are suddenly undermined—why should one finish school, go on working, plan for the future, or continue dating a special someone, go on living?[95] Finally the PWA suffers a steady demoralization that results from feeling that he or she has become a pariah, a person who cannot satisfy ordinary social and sexual needs without endangering others.

There is, at present, no weapon that is lethal to the virus that is not also lethal to humans; thus it is unfortunately true that once HIV infection has passed, by whatever means, the individual is infected and infectious for the remainder of his or her life. No direct assaults upon the virus have proved successful; the consequence is that dysfunction within the individual's immune system gradually increases until such time as the conditions defined as AIDS appear. Therapy is limited to slowing, as best we can, the rapidity of HIV's replication plus treatment of opportunistic infections as they appear. This is a losing game because, first, if one opportunistic infection is brought under control another can and will develop and, second, because the patient's system gradually becomes too weak to give natural support to medical intervention. It is like trying to put out a forest fire without being able to get to the core of the blaze.

Dr. John McGowan of the AIDS program at the National Institute of Allergy and Infectious Diseases said, "We're going to have to have alphabet soup to treat this disease."[96] Workers in the field agree. There may never be a single remedy but rather an evolving potpourri of drugs, therapies, and vaccines, the exact recipe of which might vary with the patient's age, sex, general health, and display of opportunistic infections.[97] For example, it does seem that there needs to be a different mix of both treatment and support for women who present infections unique to their sex, such as vulvovaginal candidiasis, pelvic inflammatory disease, and cervical cancer, as well as coping with AIDS in a different context. Although they are sick themselves, they may, nonetheless, still be the primary care givers of a family.[98] The IV drug user presents his or her own set of problems. Laboratory studies indicate that HIV gets high on coke too! The virus grows three times faster in cells exposed to cocaine.[99] Similarly, pediatric cases require definition and treatment distinct from adult cases; infants are especially vulnerable because they have not had time to develop their own immune systems, relying upon the antibodies transferred from the mother (who transmitted the HIV). Science is just now confronting the fact that most of the American data are derived from studies of gay men in cities like San Francisco, New York, and Chicago, while the incidence among other groups about which we know much less, such as women, is increasing rapidly.

The major weakness bedeviling the search for vaccines, more effective drugs, and better treatment protocols is the lack of knowledge about the structure and operation of HIV in the body; with all that we have learned in such a short time, there are still glaring gaps in our understanding of how HIV works in the body, as distinct from in a test tube.[100] The distinction between *in vivo* and *in vitro,* in the body and in the test tube, is one that is critical to understanding why, with all the resources of intelligence, equipment, and effort the search has so far failed, and why it may take a long time to succeed.

Human beings must be seen as incredibly complex and efficient chemical factories, each one slightly different. Everyone's body-factory processes everything put into it the instant that it is introduced, from a cookie to a drug. The result is frequently something quite different from what the maker intended or can control. The cookie might upset your stomach, the drug might not work—indeed, it might kill you instead of cure you. Ideas that fly in the laboratory, sometimes crash in the stomach or bloodstream. There is nothing that can be done about this except to keep trying; no one really knows whether something will work until it is tried. The hazards of lost time, lost resources, and lost people that are inevitably involved in the trial and error process are usually in inverse proportion to how much we know of ourselves and the virus that intrudes. Without a thorough knowledge of HIV's complex relation to the human organism, science can only grope, instead of march, toward solutions.

However, even better knowledge does not guarantee the development of a cure in the complete, popular sense of that term. In this century, it is more likely that AIDS will become a "chronic but manageable" disease, an affliction contained and managed by a much longer list of drugs than those we now have. Dr. Burton Lee of the Sloan-Kettering Cancer Center and a member of the President's Commission on AIDS put the matter this way, "There's no pie in the sky with AIDS. The sad fact is that medicine has never cured a viral disease, and AIDS is caused by an exceptionally complicated retrovirus." No one should expect a quick fix.

Notes

1. Paul Cotton, "HIV Genes Overlap with Ours," *Medical World News*, March 14, 1988, 38. Emmanuel Dreuilhe, *Mortal Embrace: Living with AIDS* (New York, Hill and Wang, 1988).

2. The chimpanzee is the only nonhuman primate that can be infected by an inoculation of natural HIV-1. Its immune system will react by the creation of antibodies to the virus, although the chimp does not get seriously ill. It can, therefore, be used as an animal model for research in vaccines. Unfortunately it is the rarest and most expensive of animal substitutes for humans. See Presto Marx, et al., "An Animal Model of Sexual Transmission of AIDS," in Nancy J. Alexander, Henry L. Gabelnick, and Jeffrey M. Spieler (eds.), *Heterosexual Transmission of AIDS* (New York: Wiley-Liss, 1989). In 1994 a team of researchers at the Southwest Foundation for Biomedical Research announced that they had fabricated a virus (called SHIV) that would infect the baboon, a much more plentiful research animal. "Hybrid Virus Tested at S.A. Baboon Center," *San Antonio Express-News*, February 6, 1994, 1B.

3. A review of the most popular origin theories is in *Natural History*, November 1992. See also the review of theories in Jad Adams, *AIDS: The HIV Myth* (New York, St. Martin's Press, 1989), chapter 7.

4. A laboratory worker was infected with the Simian virus after a blood exposure to an infected animal. His blood tests positive for SIV and, as yet (1994), he is symptom-free. *Baltimore Sun*, January 20, 1994, reporting on the report in the *New England Journal of Medicine*.

5. On the biologic origin of HIV see Robert C. Gallo, "The AIDS Virus, Part II," *Scientific American*, January 1987, 56; Max Essex and Phyillis J. Kanki, "The Origins of the AIDS Virus," *Scientific American*, October 1988, 64–71; Max Essex, "Origins of AIDS," in Vincent T. DeVita et al. (eds.), *AIDS, Etiology, [Table 2.2 Approved Medicines] Diagnosis, Treatment, and Prevention* (New York, J. B. Lippincott Co., 1988). See also the good summary in Professor A. Karpas's letter to *Nature*, December 13, 1990, 578.

6. *Nature*, December 1991.

7. Tom Curtis, "The Origin of AIDS," *Rolling Stone*, March 19, 1993. This article was based on a speculative editorial in *Research in Virology* 144 (1993).

8. Eve K. Nichols, *Mobilizing against AIDS*, rev. ed., (Washington, D.C.: Institute of Medicine, National Academy of Sciences, 1989), 109.

9. See the chilling demographic projections of R. M. Anderson and the Parasite Epidemiology Research Group, Department of Pure and Applied Biology, Imperial College, London University. R.M. Anderson et al., "The Impact of the Spread of HIV on Population Growth and Age Structure in Developing Countries," in Alan F. Fleming et al. (eds), *The Global Impact of AIDS: Proceedings of the First International Conference on the Global Impact of AIDS*, co-sponsored by the World Health Organization and the London School of Hygiene and Tropical Medicine, London, March 8–10, 1988 (New York: Alan R. Liss, 1988), chapter 12.

10. It should be noted that, although the majority of the scientific establishment seems to support the position that HIV is the causative agent in AIDS, there is a minority position. Dr. Peter H. Duesberg, Professor of Molecular Biology, University of California at Berkeley, is a major protagonist of another view

which denies that HIV is that agent. Dr. Duesberg published his challenge to conventional HIV theory in the February 1989 issue of the *Proceedings of the National Academy of Sciences* ("Human Immunodeficiency Virus and Acquired Immunodeficiency Syndrome: Correlation but Not Causation"). Dr. Duesberg contends that AIDS is caused by a combination of (1) "chronic promiscuous male homosexual activity," (2) "parasitic infection," (3) malnutrition, and (4) narcotic toxins. See the interesting comment in *Science* (February 10, 1989, p. 733) on the fight between Duesberg and the National Academy. The minority position is reviewed in Adams, *AIDS: The HIV Myth*. Another major research scientist whose work raises questions about the role of HIV is Dr. Shyh-Ching Lo who is the head of the AIDS pathology division of the Armed Forces Institute of Pathology's Molecular Pathobiology Laboratory. See his study in *The American Journal of Tropical Medicine Hygiene* 40 (1989): 213–26, 399–409. There is also the possibility that a mycoplasma organism is involved in the development of the syndrome. Mycoplasmas are the smallest known organisms which, unlike viruses, have the ability to reproduce themselves. They occupy a biological niche someplace between bacteria and viruses. A group of scientists met in San Antonio in December 1989 to explore this possibility. *San Antonio Express-News*, December 9, 1989, 14a. Brant Mittler, "Behold, AIDS Research Behind Closed Doors," *Medical Tribune*, February 8, 1990. Dr. Luc Montagnier of France, whose team discovered HIV, gave some support to the view that mycoplasmas may be co-factors in statements at the Sixth International Conference on AIDS, San Francisco, July 1990, "AIDS Drugs—Coming, but Not Here," *Science* (April 21, 1990), 287.

11. An international controversy, ultimately involving the presidents of France and the United States, developed over who discovered what and when. National and professional pride, as well as valuable patent rights, were involved in this rather degrading conclusion to a notable scientific achievement. Good summaries can be read in *Journal of the American Medical Association (JAMA)* (December 25, 1987), 3482–87; and *Chicago Tribune*, November 19, 1989. The *Tribune* ran an extraordinary pair of articles by investigative reporter John Crewdson on this controversy. See also "The French Connection, II: An International AIDS Dispute Is Reborn," *Newsweek* (April 2, 1990), 65. In October 1990, the National Institutes of Health announced that it was undertaking a full-scale investigation of "possible misconduct" (that is, copying the French discoveries rather than independently developing them) in Dr. Gallo's laboratory at the National Cancer Institute. The final result of these investigations was that, indeed, the "discoveries" of Gallo's labs were, in fact, copies of or contaminations from the French isolated virus. So credit was officially given to the priority of the Pasteur Institute's discovery. In later 1993 proceedings, Dr. Gallo was exonerated on charges of "scientific misconduct," that is, an attempt to claim the French discovery.

12. The American figure is very "soft," and very debatable. It was derived, at the 1986 Coolfont Planning Conference, by extrapolating from the assumed number of homosexuals in the United States (as projected from the Kinsey research of the 1940s). At that time there were about thirty thousand cases reported. It did not take into consideration other transmission modes like IV drug use. In 1989, California epidemiologists were stating that there might be over 2 million infected in that state alone. It is more than possible that an accurate national survey would more than triple the old 1.5 million guesstimate. The "official" estimate stated by the Federal Centers for Disease Control in 1990 is one million.

13. T4 and CD4 are different names for the same molecular receptor. HIV is capable of attaching to and infecting monocytes/macrophages, using them for transportation throughout the body including the brain and central nervous system.

14. For an excellent review article, see Giuseppe Pantaleo et al., "The Immunopathogenesis of Human Immunodeficiency Virus Infection," *The New England Journal of Medicine* (February 4, 1993), 327–35. It ought to be noted that there are a number of other diseases of the immunological system—multiple sclerosis, for example—but they are usually expressions of innate genetic deficiencies. Perhaps the most popularly known are those that produce bubble-babies, children that can only survive in a totally protected environment.

15. P. C Fox et al., "Saliva inhibits HIV-1 Infectivity," *Journal of the American Dental Association* 116, no. 6 (1988), 635–37. A. C. Varrusio et al., "Risk of Transmission of the Human Immunodeficiency Virus to Health Care Workers Exposed to HIV-Infected Patients: A Review," *Journal of the American Dental Association* 118, no. 3 (1989), 229–342.

16. Mangalasseril and Markham, "Role of Human T Lymphotropic Retrovirus in Leukemia and AIDS," in Gary P. Wormser et al., eds. *AIDS: Acquired Immune Deficiency Syndrome* (Park Ridge, N.J.: Noyes, 1987), 219.

17. Lawrence K. Altman, "Drug-Resistant Strains of HIV Linked to Tripling of AIDS," *New York Times*, December 17, 1993, A26.

18. The first reported infection by HIV-2 in the United States was in 1987. Since then sixteen additional cases have been found. "AIDS Update of Experimental Therapies," *Health Info-Com Network Newsletter*, May 16, 1990. James Brooke, "Virus Discoveries," *New York Times*, February 28, 1988, 12.

19. Adapted from a series on FIV by Dr. Philip W. Martin, *San Antonio Express-News*, January 3, 4, 5, 1994.

20. For a much more extensive description of the immune system and the molecular biology of the virus, but one which is still geared to the nonbiologist, see Mary Catherine Bateson and Richard Goldsby, *Thinking AIDS* (Redding, Mass.: Addison-Wesley, 1988), chapters 3–6; or William B. Johnson and Kevin R. Hopkins, *The Catastrophe Ahead, AIDS and the Case for a New Public Policy* (New York: Praeger, 1990), chap. 6. A more technical and extended description, but still accessible to the nonbiologist, can be read in Nichols, *Mobilizing against AIDS*, chap. 5. For those interested in professional descriptions of HIV's life cycle, I suggest William A. Haseltine and Flossie Wong-Staal, "The Molecular Biology of the AIDS Virus," and Robert Yarchoan, Hiroaki Mitsuya, and Samuel Broder, "AIDS Therapies," *Scientific American* (October 1988); Vincent T. DeVita et al., *AIDS, Etiology, Diagnosis, Treatment, and Prevention* (New York: J. B. Lippincott, 1988), chaps. 2 and 5.

21. It is likely that virus infected cells, rather than free virus, are the principal transmitting mechanism. Jay Levy, *JAMA* (May 27, 1988), 3037.

22. For the latest thinking on the process see: "HIV-Mediated Defects in Immune Regulation," Report of the Immunopathology Conference sponsored by the Division of AIDS, National Institute of Allergies and Infectious Diseases, September 29–30, 1993. Copies of the Report can be obtained from AIDS Treatment Data Network (212-268-4196). Also see Warner C. Greene, "AIDS and the Immune System," *Scientific American* (September 1993), 98–105; Wormser, *AIDS*, chaps. 9, 11; Institute of Medicine, National Academy of Sciences, *Confronting AIDS: Directions for Public Health Care and Research* (National Academy Press, 1986), chap. 6; Anthony Fauci, "The Human Immunodeficiency

Virus: Infectivity and Mechanisms of Pathogenesis," *Science*, 239: 617–21; for popularized-technical versions see William A. Haseltine, and Flossie Wong-Staal, "The Molecular Biology of the AIDS Virus"; Jonathan Weber and Robin A. Weiss, "HIV Infection: The Cellular Picture," *Scientific American* (October 1988).

23. See Alan R. Lifson, "Do Alternate Modes of Transmission of HIV Exist?" *JAMA* (March 4, 1988), 1353.

24. U.S. Department of Public Health and Human Services, Public Health Service, Centers for Disease Control, *Morbidity and Mortality Weekly Report, Supplement: Recommendations for Prevention of HIV Transmission in Health-Care Settings* (Washington, D.C., 1987). On the development of new types of surgical gloving see *Medical Tribune*, March 8, 1990, 7.

25. Many more have been exposed. Hard, reliable data are difficult to come by in this area because the virus may not evidence itself in tests until long after the presumed needle-stick incident. It is difficult to establish clear cause and effect. "Why Fear Persists: Health Care Professionals and AIDS," *JAMA* (December 16, 1988), 3481. Ruthanne Marcus, "Surveillance of Health Care Workers Exposed to Blood from Patients Infected with the Human Immunodeficiency Virus," *New England Journal of Medicine* (October 27, 1988), 1118–19.

26. *JAMA* (November 7, 1990). See the excellent special report by Elisabeth Rosenthal, "Practice of Medicine Is Changing under Specter of the AIDS Virus," *New York Times*, November 11, 1990, A1.

27. As of 1993, the data indicates that it does not stop seroconversion. However, hospitals continue using the procedure, lacking anything else to do for an exposed health care worker. Dr. Marcus A. Conant made the recommendation at the annual meeting of the American Academy of Dermatology. See "HIV, Hepatitis Continue to Pose Major Risks for Health Workers," *Internal Medicine News*, January 15–31, 1990, 1.

28. Sari Staver, "One in 250 HIV-Infected Sticks Transmits the Virus–Studies," *American Medical News*, January 13, 1989, 19–20. And see interview with Dr. Lorraine Day who resigned as chief of orthopedic surgery at San Francisco General Hospital to protest inadequate medical and hospital administrative response to the hazards of the operating room. *New Dimensions*, March 1990, 36–40.

29. The *New York Times* cites the Soviet magazine *Ogonyok* which stated that in 1988 the Soviet Union produced only 7 million disposable syringes a year against an estimated need of 6 billion, and 200 million condoms against a need of 1 billion. John F. Burns, "Outbreak of AIDS Triples: Testing in a Soviet City," *New York Times*, National Section, February 5, 1989.

30. This tragic story was told by Dr. Vladimir Pokrovsky the representative of the Soviet Union at the 5th International Conference on AIDS, which met at Montreal, Canada in June of 1989. See *New York Times*, June 3, 1989. The Soviet Union has enacted new legislation making multiple uses of syringes and other dangerous practices subject to criminal prosecution. However, the nation is still far from producing adequate supplies of antiseptic and disposable equipment.

31. *Ogonyok*, cited in *Health InfoCom Newsletter*, April 20–22, 1990. And see also *Nature*, the June 14, 1990 issue, which contains a commentary on some official Soviet reports relating the possibility of great increases in the incidence of AIDS.

32. Summary in "Transfusion-Transmitted AIDS Reassessed" (Editorial) *JAMA* 318, no. 8: 511.

33. This is the estimate of the National Federation of Hemophilia.
34. Randy Shilts, *And the Band Played On* (New York: St. Martin's Press, 1987) relates this story in detail. Also see John W. Ward, "Transfusion of HIV by Blood Transfusions Screened as Negative for the HIV Antibody," and Thomas F. Zuck, "Transfusion-Transmitted AIDS Reassessed," *New England Journal of Medicine* (February 25, 1988), 473, 5ll.
35. *Congressional Quarterly*, August 18, 1990, 2685.
36. Peter Finn, "Hemophiliacs Seek Redress for AIDS Toll," and "Farm Family's 6 Sons, Wives, Babies Fall," *Washington Times*, January 26, 1994. Sandra Blakeslee, "Blood Banks Facing Hundreds of AIDS Suits," *New York Times*, Health Section, April 27, 1989, 24. Janice Somerville, "AIDS Related Suits," *American Medical News*, February 17, 1989. The problem is not confined to the United States. *The Melbourne Star* Observer, September 8, 1989 reported that hundreds of Australian hemophiliacs may sue the Red Cross Blood Bank for receiving contaminated blood clotting agents between 1983 and 1985. The estimates are that one fourth of Australia's hemophiliacs are infected. Major problems have also surfaced in Canada, France, Germany, Romania, and other countries. In most cases, however, the governments of other nations are dealing with the problem without the need for litigation.
37. French officials refused to adopt an American patented HIV test, preferring to wait for their own to be brought on line. Further, they could not face the political, budgeting, and bureaucratic problems that would ensue from discarding $40 million worth of contaminated blood and blood products.
38. CDC Press Release, United Press International, "CDC Study Finds Five Transfusion-Related AIDS Cases per Year," October 25, 1993.
39. See John W. Ward et al., "Transmission of Human Immunodeficiency Virus by Blood Transfusions Screened as Negative for HIV Antibody," *New England Journal of Medicine* 318, no. 8 (February 25, 1988), 473–77. The risk of transmitting HIV through transfusion of *screened* blood is calculated as between 1:153,000 to 1:200,000. See *New England Journal of Medicine* 322, no. 12 (March 22, 1990), 850. There is considerable argument in the professional literature about the extent of possibility of testing negative on the Elisa or Western Blot while, nonetheless, being infected with the virus. There is also controversy about how long a person can be infected without registering same in the standard tests. Very sophisticated, expensive, and time-consuming tests approach 100 percent accuracy but are too elaborate to be used in mass operations like blood plasma collection. The *Ryan White Comprehensive AIDS Act of 1990* authorized a special study running from 1991 through 1995 as well as federal services to help protect the blood supply.
40. *Reader's Digest*, "Special Report: How Safe Is Our Blood Supply?" July 1988, 37–44. This report points out that there have been thirteen cases of transfusion AIDS *since* 1985 when screening was finally installed.
41. *American Medical News*, June 10, 1991, 13. The donor, who was shot and killed in 1985, was HIV+. However that fact was not detected in two separate testings prior to the harvesting of his skin, bones, etc., for storage and transplant. Three people who received transplants have died. In December 1993, the FDA announced that it would commence regulating the sale of bone, skin, and other tissues (as distinct from organs, already under regulation) used in transplants to help protect recipients.
42. *New York Times*, "New York Won't Tell Doctors with AIDS to Inform Patients,"

January 19, 1991, A1. See also *New York Times*, "AIDS and the Privacy of Doctors: A Touchy Issue at Bellevue," January 28, 1991, A15. Sari Staver, "Government: Guidelines Coming Soon on Managing HIV-Infected Health Workers," *American Medical News*, December 28, 1990, 3, and "HIV-Infected Doctors Should Tell Patients, Stop Surgery—AMA," *American Medical News*, February 4, 1991.

43. Hill, David, "HIV Infection Following Motor Vehicle: Trauma in Central Africa," *JAMA* 261, no. 22 (June 9, l989), 3282.

44. *Washington HIV News* 1, no. 4 (January 1990).

45. For a review of the situation, see White, Kristin, "Treating Pediatric AIDS," *AIDS Patient Care* I, no. 1 (September 1987), 5–13. Gwendolyn Scott et al., "Survival of Children with Perinatally Acquired Human Immunodeficiency Virus Type 1 Infection," *New England Journal of Medicine* 321, no. 26 (January 1990), 1791–96.

46. Malcolm Gladwell, "Pediatric AIDS Studied at Adults' Expense," *Washington Post*, October 5, 1992.

47. "Aids Boarder Babies Pose Financial and Logistical Problems," *AIDS ALERT* 3, no. 6 (June 1988), 97–102.

48. Karen deWitt, "In U.S. Ads for TV, Condoms That Dare Speak Their Name," *New York Times*, January 5, 1994, A1.

49. Giuseppe Pantaleo, Ceclioa Graziosi, and Anthony S. Fauci, "The Immunopathogensis of Human Immunodeficiency Virus Infection," *New England Journal of Medicine* (February 4, 1993), 327–35.

50. See "Researchers Gain in Mapping How AIDS Virus Enters Cells," *New York Times*, December 29, 1990, A1.

51. Strictly speaking the glial cells are not directly infected; they are disrupted by other chemical changes brought on by HIV infection.

52. For a review see Fred T. Valentine, "Pathogenesis of the Immunological Deficiencies Caused by Infection with the Human Immunodeficiency Virus," *Seminars in Oncology* 17, no. 3 (June 1990), 321–34.

53. This puzzle has led many observers, like Dr. Peter Duesberg of the University of California, for example, to question whether HIV was the cause of AIDS.

54. Gina Kolata, "Hiding Place of AIDS Virus in Confirmed," New York Times, March 31, 1993, p.B9.

55. Trials are underway on a number of such drugs; a hopeful one is a powerful toxin produced by the Pseudomonas bacteria. It can attach to actively infected (not latently) cells and kill them. If it works in vivo, it will not be a cure but will slow the infection. See Gina Kolata, "Scientists Modify Powerful Toxin to Combat Spread of AIDS Virus," *New York Times*, October 14, 1988.

56. Robert W. Finbert et al., "Prevention of HIV-1 Infection and Preservation of CD4 function by the binding of CPFs to gp120," *Science*, July 20, 1990, 287.

57. Lawrence K. Altman, "Hopes Are Dashed on AIDS Therapy," *New York Times*, June 10, 1993, A4; *Project Inform Briefing Paper*, "Overview: The Conference in Berlin," July 1993.

58. For an excellent summary of the prospects and problems, see "Vaccine Development," in *AIDS SUMMARY: In-Depth Review & Update* (Philadelphia, Penn.: Philadelphia Sciences Group Publications, March 1989).

59. Dr. Ronald Derosiers of the New England Regional Primate Center, quoted in John Capri, "The AIDS Vaccine Front Is Expanding," *Medical Tribune*, March 8, 1990, 7; "Tests of a Vaccine on Monkeys Offers New Hope in AIDS Fight,"

New York Times, December 8, 1989, A1.

60. Maurice R. Hilleman, "Conclusions: In Pursuit of an AIDS Virus Vaccine," in Jay A. Levy (ed.), *AIDS, Pathogenesis and Treatment* (New York: Marcel Dekker, 1989), 609.

61. *CDC AIDS Weekly* (Atlanta, Ga.: Charles Henderson, Publ.), November 7, 1988, 3.

62. The term "vaccine development," in the singular, is somewhat misleading. Actually research is underway on many different types of vaccines, each with its own set of problems and potentials. There are inactivated, attenuated live, recombinant DNA, hybrid virus, synthesized polypeptides, and anti-idiotype vaccines.

63. See Bradley D. Preston et al., "Fidelity of HIV-1 Reverse Transcriptase," *Science*, November 25, 1988, 1168. The findings are that HIV's extensive genetic variation and rapid evolution is due to the high "error" rate of reverse transcriptase, the enzyme that directs part of the replication process. The authors use the term "hypermutability."

64. Manfred Eigen, "Viral Quasispecies," *Scientific American* (July 1993), 48. Eigen points out that if HIV can change all its hypervariable genome sites in thirty years (which seems likely), then it can easily exhaust the human immune system in less time—seven to ten years.

65. "Merck Drops Final Bid to Develop Drug for AIDS in Face of Viral Resistance," *Wall Street Journal*, September 15, 1993, B6.

66. Scientists are using transgenic mice, that is, mice genetically engineered to express an HIV infection, not simply ignore it. Normal mice have no reaction to the virus.

67. See the report on the 3rd Annual International Conference on Advances in AIDS Vaccine Development (sponsored by NIAID) in *Science*, October 12, 1990.

68. Effective antiviral vaccines have been developed against vaccinia, poliovirus, measles, mumps, rubella, yellow fever, influenza, rabies, and hepatitis B.

69. See Nichols, *Mobilizing against AIDS*, chapter 7, for a brief coverage of the various agents now in testing and trial stages.

70. For the first long-term studies on ddI, see R. Yarchoan, et al., "Long-term Toxicity/Activity Profile of 2,3'-dideoxyinosine in AIDS or AIDS-Related Complex," *The Lancet*, September 1, 1990.

71. "AIDS Drugs—Coming, but Not Here," *Science*, April 21, 1990, 287.

72. It is not known why the period of so-called latency is as long as it is. The authors of an interesting attempt to model viral development or evolution after infection hypothesize that "the most important single factor leading to breakdown of immune control of HIV is the increase in the diversity of the virus." Charles R. M Bangham and Andrew J. McMichael, "Why the Long Latent Period," *Nature*, November 29, 1990.

73. David Ho et al., "Quantitation of Human Immunodeficiency Virus, Type 1 in Blood of Infected Person," *New England Journal of Medicine* (December 14, 1989), 1621.

74. For a description of the Walter Reed system, see Appendix C in *Report of The Presidential Commission on the Human Immunodeficiency Virus*, June 24, 1988.

75. Robert Redfield and Donald Burke, "HIV Infection: the Clinical Picture," *Scientific American* (October 1988), 93–98. This article explains the classification system

developed by the authors. Their system delineates "stages" in the progression to AIDS. They are both scientists at Walter Reed Army Institute of Research, Washington, D.C. Redfield is chief of the retrovirology section, Burke is chief of the Department of Virus Diseases at the Institute of Research. Another, perhaps more accurate, method of tracking the progression is through CD4 cell counts. See R .B. MacDonnel et al., "Prognostic Usefulness of the Walter Reed Staging Classification for HIV Infection," *Journal of Acquired Immune Deficiency Syndromes* (1988), 367–74.

76. See the excellent review article by John Mills and Henry Masur, "AIDS-Related Infections," *Scientific American* (August 1990), 50.

77. Gina Kolata, "Researchers Link Speed of AIDS Development to Age," *New York Times*, National, May 21, 1989.

78. *AIDS Treatment Issues, GMHC Newsletter of Experimental AIDS Therapies*, December 1992, 7.

79. The eleven-year estimate is documented by George F. Lemp et al. , "Projections of AIDS Morbidity and Mortality in San Francisco," *JAMA* March 16, 1990. The ten-year figures came from the San Francisco Department of Health study. Peter Bacchetti and Andrew Moss, "AIDS Incubation Time," *Nature* (March 16, 1988), 251–53. Gina Kolata, "AIDS Incubation Time Often Exceeds 9 Years," *New York Times*, Health, March 16, 1989, 19.

80. National Institutes of Health, *NIAID Summaries from the IX International Conference on AIDS*, "HIV Infection Among Gay and Bisexual Men," "HIV-Infected Men with Stable CD4+ T Cell Counts for Seven to Eight Years," and "Rapid Progression to AIDS Among HIV-Infected Men," July 1993.

81. Donald I. Abrams, Jeanee Parker-Martin, and Kenneth Unger, "AIDS: Caring for the Dying Patient," *Patient Care* (November 30, 1989), 2 et seq.

82. Emmanuel Dreuilhe, *Mortal Embrace, Living with AIDS* (New York: Hill and Wang, 1988).

83. "New Evidence that HIV Can Cause Disease Independently," *HIVNet Medical Newsletter*, available on INTERNET, April 20, 1993.

84. Peter H. Duesberg, "Human Immunodeficiency Virus and Acquired Immunodeficiency Syndrome: Correlation but Not Causation," *Proceedings of the National Academy of Sciences* 86 (February 1989), and "AIDS Epidemiology: Inconsistencies with the Immunodeficiency Virus and with Infectious Disease," *Proceedings* 88 (February 1991).

85. Robert S. Root-Bernstein, *Rethinking AIDS. The Tragic Cost of Premature Consensus* (New York: The Free Press, 1993).

86. The duality of requirement is often overlooked. It would do the CDC no good to define AIDS as "something like Flu, only worse." Such a description or definition would not distinguish AIDS from a multitude of other ailments, and make tracking and record keeping impossible.

87. "1993 AIDS Surveillance Case Definition—Answers from CDC," in *AIDS News Service*, VA Medical Center, San Francisco, September 7, 1993.

88. For a technical, but still accessible description of the entire range of infections under the 1987 definition, see Gifford Leoung and John Mills (eds.), *Opportunistic Infections in Patients with the Acquired Immunodeficiency Syndrome* (New York: Marcel Dekker, 1989). The "indicator diseases" of the *1993 Revised Classification System* (p. 15) are candidiasis of bronchi, trachea, or lungs; esophageal candidiasis; invasive cervical cancer; coccidioidomycosis,; cryptococcoses; chronic intestinal cryptosporodiosis; cytomegalovirus disease

(other than liver, spleen, or nodes); cytomgegalovirus retinitis (with loss of vision); HIV-related encephalopathy; herpes simplex with chronic ulcer(s), or bronchitis, pneumonitis, or esophagitis; histoplasmosis; chronic intestinal isosporiasis; Kaposi's sarcoma; lymphoma, Burkitt's or equivalent form; lymphoma, immunoblastic; lymphoma, primary of the brain; mycobacterium avium complex, or m. kansasii; mycobacterium tuberculosis,; mycobacterium, other species or unidentified species; pneumocystis carinii pneumonia; recurrent pneumonia; progressive multifocal leukoencephalopathy; recurrent septicemic salmonella; toxoplasmosis of brain; wasting syndrome due to HIV.

89. For the full range of pulmonary complications, see John F. Murray and John Mills, "Pulmonary Jnfectious Complications of Human Immunodeficiency Virus Infection" (in 2 Parts), *American Review of Respiratory Diseases* 141 (1990).

90.   See J. W. Conant et al., "Kaposi's Sarcoma: Epidemiology, Pathogenesis, Histology, Clinical Spectrum, Staging Criteria, and Therapy," *Journal of the American Academy of Dermatology* (March 1993), 371–95. "KS Is Not Cancer; Is It Also Not AIDS?" *AIDS Treatment News*, March 16, 1990 and the references cited there. Recent research indicates that certain of the HIV cell proteins have the effect of greatly stimulating KS cells into an aggressive growth. But KS and HIV infection can exist independently of one another.

91. Matthew Stenger (ed.), *The Management of HIV-Related Cytomegalovirus Infections*, highlights of a symposium on current therapies and future strategies in the management of CMV infections held prior to the Sixth International Conference on AIDS, San Francisco, June 1990. Newsletter published by Professional Healthcare Communications (ProHealth), One Lombard St., San Francisco, CA 94111. Also distributed as *AIDS Clinical Update*, October 1, 1990 by New York's Gay Men's Health Crisis.

92. Jacques J. Bourgoignie, "Renal Complications of Human Immunodeficiency Virus Type 1," *Kidney International* (Nephrology Forum) 37 (1990), 1571–84.

93. Peter M. Marzuk et al., "Increased Risk of Suicide in Persons with AIDS," *JAMA* (March 4, 1988), 1333–42. See also the Associated Press feature article that appeared in the first week of July 1990 in which the director of an AIDS support group in Vancouver admitted that he had helped patients take their lives by leaving fatal overdoses within reach. *San Antonio Express-News*, July 5, 1990, 8E. How much assisted and unassisted suicide goes on is probably impossible to estimate with any degree of accuracy. But that it does occur is unquestionable. *Internal Medicine News*, January 15, 1991, "Suicide Ideation Peaks Early in HIV Disease."

94. See on this aspect Dreuilhe, *Mortal Embrace*.

95. A sad story came out of Marion, Virginia. A young man committed suicide convinced that he was infected when, in fact, he was not. His doctors failed to inform him that his HIV tests were negative. The doctors, in turn, failed to act because the courier from the testing laboratory misplaced the results. "Suit Dismissed in Suicide over AIDS Test," *Washington Post*, January 14, 1993.

96. *Science* (April 21, 1990), 287.

97. See "New Eclecticism Approach to AIDS," *American Medical News*, September 23/30, 1988.

98. Review article entitled "HIV Disease and AIDS in Women, Current Knowledge and a Research Agenda," *Journal of AIDS*, May 1992. Review article entitled "A Review of Reports on Women and AIDS," *Treatment Issues, GMHC Newsletter of Experimental AIDS Therapies*, November 1992, 3. "Women with AIDS Seen

Dying Faster," *New York Times*, October 19, 1987, reporting on the research of Dr. Margaret Fischl of the University of Miami. There are some clues indicating that this effect is due to the differences in male-female hormonal components, see John S. James, "DHEA, Mystery AIDS Treatment," *AIDS Treatment News*, January 15, 1988. The substance involved in this new experimental treatment is dehydroepiandrosterone which is steroid secreted by the adrenal gland and is closely related to the male hormone, testosterone.

99. *Health InfoCom Medical News*, October 22–24, 1990.
100. "Molecule X: The Other Key to HIV?" *New Scientist* (July 7, 1990), 6. The phrase "glaring gaps" is a quote from Dr. Anthony Fauci, head of National Institute of Allergy and Infectious Diseases, National Institutes of Health.

3

Then and Now:
The Bubonic Plague and Aids

LAUNCHING AN EPIDEMIC

Every living thing has a territory in which it evolved and from which it emerged to face the world, a home-base on this planet. There are Bengal Tigers, American Bison, and unending hosts of butterflies, salmon, birds, whales, and caribou which annually migrate back to their point-of-origin. We humans, who now cover the Earth, apparently are descendants of ancient hominids who evolved in places like the Olduvai Basin of Central Africa's Great Rift Valley millions of years ago. Evidence of our dispersal is buried in the dirt of archaeological sites, painted on cave walls, incised on clay tablets, written on papyri, manuscripts, books, and now the electronic impulses of the computer. We call it the spread of human culture and civilization.

It is the same for the invisible empire of microbes that prey upon us. Some home-base areas, like India's Ganges River valley, China's Yellow River valley, equatorial Africa and America, seem to have been designed as natural kitchens serving endless varieties of bacteria, plasmodia, viruses, protozoa, and fungi. These are areas where disease pathogens develop and are endemic. They serve as the initial staging areas for epidemics. In an elegant phrase from epidemiology they are the original "geographic foci of endemicity." Sailors in the nineteenth-century British navy had a more pointed expression; they referred to a tour of duty off the coast of Equatorial Africa as the "coffin cruise." Having no independent means of locomotion, microbes generally stay home—unless, of course, they encounter people. Then, if conditions are right, rapid dispersal is possible. We call this unwanted event an epidemic.

Like human cultures, epidemics also leave their record in burial grounds across the world. Records state that twenty thousand per day perished in the Great Plague of which Bishop Cyprian wrote in the third century. The

59

bubonic plague of 1347—50 killed from 17 to 28 million, and in the four hundred years of revisitations (1340–1740s), perhaps 50 million people died all together. Ninety million Central and South American Indians died from waves of smallpox, measles, typhus, and flu introduced by the Spanish after 1520.[1] Seven million succumbed to cholera in 1910–20 and another 10–20 million died in the 1917 flu epidemic. Today we have perhaps 14 million individuals infected with the HIV. The World Health Organization projects between 50 and 100 million by the year 2000. For some microbes, but by no means all, and certainly not HIV, we have established a degree of effective medical treatment, control, and containment. We have eliminated only smallpox.

Seen as events of possibly global extent, epidemics or pandemics are the product of many interacting variables. Like earthquakes, volcanic eruptions, and great storms, their complexity is mind-boggling.[2] There are three major groups of variables: (1) the characteristics of the specific microbe, (2) the characteristics of potential hosts, and (3) environmental and behavioral conditions.

THE ETIOLOGIC AGENT

In the beginning there must be a bug. What are its characteristics, its operating parameters? Is it endemic to some remote area like the deadly Ebola Fever, or happily residing in a major population center like cholera or dysentery in Calcutta? Does it pass part of its life cycle in the essential water supply like Schistosomiasis? Is it a relatively rare fungus, or a common microorganism that surrounds us—like that which produces *Pneumocystis carinii* pneumonia in PWAs? Does it have a symbiotic, nondestructive relationship to its carrier like that of the malaria plasmodia to their carrier mosquitoes, or might it kill its host as does the smallpox virus? What is its virulence? Does it sicken (like food poisoning from the salmonella virus lurking everywhere), produce long-term debilitation (like malaria), or kill? And if it kills, what is the (natural or untreated) mortality rate—60 to 75 percent as in the bubonic plague or a 95 to 100 percent rate as is the case with AIDS?

THE HOST

Next, there must be a host or, more accurately, hosts, for one infection does not an epidemic make! The HIV has been in the United States at least since the early 1960s, but we date the epidemic from 1981. In St. Louis, Missouri, in 1969, a young man named Robert died of what now appears to have been AIDS. He had never been out of the country and was probably infected with HIV in the early to mid 1960s. But his case at the time was an isolated, unexplained infection, and, if it passed on, the numbers were so small as to escape notice.[3] Not only must there be many potential hosts, but they should be living in close proximity. Epidemics thrive only if there is sufficient density of population for the contagion to be passed on. At minimum, the time-space factors must be within the parameters established by the natural infectivity of the bug. To put it another way, in order to keep an infection going, the number of newly infected people added to the existing reservoir of infected people must balance or exceed the number dropping out through recovery or death. Otherwise the epidemic sputters out like a fire that has finally consumed all its fuel. During the Middle Ages entire religious houses were destroyed simply because the men and women, living in closed and close communities, presented ideal transmission conditions for the plague bacillus. Today we have various urban subenvironments that are conducive to the spread of many transmissible pathogens, including HIV. Heterosexual and homosexual sex emporia, drug "shooting galleries," penitentiaries, and college dormitories all present better than average transmission environments.

Dispersed agricultural populations are not generally subject to epidemics although individual infections can and do occur.[4] Data from America's HIV epidemic illustrate the point: First, between 1988 and 1993 North Dakota has maintained a low, steady rate of AIDS cases of 0.8 per 100,000. North Dakota has a population density of nine people per square mile, and its largest metropolitan statistical area contains 148,000 of a total of 638,000 people. Second, between 1988 and 1993 New Jersey watched its AIDS rate rise from 30.8 to 44.7 per 100,000. It has a population density of 1,002 per square mile and its major cities are part of a two-state megalopolis of 18.2 million people. Epidemics, at least epidemics before AIDS, have been urban, metropolitan events.[5]

There are other relevant host characteristics. The impact of an epidemic will vary with the demographic structure of the host population—adult/child, age group, sex group, and other kinds of ratios are very important. Other significant factors are the overall nutrition and health of the population, the prevalence of other debilitating infections, and whether or not the target population has, through previous visitations, built up some natural immunity.

THE SETTING

Third, there are many environmental factors that affect the initiation, duration, and severity of an epidemic. For example, the flea that carries bubonic plague prefers ground-nesting rodents; the rodents (like the California ground squirrel), in turn, prefer semiarid grasslands which provide nesting sites and grain foods. Consequently, in ordinary circumstances the spread of the microbe will be limited by the availability of rodents which, in turn, is limited by the availability of territory and food. It is estimated that the plague bacillus could not travel more than ten miles per year and would eventually be stopped as its carrier rat encountered barriers specific to it, such as the end of the grasslands. Climate, weather, and season are also factors of significance. It can get too cold for the malarial mosquito to function, or it can be the wrong season for a virus. When I was a young man, back in the 1940s, all parents dreaded the onset of the spring and summer polio season but were unconcerned the rest of the year.

The above is just minimally suggestive of the variables involved in determining whether or not epidemic possibilities exist. The actual matrix would differ with each microbe in its cultural and environmental context. It can be likened, I think, to the definition of critical mass in assessing the possibilities of nuclear melt-down/explosion, although judging whether or not all relevant factors are in proper relation to trigger an epidemic is infinitely more complex and problematic.[6] Still, when that point is reached, disaster strikes.

Before the Age of AIDS the word "epidemic" for most people evoked images of either biblical events or the bubonic plague of the fourteenth century. But it is really the latter, the Black Death, that is our archetype epidemic; it has been THE EPIDEMIC of Western cultural memory. It is enshrined in our literature from Boccaccio's *Decameron* (1350) to Camus's *The Plague* (1947), and its devastation helped bring about sea changes in the culture to which we all are heir.[7] Notwithstanding the bubonic plague's significance, AIDS may well become the archetype epidemic for future generations. A comparison is in order.

THE GLOBAL SPREAD OF BUBONIC PLAGUE

The microbe that causes the Bubonic Plague is called *Yersinia pestis*. It is a microscopic round-headed bacillus which infests the nests of ground-burrowing rodents such as the wild gerbil, the Asian marmot, and the California ground squirrel. The microbe's ancient and original home bases seem to have been Central Asia and Southern Africa, but today it is found in all semi-arid grassland areas that are the natural habitat of the host rodent population; for example, today California, New Mexico, and Texas (which posted plague warnings in 1993)[8] are major centers of endemicity.[9] As mentioned before, young rodents leaving the nest can carry the bacillus limited distances and thereby over many, many generations are able to gradually spread the infection throughout their habitat. The agent by which the bacillus is transferred from rodent to rodent is the rat flea, which gets a stomach full of the bacillus when drawing blood. The bacilli then multiply in the flea's digestive tract until they are disgorged into the blood stream of a new rodent-host. There are over two thousand varieties of fleas, of which about 120 can transmit the deadly microbe. The rodent host dies from the infection, and the flea is forced to find a new host; it much prefers a rat, but there are a few that, in a pinch, will transfer to a passing human.

A human can be afflicted with one of three varieties: (1) the standard form, which produces the classic symptoms of discolored swellings especially in the armpit and groin areas, a putrid body smell, a spastic jerkiness of action, and a 60 to 75 percent chance of death within seven days; (2) the rarer septicemic form, which results from an extra large disgorging of bacilli by the flea. Death follows within a few hours of infection, so rapidly that no symptoms have time to develop; and finally (3) the pneumonic form, the only human-to-human form, in which the bacillus is transferred from human to human through sneezes and coughs. Like the septicemic form, this is also rapidly and absolutely fatal; in fact, pneumonic plague is considered the deadliest bacterial infection known. One of the classic forewarnings of bubonic plague was and is a visible abundance of dead rodents and, less visibly, their deadly orphaned fleas.[10] But how did the microbe move out from its home-base ultimately to infect Europe, Asia, and the Americas in wave after wave of disastrous epidemics from before the time of Christ into the twentieth century?[11] The flea hitchhiked from its original home in Central Asia on the great trade routes of the ancient world. China and the Mediterranean world were linked by caravan routes that ran between the Eastern Mediterranean trading centers of Istanbul, Tyre, Antioch, Damascus, Baghdad, and Niniveh in the West to Lanzhou and Zian of China in the East. From 500 B.C. the network of caravan routes gradually became more established, safer, and more heavily used. The last links of what became known as the Silk Roads were forged by the Han Emperor Wu, who in the second century B.C. sought to extend China's influence to the West by regularizing trade with the Middle East. Two of these ancient commercial highways are of special interest. One commenced at Tyre, Antioch, and Damascus and proceeded via Hamadan and Tehran to Samarkand and Tashkent in what used to be the USSR. There it linked with another, the Steppe Route, which started at Istanbul, went to Tbilisi, Georgia, looped over the northern shores of the Caspian Sea and then preceded through the steppes of Central Asia to Tashkent. The joined routes then skirted the northern foothills of the Himalayas, crossed over mountain passes and dropped into Xinjiang, the northwestern-most province of China. These routes of the ancient world allowed East and West to exchange ideas and goods, but they also exposed both the Oriental and Occidental populations to recurring epidemics because they crossed through the central Asian grassland home of *Y. pestis*. When caravans dumped their bales of Chinese silk for the clothing of the Mediterranean upper classes, they also deposited rats and fleas. The bacillus was then spread, hopscotchlike, by trading vessels sailing from seaport to seaport around the periphery of the Mediterranean. The epidemics that ensued were the unintended byproduct of commercial intercourse. Ironically, one of the most characteristic of human activities—and the one we all depend upon to enrich our material lives—was and is the single most important method of spreading deadly microbes. The irony is compounded by the fact that war, another of our major activities, is second only to commerce as an engine spreading pestilence throughout the world. The infamous Black Death, the plague of the 1340s that prostrated Europe, may have commenced with the siege of the Black Sea port of Kaffa (now Feodosia) in December 1346 by horse-mounted Tartar troops. The chroniclers of the siege of Kaffa relate that the Tartar chieftain catapulted plague-ridden bodies from his troops over the walls of Kaffa to spread disease and force the city to capitulate. This may be the first recorded instance of germ warfare.[12] In any case, within two years the plague had spread from its point of origin to England and all of Europe. Initial transport was provided by a fleet of ten Genoese vessel carrying goods (and rats) from infected Black Sea ports to cities like Genoa, Messina, and Venice; from the seaports the plague moved inland to commercial trading centers like Paris, where so many people died that wolves moved back into the city.

The plague's spread was temporarily halted in England, Europe and Asia. From the fourteenth through the seventeenth centuries it visited and revisited England, the Continent, and the Mediterranean lands, but it did not move to other continents. European folklore linked rats, death, and evil, a still riveting combination in our cultural and literary imagination; think of the vampire Nosferatu, nightmare of God, stalking the land accompanied by his retinue of plague-bearing rats. And everyone knows the tale of the Pied Piper. The politicians of Hamelin hired him to protect the town and its children from rats. He did so. When they reneged, the Piper took all the children as payment; the plague would have left some. Perhaps there is a lesson for today's politicians in this tale of dishonor.

The behavioral engines of its spread through the seventeenth century had been commerce and war, and the technology that made it possible were the caravan and the short-hop coastal sailing vessel. It requires some stretch of the space-traveling twentieth-century imagination to recapture the technological innovations the transcontinental caravan and the coastal sailing vessel represented in their time. The caravan was a marvel of logistic organization, long-range planning, and land navigation through uncharted wilderness. It required great sums of risk capital, the cooperation and support of all political systems along the route, and no small amount of good luck. Similarly the coastal trading vessel made feasible the movement of bulky commodities, which would have defied economic land transport, particularly along the complex northern coast of the Mediterranean from Turkey to Spain. Both of these modes operated within time frames that met the biologic requirements of transmitting the plague. A coastal vessel could load goods with its accompanying rats/fleas and discharge them elsewhere before everyone on board was infected and died. A voyage of too long duration simply meant that an epidemic contained on board would sputter out before reaching port; there were many instances of ships drifting ashore with all rats and all hands dead. Only the fleas would be left on the "ghost ships" of lore.

Before *Y. pestis* could spread to the New World, a major step in transport technology had to be made, one that would shorten the passage time. This came in the late nineteenth century with the development of the transoceanic steamship. Along with the railroad, it ushered in the age of mass movement of people and goods and the rapid dispersal of epidemic agents. It made possible the spread of the bubonic plague to every spot on the globe which had been, up to that time, blessedly free of it. The steamship arrival of the bubonic plague in California, probably from Asian ports, is generally dated around the turn of the twentieth century. In March 1900 San Francisco had its first panicky brush with the Black Death after the body of a Chinese man, dead from plague, was found in the basement of a Chinatown hotel. The Board of Health, backed by the mayor, cordoned and quarantined twelve square blocks of Chinatown and stationed police to keep Chinese inside. When the epidemic spread anyway, federal authorities were called in to help with the containment. They set up roadblocks and inspected railroad passengers at the state line in an attempt to keep the Chinese and "their Plague" in San Francisco.

California's governor refused to admit that the Plague existed; it would be bad for business. He secured the backing of the State Board of Health and the Chinese community (which was hiding its sick). San Francisco's newspapers, at the behest of advertisers, ignored proved cases and lampooned city health workers. There was a political stalemate with the Republican governor on one side and the city's Democratic mayor on the other. Oblivious to human politics and foibles, the plague spread. Finally the national government sent in a team of investigators, and in 1901 the governor was forced to capitulate. He stated four conditions for his "cooperation": (1) that the entire operation be kept quiet, (2) that neither the state nor its cities be quarantined, (3) that containment be "pursued with the least possible detriment to our commercial interest," and (4) that the federal authorities not bill the state for costs.[13]

Thus, in an appropriately disruptive way, *Yersinia pestis* completed its world tour. From the steppes of Central Asia to China and the Mediterranean, thence to Europe, and finally to the New World was a journey that took over two thousand years. During the passage the bacillus played a role in some of the great changes of history at a cost of untold millions of dead along the way.

THE GLOBAL SPREAD OF AIDS

Current evidence indicates that the home base of the HIV is Central Africa.[*] Understandably African politicians in 1985–87 responded to this ascription with countercharges of "Western Imperialistic Lying and Anti-Black Racism"; after all, who wants credit for a new pestilence? But this political phase has passed, and there is general agreement on the epidemiological data that points to Equatorial Africa as the home base of HIV-1 and West Africa as the base of HIV-2.[14]

AIDS was endemic to remote African villages long before it was known or named by Western science. The natives called it the Thin Sickness and were familiar with its ravages. In the Ugandan village of Kytera the rate of infection may be as high as 20 percent, and most of the children are orphans.[15] In 1985 a research team demonstrated that the HIV seroprevalence rate had remained stable since at least 1975 in the village of Yondongi of northwestern Zaire, and this stability might be characteristic of remote rural settings for as long as they remained unaffected by contemporary war and/or commerce.[16] Exactly how long the two major types of the virus have been endemic can only be estimated by various methods. Genetic sequencing analysis estimates viral age by computing backward in time from the current viral structure. It answers the question, "Given the known rate of change in the HIV genome, how long would it have taken for the virus to reach its present state?" Epidemiological analysis asks the question, "Given a known doubling-rate (the time needed to double the number of people infected), how long would it have taken to produce the estimated 14,000,000 infected now?" Genetic sequencing suggests that HIV emerged as a separate entity between six and twelve hundred years ago,[17] while epidemiologic data indicate that it had been spreading in Africa for a century or more before going global.[18] In any case, by the 1970s upper-class Zairians were traveling to European hospitals to get help for a puzzling new "tropical disease." The first authenticated European case from African exposure was the death of Dr. Grethe Rask, who worked at a hospital in Abumombazi in

---

[*] It should be emphasized at the outset that what follows this is intended to be a *plausible* description of HIV's spread throughout the world. However, its diffusion was so fast and the disease-tracking agencies were so slow to focus on it, that well-documented time/space maps of its original spread cannot be drawn. For interesting computer-generated maps of HIV's spread in Africa and the United States, see Peter Gould, *The Slow Plague: A Geography of the AIDS Pandemic* (Cambridge, Mass.: Blackwell, 1993).

northeastern Zaire near the border with Sudan. Dr. Rask collapsed on Christmas Eve 1976 in Kinshasa, Zaire, and returned to her native Denmark to die in 1977. At that time no one knew what had killed her; now all the symptoms of AIDS are recognizable.

HIV did not stay in the villages. The withdrawal of European colonial power from Equatorial Africa, commencing with Ghana's 1957 declaration of independence from Britain followed by Guinea's separation from France in 1958, began a period of war, revolution, and socioeconomic disruption which continues to the present day. The stability imposed by European power since 1884 dissolved as various African groups vied to seize the reins of power.[19]

The significance of these tumultuous political events for AIDS is that a population that, up to that time, was rural and stable became urban and mobile. People moved, and they carried their infections with them. For example, Angolan officials estimate that, in the period just before independence from Portugal in 1975, one million people migrated into Zaire. Despite continuing strife in northern Angola, masses of people continue to flow freely back and forth across the border carrying the virus with them. The highest Angolan seropositive rate is found in precisely those northern border areas. Congo, just north of Angola and sharing a long border with Zaire, has an estimated 10 percent rate of infection in its urban sexually active age groups (40 percent of the Continent's population is in this age group). On the other hand, Gabon, the Western neighbor of Congo, enjoys a comparatively low infection rate. Apparently it is protected by jungle covering so thick that population movement is impeded.[20] Accurate epidemiological studies are hard to complete in specific African locales, but the larger picture painted by World Health Organization data is grim. Sub-Saharan Africa, which has about 10 percent of the global population, accounts for 66 percent of adults and 90 percent of children with AIDS. The high AIDS rates found throughout Central Africa are indirect evidence that the virus has been spreading for a long time, at first slowly within villages and later at the accelerated rate produced by population movement.

Equally important is the fact that, unlike America and Europe, it has been spread largely through vaginal intercourse. Estimates are that three fourths of the cases result from male/female infection, and the ratio between the sexes is approximately even, as compared to the 12:1 male/female ratio in the industrialized nations. Rapid and disruptive changes in the politico-economic systems have forced men to leave their villages to find work in the cities. Once there, they are separated from both their families and the restraining force of traditional tribal values. In many, many cities throughout Africa, Asia, and Latin America, one result of urbanization has been the emergence of a large prostitution industry servicing the sexual needs of this army of displaced men. The shambles of the Central African economy are such that the women have no means of support, nothing to sell but their bodies. As an example, all these and other factors merge to make the great highway between Kinshasa and Mombasa—crowded with truckers and prostitutes—a veritable expressway of infection. A century ago a similar process occurred in America, also a byproduct of industrialization and urbanization, resulting in a consequent dramatic increase in the rate of syphilis and gonorrhea. Now, however, the disease being spread via the route of prostitution is AIDS. In some places AIDS is known as "The Disease of Shame" referring to the fact that it is acquired by consorting with or being a prostitute—an African heterosexual stigma, rather than an American homosexual one. Retrospective studies of HIV infection in Nairobi prostitutes indicate that between 1981 and 1985 the rate rose from 8 to 61 percent. Surveys of the urban prostitute populations of Rwanda, Kenya, and Zaire indicate HIV-1 prevalence rates of from 25 to 88 percent.[21] By comparison, 1988 data indicated that the rate among New York City prostitutes was 12 percent, and among northern New Jersey prostitutes it was about 49 percent, while southern Nevada, where prostitution is state regulated, registered the lowest rate.[22]

Other agents strongly implicated in the African spread of HIV are multiple use of unsterile hypodermic needles and a contaminated blood supply. All observers agree that "disposable" needles are simply not thrown away as they should be; the needles are sharpened and reused. This dangerous practice is not the result of ignorance; it is the result of economics. Large city hospitals are underfunded and ill equipped, rural hospitals are primitive—in neither is anything "disposable." Similarly even after it became clear in the industrialized nations that the blood supply had to be screened, Africa could not afford the $6 to $8 cost per unit. The United States is spending at least $100 million per year to screen the supply to diminish the risk of spreading AIDS through transfusion; that amount exceeds the total public health budget of all the Central African nations, which have also to cope with endemic malaria, bilharzia, many enteric ailments, ulcerative venereal diseases, chancroids, and many others.

By whatever mode, the major cities of central Africa became "geographic foci of endemicity" in the 1960–80 period, bases from which AIDS could spread to the world. The technology of that spread was air commerce; AIDS is the first airborne epidemic. A traveler could enplane in Kinshasa or Nairobi, arrive in Paris, London, or New York not many hours later, and then, for example, fly on to St. Louis, Missouri. Actually HIV does not need jet travel. With an incubation period of a decade it is not subject to the time-space limitations that restricted *Y. pestis*, but clearly the airplane made possible HIV's global dispersion in a stupefyingly short period.

Just as it was possible to trace the movement of the bubonic plague from

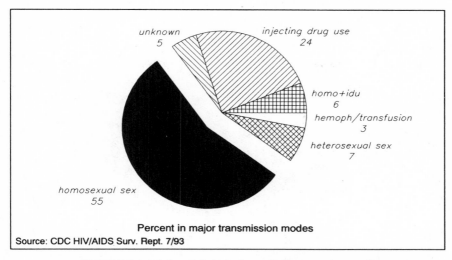

FIGURE 3.1 Adult AIDS, U.S. (cumulative to June 1993)

seaport to seaport, it is possible to trace AIDS from airport to airport. For example, AIDS came into Haiti during the late 1960s from two sources: American and European travelers, and Haitians returning home after working in Zaire.[23] Travelers, some infected, arrived by plane. Haiti provided conditions for the spread of AIDS similar to those in Africa—poverty, poor medical facilities, poor general health, and an exploited, prostituted underclass in which any communicable disease could spread rapidly. AIDS statistics from Haiti to the World Health Organization are usually more than a year in arrears and notoriously low in their estimates. Even so, the AIDS rate of the tiny half-island is the highest in the Caribbean.[24]

From Haiti, and in sufficient volume to boast epidemic potential, HIV traveled to the United States. First, Haitians escaping the corrupt and brutal Duvalier regime brought AIDS with them to America. However, it is not likely that once they were here they were important sources of its spread since they tended to remain in their small, closed refugee communities. Their heterosexual/vaginal infection became an anomaly in the American pattern, which epidemiologists were hard pressed to explain in the early days of the epidemic. The first reports of the CDC simply lumped all Haitians into a "high risk group." The "high risk" designation of an entire nationality was later dropped for political reasons. Second, AIDS was brought back by vacationing Americans. Here the CDC designations did point to an undeniable truth—the accidents of history made the gay community the primary instrument by which the virus was introduced into America in epidemic-level quantities. Haiti was a favored vacation spot for East Coast gays. It was

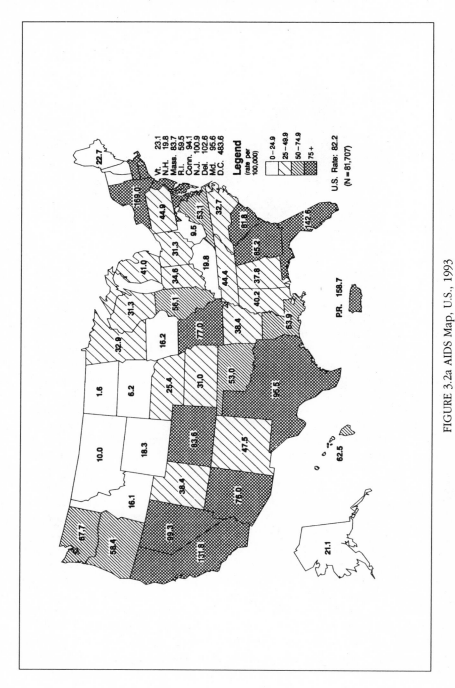

FIGURE 3.2a AIDS Map, U.S., 1993

Adult/Adolescent AIDS Annual Rates per 100,000 Population, Cases Reported October 1992 through September 1993, Males.

Source: Centers for Disease Control, "HIV/AIDS Surveillance Report," October 1993, Figure 1, p.15.

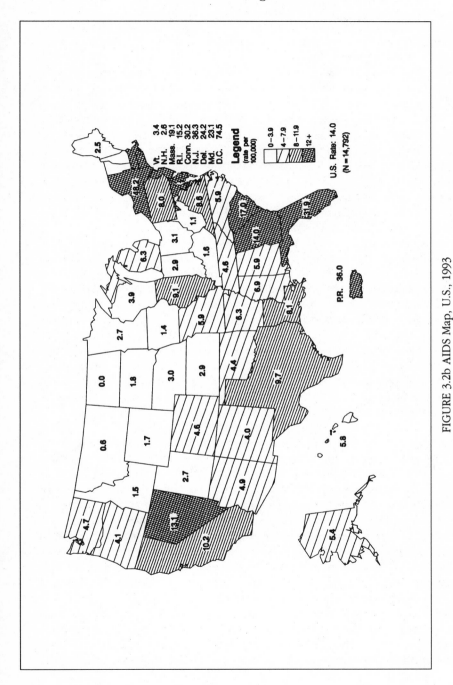

FIGURE 3.2b AIDS Map, U.S., 1993

Adult/Adolescent AIDS Annual Rates per 100,000 Population, Cases Reported October 1992 through September 1993, Females.

Source: Centers for Disease Control, "HIV/AIDS Surveillance Report," October 1993, Figure 2, p.15.

exotic, inexpensive, and just a short flight from New York. The HIV that surfaced in New York's gay and IDU communities in the 1970s was at least partly an Haitian import.

From New York, Florida, and the Caribbean the virus could spread rapidly to other parts of the nation. But as was the case with the bubonic plague, it did not spread evenly. The plague hit the seaports immediately and then the inland cities that were the most closely connected by commercial ties. In like fashion, the American areas with the highest number of cases are all major hubs of national and international air traffic (the top ten cities are: New York; San Francisco; Los Angeles; Newark, New Jersey; Houston; Chicago; Washington; Miami; Philadelphia; and Atlanta).[25] As the computer-generated maps developed by Professor Peter Gould show, HIV then spread in the United States much as it had already spread in Africa—along highways from major centers to smaller satellite communities.[26]

The most dramatic example of this process in action comes from the story of the infamous "Patient Zero," Gaetan Dugas.[27] Dugas was an Air Canada flight attendant whose travels during the period 1979–84 took him frequently to France (the nation most affected by the early spread of AIDS prior to its surfacing in America) and at least ten American cities; CDC's *Morbidity and Mortality Weekly Report* (June 18, 1982) clearly showed that he was the center of a miniepidemic, and that fully one-sixth (40) of all reported cases of AIDS up to that time were connected to his coast-to-coast homosexual exploits. No one knows how many others were infected by individuals from this early infected group. Dugas died, appropriately somehow, while on a flight from Quebec to British Columbia at the age of thirty-two. The infection that he helped spread so widely is still very much alive.

While Dugas was spreading AIDS among homosexuals, Elizabeth Prophet was doing the same among San Francisco's heterosexuals. Ms. Prophet's arrest record for prostitution commenced in 1974 when she was twenty-two. In 1978 her infant daughter was hospitalized with what we now know was pediatric AIDS; her second (1979) and third children (1982) were also born with AIDS. She died in May 1987 of *Pneumocystis carinii* pneumonia, an opportunistic infection associated with HIV infection; her children have also died. Given present knowledge regarding the course of HIV infection and her personal history, it is likely that she was infected in San Francisco in the mid-1970s. How many men she passed the virus to during her ten-year career will never be known. Two weeks after her death the father of one of her three children also died of AIDS.[28]

Similar stories about the spread of HIV from Central Africa could be told about Europe, Asia, the Pacific, and Latin America. The virus is rapidly spreading into areas that, only a few years ago, reported little or no incidence. Asia has been pointed to by epidemiologists as one of the explosive areas for the

1990s. World Health Organization officials at the 1993 Berlin AIDS Conference stated that "the most alarming trends of HIV infection are in south and southwest Asia where the epidemic is spreading in some areas as fast as it was a decade ago in sub-Saharan Africa." But Asia presents difficult problems of epidemiological analysis. The 1993–94 reports of Asian AIDS cases are not, in themselves, startling in proportion to the populations involved. Further, most of the data comes from major urban centers that are already pockets of endemicity—cities like Bombay, India, Bangkok, Thailand, and provinces like Ruili, China. Nothing is known about either the sexual practices or the seroprevalence of the vast millions that occupy the rural hinterlands of Asian nations. Yet, Asia may well provide proof for the advice that, "If you wait until you see AIDS, it's too late to do much about it."

However, there can be no doubt that HIV, by whatever route, has arrived in Asian cities. Data from Bombay and New Delhi (1993) indicate that there are already one million Indians infected, and Indian scientists expect that number to rise to six million by the year 2000. Between 1988 and 1993 the rate of infection in prostitutes doubled, with approximately one third of them already infected. The chief routes of transmission have been heterosexual sex (80 percent of cases) especially in India's brothels, injecting drug use, and a contaminated blood supply. Thirty percent of India's blood supply comes from professional donors who sell their blood (and sometimes body parts) in order to stay alive. As a class they are poverty stricken and have a high incidence of sexually transmitted diseases. Officials admit that most Indian blood banks do not have, and cannot afford, the necessary kits to screen the blood they receive.[29] A better scenario for the staging of a major epidemic can hardly be imagined.

Similar information is coming out of Thailand with its flourishing sex and drug tourist industry. Thailand already has one of the highest HIV infection rates in the world; projections to 2000 estimate two million or 10 percent of the entire population. The government and business community of Thailand are now united in a high profile, ambitious program to contain the spread of HIV, but, as I just said, they may prove the point—waiting until you see AIDS may be too late. Japanese officials charge that most Japanese cases come from vacation sex-tours of Thailand booked for Japanese men by Japanese agencies. Perhaps this is true, but some could also come from their travels in the United States, the Philippines (whose officials are locked in a bitter struggle with the Catholic Church hierarchy over the distribution of condoms), and Europe. The Japanese businessmen's practice of offering sex as part of an evening's dining and entertainment (a corruption of the Geisha tradition), may be their undoing in an STD epidemic.

Evaluating the extent of HIV's spread in Latin America presents similar problems of data integrity and adequacy, but the reality of the epidemic's arrival is

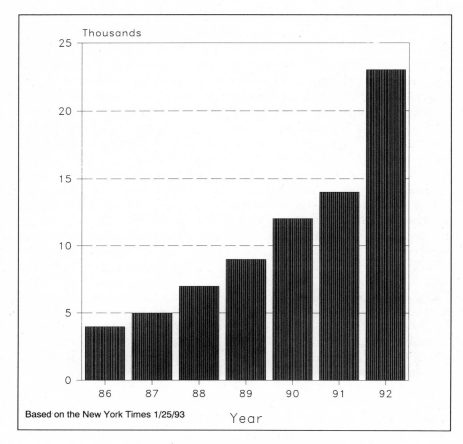

FIGURE 3.3 AIDS Cases, Latin America

unquestioned. A major problem in Latin American reporting is the homosexual stigma attached to AIDS throughout the Americas; it is estimated that as many as 50 percent of the diagnosed cases are not reported because of it. The Latin American pattern of spread may be more complex than that of either Africa, the United States, or Asia in that it has a heavy complement of bisexual males getting infected through sex with males, then transmitting it to wives and mistresses (and children) through sex with women. Rio de Janeiro's major AIDS hospital reports that 30 percent of the men seeking counseling report themselves as bisexual; the percent of Brazilian females with AIDS has risen from 3 to 20 percent of the AIDS total from 1985–93.[30] In late 1991 the PanAmerican Health Union estimated nearly one million infected.[31]

The precise epidemiological tracks of HIV's spread will never be known as paths cross and backtrack on other paths in this age of rapid, mass transit. The detail we have on Patient Zero in America is exceptional; the result of intensive contact tracing in the early days when epidemiologists were trying establish the nature of the outbreak. Many questions will never be answered. For example, was Europe an important staging area for the further spread of AIDS, or was it mostly a recipient? Perhaps at this stage, over a decade into the epidemic, there is no point in trying to determine who got what from whom. However, there can be no doubt that, in the 1980s, the United States became a most important link in the chain of transport which helped spread AIDS from its original home base in rural, central Africa to the rest of the world.[32] Criticisms of the reluctant and sluggish response of the Reagan administration gain some credence when it is realized that vigorous presidential leadership—the kind elicited by the appearance of Legionnaires disease, the mistaken fear of Swine Flu, or the recent San Francisco earthquake—might very well have helped slow and contain what is now a major and unstoppable world epidemic (see AIDS dispersion maps, Figures 7.1, 7.2, and 7.3).

THE BUBONIC PLAGUE AND AIDS: A COMPARISON

The bubonic plague and the AIDS epidemic share some features. Each disease was taken from its limited home base and spread throughout the world by the human engines of war and commerce, traveling on the most modern transport of the day. The difference in time that each took to encircle the globe—2,000 years and 35 years, respectively—was partly a function of the organisms themselves and partly a reflection of transport technology. Each was and is seen by many people as an act of divine retribution, God's punishment for the various sins of the people. And each disease reactivated ancient prejudices as people sought explanations for their fear and suffering. For the medieval European, the Jew was the answer. The plague came from Jews' poisoning the wells, and was God's punishment for tolerance of heresy within the Christian community. So Jews were walled up and burned. For the "medieval" American, homosexuals are the real authors of the epidemic, and everyone is suffering God's wrath for not rooting out this damned minority. In the earlier years of the epidemic, there were calls for branding and for rebuilding of the old leprosaria, ghettoes for the sick.

They are similar also in emphasizing the need for humans to calculate their behavioral risks. The plague is caused by a fast-acting bacillus, while AIDS is caused by slow-acting virus, but for both the principal forms of protection were and are behavioral and environmental rather than medical. For most of *Yersinia pestis'* 2,500-year history it was incurable. Only in the mid-twentieth century did it bow to antibiotics, but even with antibiotics the diagnosis must be quick and accurate. Primary protection lies in personal

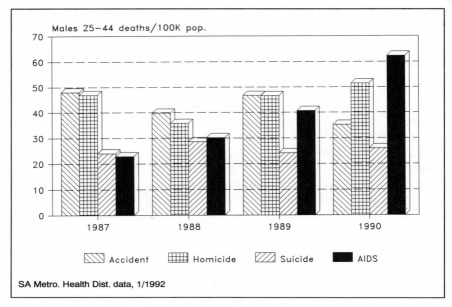

FIGURE 3.4 Causes of Death, Males, San Antonio

avoidance of contact with rats, and the construction and maintenance of such areas as harbors, rivers where they flow through cities, residential areas, trash dumps, and so on in such a way as to discourage rat colonies. People must be periodically reminded of the dangers by public health warnings such as those issued by the Texas Department of Health in connection with the 1993 outbreak.

Similarly, HIV infection is incurable; all medicinal interventions are palliative at best. The only answers are avoidance of risk and/or thoughtful risk management. One should avoid high risk behaviors where possible and use what protections as are available to make unavoidably risky behavior less risky. "Plague warnings" find their AIDS counterparts in governmental "Safe Sex" and needle exchange programs. However, the very phrasing I have used, "One should avoid high risk . . .," points to one of the central problems of the HIV epidemic and its contrast with those of the plague. The manner of HIV's transmission automatically targets the very age group that is still in the early adult phase of risk-taking, not conservative risk management, and the rising AIDS mortality rate in the young adult is sad proof.

THE VARIABLE IMPACTS

Similarities stop when the diseases themselves are compared, and it is this level of comparison that provokes me to consider the possibility that AIDS will supplant the Black Death as the archetype epidemic, the new standard for natural catastrophic challenges to the human community. The bubonic plague, in common with most other epidemic-prone afflictions like small-pox, cholera, and measles, culled the weak from the population. The old and the young were especially vulnerable, the first to die, the least likely to survive.[33] The older graveyards of America's East Coast are filled with tiny headstones of eighteenth- and nineteenth-century children who did not survive the childhood epidemic diseases. But AIDS develops primarily in the sexually active age groups that comprise the workforce; those under thirteen and over sixty-five together constitute only 5 percent of AIDS cases in the United States. In Zambia, for example, 68 percent of the male HIV+'s are skilled mineworkers essential to the economy of the nation. In the United States approximately 86 percent of the three hundred and fifty thousand reported AIDS cases are in the age group of twenty to forty-nine for both men and women.[34] Comparing the United States, Texas, and San Antonio charts (Figure 3.5), one can see the virus expressing the laws governing its nature regardless of the size or demographic mix of the human group infected. The age-specific focusing of AIDS is the source of much popular misunderstanding about the risks of infection. Rates of infection are generally stated as a ratio like 1:100,000, but those general population ratios do not, in fact, reflect the risks within the population most affected by AIDS. After deducting those over sixty and those under fifteen, the ratio for the remainder becomes much grimmer.

For example, in Uganda the general rate of infection for the entire population is 1:16; however, if counting is limited to those over fifteen years old, the ratio becomes 1:8 infected Ugandans, or 12.5 percent.[35] It also should be noted that, although AIDS is a disease of the sexually active age groups, it is, by the same token, a disease that targets parents. Even though it does not directly attack children (unless they are born to an infected mother), as did the plague, it does devastate their lives. In just one area of Uganda, Rakai County, with a population of about three hundred thousand, it is estimated that forty thousand children have lost one or both parents to AIDS.[36] These targeting characteristics become more pronounced as the epidemic takes hold and make AIDS, as compared to the bubonic plague, an infinitely more costly epidemic.

Another factor to be considered is that the standard form of plague had a mortality rate of about 60 to 75 percent and survivors were left with a natural immunity to further infection. Consequently, like other epidemic-prone pathogens, the plague bacillus gradually killed fewer people as a larger number of resistant adults developed in the population. AIDS, however, attacks the very system that evolved in humans to provide immunity to

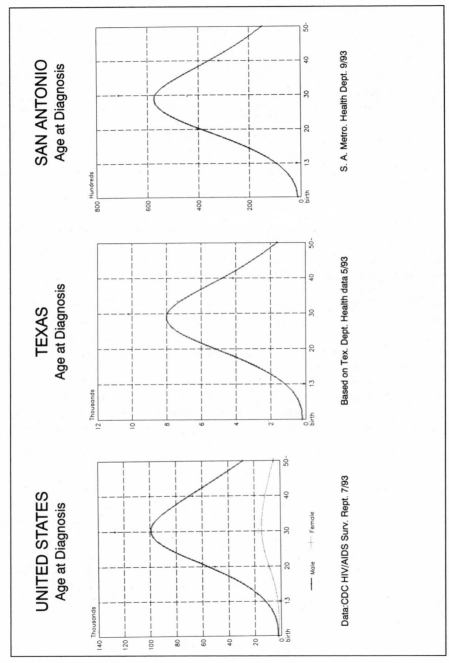

FIGURE 3.5 Age at Diagnosis

invading organisms; consequently, without effective drugs, AIDS is nearly 100 percent fatal.[37] No natural protection can develop except through mutation of the virus itself to a less deadly form. This, in turn, is unlikely unless at-risk people adopt sexual and drug use behaviors that biologically reward and select (in terms of viral evolution) less virulent strains[38]—a difficult and long-term proposition.

SPREADING THE PLAGUE AND AIDS

The pattern of each affliction's transmission and spread is also quite different. An episode of plague was triggered when various factors were coincident. Among many others, these played a part: (1) population densities of specific kinds of rodents and humans, and the relationship of the two densities in a particular site—for example, the crowded living conditions of medieval monasteries—made those residing in them especially vulnerable; (2) the construction of human habitation (brick buildings were less prone to rat infestation than others); (3) the extent of population movement between infested areas and other areas; (4) the effectiveness of urban or ocean quarantine systems; (5) finally and importantly, the progress of a particular episode of the plague would itself change the parameters that made it possible in the first place. Thus the plague recurred episodically and unpredictably, like storm waves breaking upon a shore, until, eventually, other natural forces exerted themselves to suppress it. The characteristics of the plague, of course, were rooted in the fact that the disease was primarily transmitted from rats through fleas to humans.

On the other hand, AIDS is transmitted entirely within the human community and generally through some of its most intimate, compelling, and essential behaviors. Unlike the plague, there are no longer any "geographic foci of endemicity." AIDS can exist wherever people exist; the human habitat, not some grasslands area, is the natural reservoir. There are no safe areas. For example, Canadian authorities are much concerned about the spread of AIDS among Alaskan Eskimos, who already have a high incidence of STDs and whose many languages do not even have an acceptable word for the danger, but whose sexual traditions make them very vulnerable.[39] Triggering an HIV epidemic merely requires the introduction of the virus into a human group whose patterns of behavior favor transmission. No other factors are really necessary.

This is not to say that the AIDS spread is uniform around the globe, anymore than the spread of the plague was. Biologically speaking, susceptibility to infection seems to be well-nigh universal. No one appears to have a natural ability to nullify the effects of either *Yersinia pestis* or HIV (excepting survivors of *Yersinia*) upon infection.[40] However, behavioral and environmental susceptibility is a different matter. Both the bacillus and the virus respond to environmental and human behavioral conditions that biologically favor their transmission and, therefore, their survival—just as humans flourish in the more moderate climes and fertile regions. Parish death registers during plague times in London clearly show a skewed geographic pattern of infection. Poor people living in rat-infested wood houses along the Thames River died by the wagonload; rich people living in brick country houses did not. In like fashion, one is more likely to encounter HIV in Newark, New Jersey, and Castro, San Francisco, than in Fargo, North Dakota. The first has a high incidence of drug use, and the second has a high incidence of risky sexual behavior; the AIDS rate of the third indicates that Fargo has a low incidence of both.

Looking back over the decade of tracking HIV from its rural African home base, there appears to be two behavioral patterns of spread. The African pattern: in Africa AIDS has overwhelmingly been spread through a combination of (1) vaginal intercourse in an environment with a high incidence of sexually transmitted diseases, (2) an unscreened blood supply, and (3) the use of unsterile hypodermic syringes. Globally speaking, the vast majority of those who have been infected have been infected in these ways. The American-Western European pattern: in Europe and America HIV has been spread largely through anal intercourse, the use of unsterile needles in IV drug use, and vaginal intercourse where one or both partners are IV drug users. In addition, a contaminated blood supply played an early role.

Asia mimics Africa's pattern in that it is primarily a heterosexual spread fueled by a flourishing sex industry in India, Thailand, and elsewhere. The difference with Africa is that drugs play a larger role, particularly in the Golden Triangle area of Burma, Laos, and Thailand.[41] The most severely impacted area of China, Ruili Province, borders this area and serves as a drug and HIV route into China. The Central and South American scenario echoes that of the United States and Europe, with a contaminated blood supply and bisexual cross transmissions between the gay and straight sexual worlds playing a larger role.

It should be noted that these very gross generalizations conceal the fact that within the large patterns there are numerous micropatterns, the existence of which severely complicate the problem of containing spread through public education and programs like condom distribution. A study on mathematical modelling of the epidemic provides an example:

> When [sexually] high-activity men (such as migrant male laborers in urban [African] centers) have greatest contact with high-activity women (such as female prostitutes) but also have some contact with low-activity women (wives or girlfriends), a multiple epidemic may occur. First comes a rapidly developing epidemic in the small proportion of high-activity men and women. A more slowly developing, but much larger,

epidemic follows the initial outbreak. The second epidemic involves the low-activity men and women who constitute the majority of the population. The epidemic in the high-activity classes serves to seed the slower-growing epidemic, and the two classes may be separated by a decade or more.[42]

Another micropattern can be seen in the growing American infant-AIDS problem. The epidemic of infected births ties back, of course, to an epidemic of drug use, sex, and consequent viral transmission, but it produces a completely different set of problems requiring their own approaches. AIDS is an inordinately complex phenomenon. The difference in the complexity of the two diseases, bubonic plague and AIDS, both in and of themselves, and in their social impact, is akin to the difference between checkers and chess. Except as equally efficient killers, they are not in the same league at all.

Another major distinction between HIV infection and *Yersinia* infection lies in the exponential character of HIV's spread. *Yersinia* had the potential of exponential spread through its pneumonic mode, but the bacillus never really evolved a major reliance upon this mode of transmission. It always remained a relatively rare variant, probably because it killed people so fast that it curtailed the possibility of further transmission and, thus, adversely affected the bacillus' overall survival chances. If everyone drops dead too quickly, then so does the bug.

However, with a decade (as distinct from *Yersinia*'s one week) to do its killing, HIV is not subject to the same limitations. Its union of blood-borne transmissibility with years-long pathogenicity made it an ideal agent for exponential development. Exponential spread is geometric, rather than arithmetic. Arithmetic expansion means that "A" infects "B" who infects "C" who infects "D"; the process is additive. This kind of chain can usually be broken with simple and acceptable measures. Exponential means that "A" infects "B" who infects "C" and "D" who then infect "E," "F," "G," and "H", *ad horrendum*. Dr. Stephen J. Gould of Harvard University reminded his readers of an old children's riddle as a way of visualizing exponential spread. "If you place a penny on square one of a checkerboard and double the number of coins on each subsequent square . . . how big is the stack by the 64th square? The answer: about as high as the universe is wide."[43] Another way to see exponential effect is to take out your pocket calculator and observe how rapidly you go into "overload" when multiplying by the constant 2: $2 \times 2 \times 2 \times 2$ . . ., my calculator ran over one billion on the twenty-sixth pass and gave up. In the African AIDS context, and assuming a doubling time of three years, then "it would take thirty years to change from a thousandth of a percent [of infection] to a detectable

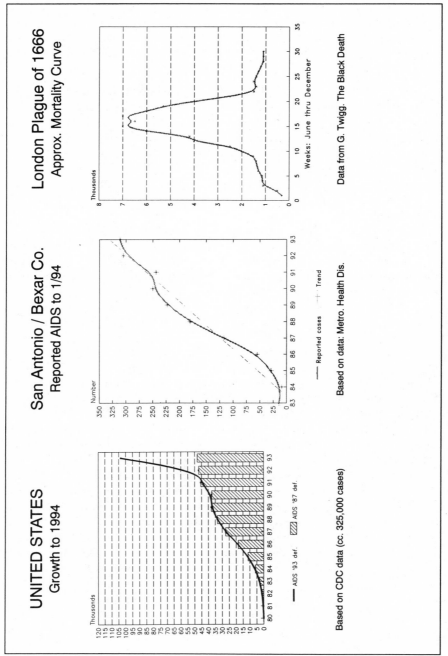

FIGURE 3.6 HIV and Plague Bacillus: Their Natural Progression in a Population

level of 1 percent, but only three years to change from 10 to 20 percent."[44] In the American context, exponentiality means that it took ninety-six months for the Federal Centers for Disease Control to register the first one hundred thousand diagnosed cases of AIDS, but only twenty-six months more (to 1992) to count the next one hundred thousand! The exponential curve will display similar characteristics whether for the nation as a whole or one city within it, such as San Antonio, Texas. These can be compared with the nonexponential mortality curve for the London Plague of 1666 (Figure 3.6).

Theoretically all people-to-people transmissible diseases (like tuberculosis, for example) are spreadable exponentially until such time as they completely destroy the host, but in the real world this does not happen; the stack of pennies falls over, something interrupts the progression. However, sexually transmitted diseases are especially likely to meet the theoretical requirements of exponentiality for the simple reason that we are not, by nature, sexually seasonal nor limited to monogamous relationships.

Other than injecting drug use, the two major behavioral factors involved in calculating the potential severity of an HIV epidemic are the frequency of intercourse, and the frequency of partner change. In Belgium one man infected eleven of the nineteen women with whom he had sex over a period from 1983 to 1985.[45] Magic Johnson has (to use his own word) "accommodated" many women, with unknown results. In the same fashion, less newsworthy people have been, or currently are, centers of their own miniepidemics.

The American Christian tradition insists that we ought to be monogamous, but many other traditions disagree. In any case, Americans have seldom practiced what they preached. The divorce and remarriage rate, to say nothing of the existence of abundant extramarital affairs, make it clear that we practice serial as well as simultaneous polygamy in both the heterosexual and homosexual world. And the linkage of our behavior with HIV's attributes produce a deadly exponentiality.

All these considerations point to one of the most interesting and difficult differences between the bubonic plague and AIDS. In the case of plague, once folk wisdom and science evolved sufficient information about the pestilence, people could slow transmission and lower risk with relatively common-sense measures requiring no great behavioral changes. In the Texas pockets of endemicity, people are cautioned not to have any contact with dead rodents and to report their appearance to public health authorities. In the medieval period most people understood that life would be safer in the country, and the rich moved out of the cities if they could. They also understood that population movement had to be curtailed, going so far as to burn at the stake those (poor, not rich, folk) who were caught running from an afflicted city and thereby spreading the contagion. Queen Elizabeth I fled the London Plague of 1563 to Windsor Castle in the country, and she had gallows erected on the access roads to the castle with standing royal orders "to hang all such as should come there from London."

But not picking up a dead rat is not of the same order of magnitude in our behavioral portfolio as not picking up that attractive number at the bar. Clearly a sexually procreated species cannot "Just say NO" to sex without perishing; we *could* radically change the nature of AIDS spread by somehow separating the infected and uninfected populations, by becoming strictly monogamous, mating for life, by always using barrier protection until it was established that both partners were free of the virus.[46] I suspect it will be a cold day in hell before such changes are in effect—though it is conceivable that someday we may be forced to use them. Even if we were able quickly to bring about such a striking revolution, the existing worldwide pool would have to be exhausted by death before we could rest easy.

PUBLIC POLICY IMPLICATIONS

The idiosyncratic features of the two diseases have many, many implications for how we react to them and shape our resulting public policy. I want to make a few observations at this point. The plague was an open, obvious, fast-acting illness. As the old chronicles record, people could and did track its deadly march from city to city across the nation and tried desperately to impede its progress by quarantines, roadblocks, and other means. The symptoms were blatant, and when it took hold, it moved like wildfire; people died in the streets. Very gradually over the centuries, it lost its association in the public emotions with outcast groups like the Jews, and rational methods from public education to rat abatement programs came into use. In our age of antibiotics it no longer presents an epidemic threat although individual infections do occur. History has taught us the hard way that we must move fast, intelligently, and decisively at the first hint of trouble.

AIDS is an altogether different story. Far from being open and obvious, AIDS spread quietly in Africa, Europe, and the United States for decades before alarms sounded. This is one of the qualities of an exponential spread combined with a long incubation period. The virus very slowly establishes a base of one, two, or three cases and then at take-off moves like the Concord, straight up. In 1982 there were only 248 cases reported in the United States; now only twelve years later, in January 1994, we have over three hundred fifty thousand cases of defined AIDS, as well as a larger number of cases (ARC) that fall short in some measure of the official definition.[47] Further, when it did come to public notice, it was so thoroughly

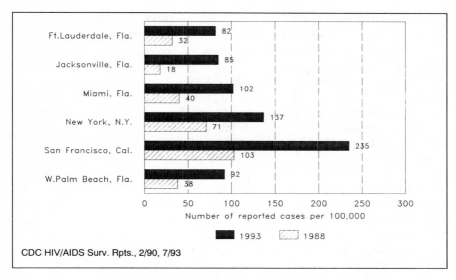

FIGURE 3.7 Increase in AIDS Rate: Top Six Cities

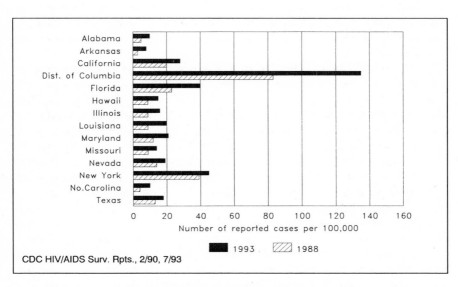

FIGURE 3.8 Increase in AIDS Rate:
States Posting a 5 pt or Greater Increase in AIDS Rate

associated with the gay community that decisive political action was aborted. As one commentator put it in 1987, "If AIDS had first been imported from Africa into a Park Avenue apartment, we would not have dithered as the exponential march began."[48]

It was impossible to ignore the plague—there is nothing like a large sup-purating abscess, foul odor, and spastic behavior to attract attention; but it was very possible to ignore AIDS, to refuse it the status in public policy that its danger warranted. It is sadly, but incontestably, true that it is difficult to develop and maintain a sense of public urgency when people are not dying in the streets.[49] The great Flu Epidemic of 1918 flooded hospitals with patients, on every block someone was sick, relatives were dropping; every-body was at risk and *knew* that they were at risk. My ninety-six-year-old mother-in-law was one of the lucky survivors of both the flu and the 1918 medical treatment for it. HIV, on the other hand, can lie quietly in the body for a decade.

Only during late 1986 and 1987 was the public seriously anxious about AIDS and that was the result of a media blitz on the subject. The blitz was, in turn, tied to circulation, sales, and TV ratings; AIDS was new, just like herpes had been before it. Now, even though the actual epidemic is far more serious, and daily becoming more so, it is just yesterday's news.[50]

Clearly President Clinton hopes to change this and heighten public understanding with the various facets of his AIDS Awareness campaign; whether he will succeed or not, only time will tell (see "Clinton and AIDS," in chapter 6).

Finally in the consideration of policy impact, as well as my suggestion that AIDS may well supplant the bubonic plague as our archetype epi-demic, we have to face the fact that there are no easy and obvious AIDS control programs. The plague was spread by a bacillus; AIDS is spread by a virus. Twentieth-century research has scored one triumph after another in confronting bacterial-based illnesses, but it has yet to cure a virus-based one.[51] Viruses may be even more successful survivors than we are. Control programs, other than biomedical ones, also face special difficulties. A rat abatement program to contain the plague and a "people abatement" pro-gram to contain HIV are very different matters. Authoritarian measures such as the general quarantine that Cuba has instituted are not available in the democracies unless we want our constitutions to fall victim to AIDS.[52] In any case, how does one quarantine 14 million people? In terms of the United States, those who have proposed mass quarantine, branding, imprisonment, public lists of infected, and other draconian measures, must consider whether, to paraphrase Lincoln, our nation could long endure part free and part quarantined.

Notes

1. McNeill, *Plagues and People* (New York: Anchor, 1976), chap. 5.
2. When epidemics become multinational events, they are sometimes called "pandemics" rather than epidemics. Biologically they are the same events; politically, economically, culturally, and epidemiologically they may be quite different. For example, the epidemiological expression of AIDS in Zaire and the United States is quite different. The male to female infected ratio in Zaire is about 1:1, while in the United States the great majority of infected are male homosexuals and/or IV drug users. At another level, AIDS will be economically costly to every nation. Although it is potentially devastating to third world economies, it is merely burdensome to an economy as powerful as America's.
3. Huminer, Rosenfeld, and Pitlik, "AIDS in the Pre-AIDS Era," *Review of Infectious Diseases* 9 (1987), 1102–8. Letter to the Editor, *JAMA* (April 21, 1989), 2198. Because Robert died of "unknown causes," his blood was stored pending later examination. When that examination was made years later, by scientists at Tulane Medical School, all indications were that he died of AIDS. See R. F. Garry, M. H. Witte, A. A. Gottlieb et al., "Documentation of an AIDS virus infection in the U.S. in 1986," *JAMA* 260 (1988), 2085–87.
4. But see Leigh Page, "Rural AIDS," *American Medical News*, June 3, 1988, p. 3; Randolph Wykoff et al., "Contact Tracing to Identify HIV infection in a Rural Community," *JAMA* (June 6, 1988), 3563–66.
5. The HIV epidemic may change this general understanding that epidemics are primarily urban. HIV has heavily infected parts of rural Uganda, Zambia, and Zaire, and Congress has authorized a study in the Ryan White Act of 1990 to track the movement of the virus into rural America. Since people are the carriers, and sex/drugs are the vectors, HIV can go anywhere. If the large numbers still come from the cities, it will simply reflect the fact that is where the large numbers are, rather than reflect a characteristic of the HIV epidemic. Robert S. Gottfried in his excellent and detailed study, *Epidemic Disease in Fifteenth Century England: The Medical Response and the Demographic Consequences* (New Brunswick, N.J.: Rutgers University Press, 1949) argues persuasively that too much as been made of the urban/rural distinction anyway. He points out that the distinction between the two kinds of area was much less sharp in the Middle Ages than it is now. During the Black Death, London was the only city of England that would rate as a city today.
6. See Per Bak and Kan Chen, "Self-Organized Criticality," *Scientific American* (January 1991), 46–53 for a very suggestive approach to a theory of catastrophic events.
7. Barbara Fass Leavy, *To Blight with Plague: Studies in a Literary Theme* (New York: New York University Press, 1992).
8. The State Department of Health noted outbreaks around Dallas and other locations. The rise in cases was attributed to higher-than-average rains, thus more grassland crops of wild grains, and thus a larger rodent population. *San Antonio Express-News*, "Plague Warnings Issued," August 30, 1993, 1a.
9. Southwestern Texas had its last outbreak in late 1987-1988. Joe Fohn, "Farm and Ranch Report: Plague Hits West Texas Rodents," *San Antonio Express-News*, February 25, 1988.

10. See Nicola Duplar, "Fleas, the Lethal Leapers," *National Geographic* 173/5 (May 1988).

11. The epidemics that hit the Mediterranean and Europe were not evenly spaced. There was a series that ran from about the time of Christ through the eighth century. Following those there was a long pause until the mid-fourteenth century when the Black Death inaugurated a new series which continued into the seventeenth century. Finally, a modern series commenced in 1903, starting in India moving to China, Japan, Philippines, Hawaii, and, lastly, California and the Southwestern states. This series seems to have burned out in the 1930s but only after killing some 12 million people.

12. Actually the source of Kaffa's plague was probably the city rats, not the bodies catapulted over the wall. See Graham Twigg, *The Black Death: A Biological Reappraisal* (London: B. T. Batsford Ltd., 1984), 47–51. For a very readable account of this fourteenth-century plague complete with contemporary artistic rendering of its devastation, see Charles L. Mee, Jr., "How a Mysterious Disease Laid Low Europe's Masses," *Smithsonian* (February 1990), 67–79.

13. Geddes Smith, *Plague on Us* (New York: Commonwealth Fund, 1941), 323–25. Chester David Rail, *Plague Ecotoxicology* (Springfield, Ill.: Charles C. Thomas, 1985), 24–29. This latter work contains summary descriptions of many twentieth-century plague episodes.

14. Max Essex and Phillis J. Kanki, "The Origins of the AIDS Virus," *Scientific American* (October 1988), 64–71.

15. Jonathan Mann, James Chin, Peter Piot, and Thomas Quinn, "The International Epidemiology of AIDS," *Scientific American* (October 1988), 82–89. The story on Kytera was filed by Robert Brazell, veteran AIDS reporter. See Lori Heise, "AIDS New Threat to the Third World," *World Watch* (January-February 1988).

16. Nzila Nzilambi et al., "The Prevalence of Infection with Human Immunodeficiency Virus over a 10-Year Period in Rural Zaire," *New England Journal of Medicine* (February 4, 1988), 276–79.

17. Manfred Eigen, "Viral Quasispecies," *Scientific American* (July 1993), 42–49.

18. Roy M. Anderson and Robert M. May, "Understanding the AIDS Pandemic," *Scientific American* (May 1992), 58–66.

19. In 1884 the various European governments competing for African territories divided up the continent as colonial appendages of their nations. Belgium, France, and England were the major beneficiaries.

20. See James Brooke, "Virus Discoveries Help an African Outpost of AIDS Research Gain Notice," *New York Times*, February 28, 1988, 12. Gabon reported less than 10 percent of the cases of Congo, its neighbor.

21. Peter Piot et al., "AIDS: An International Perspective," *Science* 239, no. 4848, 574.

22. Bruce Lambert, "Aids in Prostitutes Not as Prevalent as Believed, Studies Find," *New York Times*, September 20, 1988.

23. The Zaire government hired many French-speaking Haitians to fill the posts vacated by departing Belgians.

24. For example, see any issue of World Health Organization's *Weekly Epidemiological Record.*

25. On December 21, 1987 Washington columnist Jack Anderson published a mapping of the United States according to the number of HIV+'s per 1,000 population levels. The reporters state the map was developed by the Central Intelligence Agency:

2/1000	1.5/1000		1/1000		> 1/1000	
CA	AL	MA	AZ	NM	AK	UT
MD	CO	MI	AR	OK	KY	VT
NV	CT	MO	ID	SD	ME	MN
NJ	FL	NC	IN	WA	WV	MT
NY	GA	PA	IA	WI	WY	ND
DC	HI	RI	KS	MS	OH	OR
	IL	SC	NE	NH		
	LA	TN				
	TX	VA				

The columnists' view of things is fairly well substantiated by current data from the Federal Centers for Disease Control. See the seroprevalence mapping of the nation in U.S. Department of Health and Human Services, *HIV/AIDS Surveillance* (U.S. AIDS cases reported through January 1990) February 1990, 3, 6–7.

26. Peter Gould, *The Slow Plague A Geography of the AIDS Pandemic* (Cambridge: Blackwell, 1993).

27. Randy Shilts, "Patient Zero: The Man Who Brought AIDS to America," *California Magazine* (October 1987), 69.

28. Randy Shilts, "S.F. Hookers Who Made AIDS History," *The San Francisco Chronicle*, August 27, 1987, 4.

29. See the summary of Indian reports in Centers for Disease Control, *AIDS Daily Summary*, December 20, 1992.

30. "An AIDS Epidemic in Latin America Looms Amid Deception and Denial," *New York Times*, January 25, 1993, A1.

31. Lindsy Gruson, "AIDS Spreading in Central America," *New York Times*, October 19, 1988.

32. Dennis L. Breo, "Interview with James Chin, MD: WHO Official Says He Is Still Mobilizing for the Global AIDS Battle," *American Medical News* (November 11, 1988), 9.

33. See the age-specific mortality statistics for the four fourteenth-century epidemics in Graham Twigg, *The Black Death: A Biological Appraisal* (London: B. T. Batsford, Ltd., 1984), 63.

34. *AIDS Surveillance Report*, June 1989, San Antonio Metropolitan Health District. The national figures are from the bulletins of the U.S. Centers for Disease Control.

35. "AIDS in Africa," *New York Times*, September 19, 1990, A10.

36. "In AIDS-Stricken Uganda Area the Orphans Struggle to Survive," *New York Times*, June 10, 1990, A1.

37. There is argument about the mortality rate. The AIDS picture is complicated by the fact that there are viral strains of differing levels of pathogenicity, although none discovered so far are completely benign. For this reason and perhaps others, there are a number of long-term survivors—people who have lived ten years after a diagnosis (most die within two). It is usual now (1993–94) to place the mortality rate at 95 percent.

38. Paul W. Ewald, "The Evolution of Virulence," *Scientific American* (April 1993), 86–93.

39. John F. Burns, "Quick Spread of AIDS Seen for Eskimos," *New York Times*, July 24, 1988, 12.

40. There is some debate on this point as regards HIV. Some African prostitutes who, by any measure of lifestyle, should have been infected, apparently have not been. If they have avoided infection, then the question of natural immunity becomes a possible explanation.

41. Steven Erlanger, "Thriving Sex Industry in Bangkok Is Raising Fears of an AIDS Epidemic," *New York Times*, International, March 30, 1989, 3. Lawrence K. Altman, "AIDS Reported Rising in Thai Drug Users," *New York Times*, April 18, 1989. Barbara Crossette, "Bangkok Awakens to the Fears of AIDS," *New York Times*, November 8, 1987. "AIDS Homes In: Thailand," *The Economist*, February 4, 1989, 37. See also the lecture by Dr. Anthony Fauci, Director of the National Institute of Allergy and Infectious Diseases, "Portrait of AIDS in the 1990s," delivered at the Clinical Center of the NIH on December 6, 1989. The lecture was summarized in *Washington HIV News* 1, no. 4 (January 1990; (distributed electronically through the InterUniversity BITNET system).

42. Roy M. Anderson and Robert M. May, "Understanding the AIDS Pandemic," *Scientific American* (May 1992), 58–65 at p. 65.

43. Stephen Jay Gould, "The Terrifying Normalcy of AIDS: The Exponential Spread of AIDS Underscores the Tragedy of Our Delay in Fighting One of Nature's Plagues," *The New York Times Magazine*, April 19, 1987.

44. Roy M. Anderson and Robert M. May, "Understanding the AIDS Pandemic," *Scientific American* (May 1992), 59.

45. The case is reported and analyzed by Nathan Clumeck et al., "A Cluster of HIV Infections Among Heterosexual People without Apparent Risk Factors," *New England Journal of Medicine* (November 23, 1989), 1460–62.

46. Review the recommendations in this regard made by William B. Johnston and Kevin R. Hopkins, *The Catastrophe Ahead, AIDS and the Case for a New Public Policy* (New York: Praeger, 1990; published in cooperation with the Hudson Institute).

47. The distinction between AIDS and ARC has to do with original CDC definitions. AIDS is a strict and elaborate clinical definition (it runs three pages), while ARC (or AIDS Related Conditions) is a collection of ailments that in some measure fall short of that definition, although both AIDS and ARC individuals are infected with the virus. The strict CDC AIDS definition makes sense in terms of epidemiological reporting but has been found to be too strict for clinical use. It has had to be considerably modified for use in Africa and other countries, for example. ARC has been largely discarded as a useful category.

48. Gould, "The Terrifying Normalcy of AIDS."

49. See the article by Gina Kolata, "AIDS Advocates Find a Decline in Private Funds," *New York Times*, August 7, 1990, A11.

50. Appendix: "Cities Posting HIV Infection Increases." On the media and AIDS see James Kinsella, *Covering the Plague: AIDS and the American Media* (New Brunswick, N.J.: Rutgers University Press, 1989).

51. Some viral diseases are kept in check by vaccines (like smallpox, hepatitis B, and polio), but that is not the same as a postinfection cure.

52. Cuba has tested about 80 percent of the 3.5 million in the sexually active age groups of its population. This has produced 268 HIV+'s who are housed in a camp in an isolated part of the island. All Cuban soldiers and citizens who resided in African stations are tested before returning home, and the Cuban government strongly discourages any personal contact between Cubans and the native population. The policy is summed up: "Cubano con cubana." See the

story by James Brooke, "AIDS Begins to Spread from War-Riven Angola from Central Africa," *New York Times*, February 19, 1989, 4. See "Soviets Introduce World's Toughest Anti-AIDS Measures," *Washington Post*, August 26, 1987.

4

Conflicts in Caring

In the spring of 1986, I visited a friend being treated for AIDS at San Antonio's Methodist Hospital. I remember his hospitalization as one long period of uncertainty and pathos. On Monday Teddy would be looking and feeling so well that it seemed likely he would be discharged by Friday. When Friday came, he would be in intensive care barely breathing. Then, within a week, he was back to a regular room, and back to hope. So it went for almost the whole of his last three months. His care was superb, and the physicians and nurses were obviously skilled and caring. But AIDS treatment was all so new. I can still recall the hushed and worried conferences in the hall as the attending staff asked each other, "What do we do now? What do we do next?"

Things have changed since then, and for the better. I doubt whether the history of medicine presents another example of so much advance in so short a time as there has been in the care of people living with AIDS. The epidemic is like a river that has loosed a veritable flood of activity in all areas of our national life—basic research, medical treatment and procedures, politics and public funding, private organization and lobbying, religion, arts and entertainment, and information dissemination. For example, ten years ago there was virtually no information on HIV and AIDS, today there are over one hundred fifty journals and magazines focusing on the various ramifications of the epidemic, and by 1994 there were 90,000 mostly technical papers listed in the AIDS database of the National Library of Medicine.[1] Indeed, there is such an abundance of activity on all fronts that no one can possibly keep abreast of everything (see Appendix 1, Bibliography).

For the PWA, of course, the most important developments relate to treatment and care. Before 1987 receiving a diagnosis of AIDS was tantamount to being sentenced to a rapid and tormented death, usually by way of *pneumocystis carinii* pneumonia (PCP). Today the use of life-saving drugs like pentamidine and bactrim that fight PCP are among the many signs

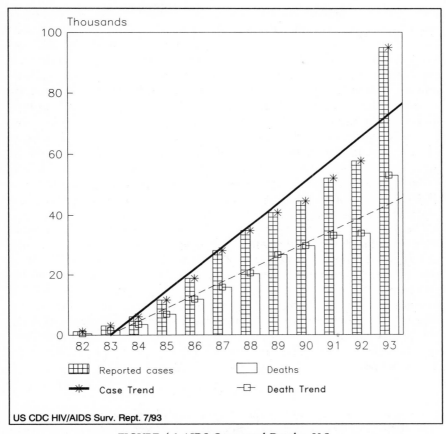

FIGURE 4.1 AIDS Cases and Deaths, U.S.

that indicate that physicians are developing effective techniques. New and more effective treatments are resulting in increased survival time for larger numbers of PWAs as well as an improved quality for the individual's remaining life.[2] An editorial in the *Journal of the American Medical Association* put it this way:

> The perception of AIDS as a medical disease is changing. Previously considered fatal in the short term . . . AIDS now is viewed increasingly as a long term disease . . . in which therapy might significantly prolong life and some complications might be totally preventable.[3]

The effect of better medical intervention can be seen in a comparison of trend lines plotting the number of cases and deaths (Figure 4.1). After 1987 the two trends begin to diverge in a striking fashion indicating that people are living longer even though the number infected is increasing—in 1985 about 31 percent lived longer than two years after diagnosis, by 1987 that figure had reached 49 percent, and in 1989 approximately 71 percent were surviving more than two years. By the early 1990s it was apparent that a small number of people with AIDS diagnoses were living in reasonable health for a decade after the appearance of an AIDS defining illnesses such as PCP, instead of the usual two years.[4] The existence of this small group of "long-term survivors" raises a multitude of so-far unanswered questions relating to natural resistance, the pathogenicity of various strains of the virus, and the impact of an individual's emotional state upon the progress of the syndrome. In any case, PWAs are living longer, and just as important, living better partly because knowledge is displacing ignorance, and proved technique is replacing trial and error.

The metaphor of a flood—even a flash flood—is useful to help visualize the extraordinary activity that AIDS has inspired. It is also useful in another way. A flood probes and exploits with searching, unrelenting fingers every fissure, every indentation, every weakness of the environment. It will find and amplify them all. So it is with AIDS in the scientific-medical sector of America's health care industry. I do not think the epidemic has really created any altogether new professional, organizational, or financing problems, but it has revealed and aggravated those that existed. This process is very evident when we examine the relations between the main actors in the drama of finding and delivering a cure for AIDS.

THE PRINCIPAL WORKERS

Not since the development of the atomic bomb in World War II has there been such a rapid deployment of intellectual and technical energies to focus on one scientific problem. At the 8th International (Berlin) Conference on AIDS, which met in 1993, five thousand papers on various aspects of the disease were presented by researchers from around the world. Each of the seven previous global conferences likewise established records in concentrated and focused research. That all this effort has not yet borne fruit with curative or long-term controlling medical routines is mute testimony to the biologic complexity of the virus, as well as the novel clinical problems that arise in treating the many manifestation of this first fatal human retroviral disease.

However, there are also nonscientific factors that have negatively influenced the character and speed of our attack on AIDS. Those who are directly involved in fighting the epidemic do not constitute one homogenous group, and do not necessarily share compatible methods or goals. On the contrary, there has been a great deal of disarray among the medical, scientific, pharmaceutical, and care groups involved. Complicating matters further is an ongoing antagonism between the bureaucracies of the medical, scientific, and pharmaceutical communities, on the one hand, and the nonestablishment ASO groups on the other. In itself there is nothing unusual in this situation. One of America's strengths is its competitive, pluralistic society, one in which a certain amount of disorganization is normal. However, fighting an epidemic requires speed of action and maximal use of resources. An epidemic is an extraordinary occasion calling for extraordinary and cooperative action. Business as usual prolongs suffering.

THE CLINICIAN

Among the professional groups involved in the care and cure of AIDS, the front-line troops are, of course, the clinical physicians engaged in what can only be called a frustrating, no-win trench warfare against the virus. Clinicians are the persons to whom patients look with hope. As a group they are the ones professionally most interested in gaining access to new techniques, new drugs, new treatments to alleviate the suffering of the real human beings in their offices. Compared with their laboratory colleagues they are more willing to accept anecdotal or clinical observations that do not meet the strict evidentiary requirements of bench science. They are more willing to try new and unproved approaches and chafe at the slowness and deliberation of their laboratory colleagues and pharmaceutical and governmental bureaucracies. As one clinician, Dr. Jay Lalezari, put it, "When you stand at a patient's bedside at two in the morning and he can't breath because he's suffocating with PCP, you'll try anything."[5] It is this group that most clearly expresses the classical humanitarian, caregiving role of the physician, a role that we mistakenly tend to attribute to all scientists in health care and related fields.[6] Many have actively collaborated, at hazard to their professional careers, in the creation of the large underground network for delivering federally unapproved treatments.[7] It is their clients who are dying right now; each death is a defeat.

The character of practicing physicians, indeed their very virtues, make it unlikely that a solution to AIDS will emerge from their collective efforts. The clinicians are too much on the front-line, too involved with their patients, and too reliant on their own unique, nonreplicable observations emerging from their particular patients (who may or may not be representative of all PWAs). On the other hand, the clinician may become aware of the efficacy of a new treatment (such as aerosol pentamidine for pneumocystis) long before their more cautious laboratory colleagues are willing to "certify" it. Even though multimember clinical practice has now become the industrial norm, individual physicians are still remarkably alone with their patients; one of their greatest needs is some kind of informational network so that a physician in Kansas City can quickly access possibly relevant observations of a San Francisco colleague with wider AIDS experience.

In July 1989, Louis W. Sullivan, then Secretary of Health and Human Services, announced the completion of a computerized database through which AIDS patients and their physicians will be able to get up-to-date information on clinical trials of new drugs and vaccines.[8] This represented a major innovation in networking among health caregivers, and a hint of ongoing restructuring in the fields of drug development, testing, and distribution. From the late 1980s a complex new set of institutions and procedures have been forged by AIDS activists, clinicians, laboratory researchers, and government people involved in biomedical administration and/or research. A whole new chapter in the design and administration of drug development and trials is being written under the lash of AIDS. The rapidity and complexity of organizational development makes it a bewildering thicket to enter, and it is too soon to evaluate the long-term impact on the progress of medicine. Nonetheless, new government agencies such as the AIDS Clinical Trial Groups and private community agencies like the San Francisco bay area's Community Consortium of HIV Care Providers or the San Diego Community Research Group have achieved some notable successes in efficient drug-trial procedure and are having an indelible impact on the way America will conduct trials of efficacy in the future.[9] These attempts to tap into the massive aggregate experience of the front-line physicians and local, nongovernmental researchers may be one of the most significant institutional changes wrought by the effort to deal with AIDS.[10]

BIOMEDICAL RESEARCHERS

Laboratory scientists, be they M.D.s or Ph.D.s, the so-called hard scientists, are a different breed. Ordinarily they are removed from the immediate pathos and indignities of death, visiting patients rarely, if at all. Their job is to provide the clinician with the necessary drugs and procedures to prevail. Their primary commitment is not to a particular patient but to a set of protocols called "scientific method" which, if followed rigorously, achieves the closest approximation to objective truth humanly possible. The hard scientist is dedicated to good science, not good medicine. Compassion is institutionalized, not particularized; better caregiving is the hoped for, but not the immediately necessary outcome of the work. The personal motivation is not the gratitude of a patient, but the personal satisfaction at having solved a puzzle and discovered new knowledge. The highest accolade for this form of science is the Nobel Prize. This is not to say that the bench scientist is cold, unfeeling, and lacking in human warmth—far from it. We are dependent upon laboratory scientists for those advances in modern medicine which eventually benefit us all. It is just that their priorities, targets, standards of reference are different, more long-range, more targeted to the overall problem than to the specific patient.

Like the clinical physician, the hard scientist can fall victim to his very virtues. He has been the butt of the mad scientist parody in a century of literature (Dr. Frankenstein, Dr. Jekyll), the scientist who has forgotten, in pursuit of knowledge, just who that knowledge is to serve, and what limits our common humanity impose upon research.[11] An example of a genuine dilemma in the AIDS context involves the issue of proper drug testing protocols. For example, are double-blind, placebo controlled studies ethically justified in the case of a fatal illness, even though they do provide the most complete evidence of drug effectiveness? In the context of the AIDS epidemic there has been much criticism to the effect that if one is dealing with a doomed patient, then careful and time-consuming adherence to standard protocols for the testing, evaluation, and approval of promising drugs may well be inhumane science, that is, "mad science," perverted hard science.

The literature on AIDS is filled with bitter complaint about the snail-like bureaucratic slowness of the National Institutes of Health, the Federal Drug Administration, and the pharmaceutical industry in releasing new drugs. A recent example involved a panel of AIDS experts convened by NIAID to assess a promising new steroid treatment for *Pneumocystis carinii* pneumonia. In May 1990 the panel reached the conclusion that the new treatment was an effective, life-saving therapy. However, it delayed notifying physicians. Bulletins were not issued until October 10, 1990, five months and many respiratory-failure deaths later. Even then the notification process was so flawed that many physicians with an AIDS practice did not get the word.[12]

On the other hand, there are clear dangers in clinical studies not bound by laboratory controls.[13] Indeed, as the deaths resulting from the recent testing of the experimental hepatitis drug fialuridine (FIAU) remind us, there are significant dangers even in tests where presumably classic controls are in place.[14] At least part of the criticism about delay can be attributed to the fact that the organizations representing the "laboratory perspective" have never addressed the task of educating the public on the need for the complex multistage, ten-year program ordinarily required for the thorough testing and distribution of a new drug.[15] But there is a point also to the argument that an epidemic is no time for business as usual.[16]

People wiser by far than I am have tried to resolve the ethical dilemmas flowing from the clinical and the laboratory perspectives without notable success.[17] But one thing is clearly true: the longer medical advances stay in the pipeline of review and clearance, the more people will suffer and die. John James, editor of *AIDS Treatment News*, estimated that the cost of delay or failure in the delivery of new, effective treatments at this stage of the epidemic is about fifty thousand deaths worldwide every eighteen months.[18]

DRUG MANUFACTURERS

Although there are disputable equities and arguments on both sides of the clinical/laboratory debate, there are none that I can fathom in any collision of values between saving lives in an epidemic and making money from an epidemic. It is immoral, basely immoral, to concede priority of claim to the profit motive over that of life itself. Yet there is no question whatever that such moral skewing takes place in the marketplace. Some of our great automakers have knowingly distributed cars that were, to use Ralph Nader's phrase, "unsafe at any speed"; our tobacco industry hawks an addictive carcinogen that has been a subject of condemnation since the time of England's King James I who wrote a tract on the "stinking weed"; most of our patent medicines at one time were largely alcohol fortified with opium derivatives; and there is no question but that many thousands of hemophilia and surgical patients were infected as a result of the unwillingness of the blood bank industry to incur the additional costs of screening their supply. In the seventeenth century, America was founded by merchant-adventurers seeking both material and divine profit. Their entrepreneurial descendants have tended to confuse the two ever since.[19]

The pharmaceutical industry, like all others, is dominated by the profit motive. The skillful caregiving image projected by its advertising tends to obscure the fact that it is an industry that is dedicated to the "bottom line." Like other industries it has its own catalog of disastrous products that were potentially profitable but unsafe, such as thalidomide and the Dalkon Shield IUD. One experienced observer of the scene, John James of *AIDS Treatment News*, doubts that, even in the event of a major breakthrough such as the discovery of a "penicillin" for AIDS, the drug would enter the market until time-consuming patent processes had consumed thousands of lives. He cites in this connection the history of a promising drug called "Compound Q" derived from the root of the Chinese cucumber, *Trichosanthes kirilowii*.[20] Laboratory development in the United States was kept a dark secret for two years. The developers insisted that they wanted to avoid raising false hopes. However, as James pointed out, their concerns on that score dissolved the day their final patent applications were approved and potential profits were protected.[21] Similar stories of profit-motivated delays rather than health-motivated efficiency could be told of fluconazole, aerosol pentamidine, and AL-721.

However, in fairness it should be added that our present patent, liability, and licensing laws offer no incentive to the pharmaceutical industry to make potentially life-saving, but still experimental, drugs quickly and widely available. As one observer has said, "In the United States today, allowing physicians to use any experimental drug is all cost and no benefit to the company which holds the patent rights."[22] The drug licensing laws under the 1962 Kefauver Amendments to the Food and Drug Act (which were enacted in response to the thalidomide disaster) encourage extreme caution, and the economy offers no money incentive until the number of the sick (and therefore potential users) reaches a level where production and distribution is profitable.

The base concern, the fundamental question acutely raised by the AIDS epidemic, is "Should we, as a nation, leave control of our national health policy and products in the hands of profit-oriented private associations—be they hospitals, insurance companies, pharmaceutical corporations, or partnerships of physicians in private clinics?"[23] If we do, then we support a policy that virtually guarantees that either only the well-to-do will have adequate access to good medicine, or that in order to provide more equal access, private corporations will be given a blank check on the federal treasury through national subsidies. An example of the latter would be the federal funding of the anti-HIV drug AZT (Retrovir). Few individuals could afford the very high price charged (originally about $9,000 per year, now about $2,500 after much political activism), so Congress allowed the taxpayers to pick up the tab. Burroughs Wellcome Corporation made extraordinary profits, even though the drug was actually developed by the government itself. AZT's profitability is, of course, a corporate secret; however, it has been estimated to be between 900 and 1,800 percent.[24] In November 1990 Congress unanimously amended the 1983 Orphan Drug Act, which had the unintended effect of making such windfall profits possible. President Bush vetoed the bill presumably because he believed that such usurious margins of profit were needed and acceptable in order to encourage drug manufacturers to make the medicines we need.[25]

There is nothing wrong with profit, but in the health area it is lamentably easy for profiting to become profiteering. This is due to the fact that there is no way to establish a market value on life or "health," and because the key personnel and products cannot really be evaluated by the consumer. These facts, and others, allow those in the health care field to escape the public scrutiny devoted to other services and products. Why should, for example, pentamidine, when distributed by a Japanese company (Fujisawa Pharmaceutical) to American AIDS patients, cost from $105 to $300 a vial, when exactly the same drug is distributed in Europe by a French pharmaceutical firm for $30?[26] In the case of AZT, why should a drug developed at taxpayer's expense be used for the profit of one company?[27] A recent case involving extraordinary treatment cost involves Foscavir. About 40 percent of PWAs develop an opportunistic infection that causes blindness. It can be effectively treated with Foscavir—if the patient can raise the $50,000 annual costs ($59.00 per day for the drug, plus administration). Foscavir's maker, Astra USA, Inc., has suggested that it might cut the prices a bit, but only after the drug exceeds $50 million in annual sales![28] Whatever our final answers to the issues involved in medical costs, there is no question but that AIDS is forcing the nation's policy makers to look at the industry with a new and more critical interest.

Prominent medical and business figures are now publicly stating that our present health care delivery system is slow, chaotic, undependable, over-priced, and economically very discriminatory—a sentiment seldom heard before HIV spread through the land. In 1989 then Surgeon General Koop said:

> the health care marketplace, although laissez-faire, is not freely competitive and has virtually no moderating controls working on behalf of the patient. So we seem to have a system of health care that is distinguished by a virtual absence of self-regulation on the part of those who provide that care—hospitals and health-care workers, primarily physicians—but distinguished as well by the absence of such natural marketplace controls in regard to price and quality of service.[29]

In 1993 President Clinton gave specific point to Koop's statement when he denounced drug companies for profiteering on vaccines used to immunize children. He pointed out that U.S. parents must pay $10 for a polio vaccination that costs only $1.80 in England and even less in Belgium.[30] This is a sad litany for what was once the finest and fairest health care delivery system in the world. Whether the Clinton administration's health care proposals will begin the process of curing the sickness in our health care system only time and legislation will tell.

AIDS SERVICE ORGANIZATIONS

In addition to the information explosion and its organizational consequences, there has been a weedlike growth of private agencies addressing various facets of the epidemic. In the best American tradition, the first on the scene were voluntary community care groups, privately organized and funded. Most of those operating today were established in the four-year period 1982–86.[31] As one might expect, the beginning efforts were made in the nation's two most affected cities with the founding of New York's Gay Men's Health Crisis and the San Francisco AIDS Foundation. Both are now large, successful associations with multimillion dollar budgets, and all the problems typical of middle-aged organizations—complex agendas, internal divisions, and bureaucracies.[32] From this beginning, private voluntary organizations focusing on nursing, food, and living assistance, counseling and preventive education spread across the country (generally called ASOs—AIDS service organizations). There are now over twenty-five hundred such groups, supplemented by about eighty organizations representing people with AIDS, as well as many AIDS targeted fund-raising groups.[33] Collectively these private associations annually raise and spend hundreds of millions in private money.[34] In Texas there are 177 private groups; my home city, San Antonio, lists fifteen private ASOs (as well as six public ones). I doubt that there is any historic parallel to this explosion of private initiative and organization. The still-to-be-written chapters of this grass-roots response will be among the finest in America's long and proud history of self-help and compassionate care.

However, the picture has its troubled spots. I can think of no social agency that attempts to serve a more culturally disparate clientele and one with a greater range of problems. The clients of most ASOs are frequently bound by no more than a common affliction, and one, moreover, that has many different stages, each calling for separate approaches and services.[35] I will speak only of the agency with which I had some connection, but the problems faced by the San Antonio AIDS Foundation are found commonly throughout the ASOs serving major metropolitan areas.[36] In our agency you could meet people radiant with glowing health and others on a final countdown. SAAF's clientele ranged in income from homeless and penniless to comfortable upper-middle class, in education from illiterate to graduate degrees, in sexual practices from sado-masochists to conservative "missionaries," in sexual orientation gays, straights, bisexuals, celibates, and variations I never knew existed. The mode of HIV transmission ran the gamut from gay and straight sex, assault/rape of both adults and children, drug injection, medical mishap in organ transplant or transfusion, to simply being born to an infected mother.

The members of every subgroup seemed to agree that SAAF was paying too much attention to the needs and problems of other groups, and neglecting them. Even with a director who was very conscious of the problem and tried to bring together people of different backgrounds, there was, in fact, no understanding, and little tolerance or empathy between the various client groups—drug users and others, gays and straights, middle- and lower-class clients, and so on. Only the children were able to bridge the gaps. Speaking personally, I found to my chagrin that, with all my education and experience in communicating, there were whole groups of people to whom I could not comfortably relate and with whom I could talk only on the most superficial level.

There is really no solution to this problem. It flows from the nature of the epidemic itself, the pattern of infection. There are no historical models, no guidebooks for community service agencies that fit the needs of the current epidemic. People working in the field have to improvise as best they can and improvise within a very high stress environment where all conflicts of

client and agency interest are played out against a background of accumu-
lating deaths.[37] Bill Bearden, the former director of a local ASO, put his job
in perspective when he tendered his resignation, "No sane person should
try to do this job for more than two years."

Another problem area arises from the demands of federal policy as
expressed in the Ryan White Act (see chapter 6). This act promotes the
development of multiple agencies gathered under the hopefully coordinating umbrella of a communitywide consortium. Viewed from one angle, the
proliferation of AIDS agencies, consortia, and committees is good; it means
that people who want access to AIDS policy can be heard and (especially
important for PWAs) can feel that they have some control over all the apparatus and policy that focuses on AIDS. It is American democratic pluralism
in action. The downside is that fifteen agencies give birth to fifteen directors
and staffs supported by fifteen payrolls which inevitably consume a large
portion of the money made available to alleviate problems encountered by
people living with AIDS. AIDS services in San Francisco after 1985 became
an object lesson in the dangers of fragmentation. Every minority group
demanded and got its own program; the result was a plethora of underfunded, squabbling, inadequate programs.[38]

In the case of San Antonio, I do wonder whether an area of about one
million, with perhaps ten to thirteen thousand seropositives, can afford so
many agencies.[39] How much of the federal, state, and private money will
resurface in the form of meaningful services? A multiplicity of agencies also
dilutes the authority that any single agency can claim; in a policy area that
needs a strong advocacy arm to speak on behalf of embattled PWAs, the
organizational basis for it is swallowed in a quicksand of committees and
possible conflicts of interest.[40] In any case, clearly from 1992, a major
accountability problem for our AIDS programs is shaping up. The entire area
will need close surveillance lest the War on AIDS recapitulates President
Johnson's War on Poverty, which spent billions, helped launch a more vigorous minority-based middle class, enhanced my personal income as a con-
sultant, but did nothing to alleviate poverty in America.

PROFESSIONAL ETHICS

The epidemic has also revealed an underlying, and surprising, weakness in
the ethical underpinnings of the health care industry. Like most people, I
grew up thinking of physicians as motivated by more altruistic standards of
service than those which informed other professions. From the early "Dr.
Kildare" TV series to current health care oriented TV shows, the physician
is portrayed as a person striving to be a bit better and a bit more compassionate than most of us. But AIDS has revealed more fear, more prejudice,
and more greed than we have wanted to associate with the profession.[41] It

has raised anew questions of medical ethics that had long been thought resolved, questions involving the ethical obligation of the practicing physician to accept risk as an unavoidable accompaniment of the profession.[42]

In 1846 the American Medical Association adopted its first code of ethics; it stated clearly:

> . . . and when pestilence prevails, it is their duty to face the danger, and to continue their labors for the alleviation of suffering, even at the jeopardy of their own lives.[43]

But about one hundred years later the age of antibiotics began, and we were all, patient and physician alike, lulled into a false sense of security. The grave risks that had always attended the treatment and care of the sick seemed to be reduced to negligible proportions. Among the general population the fear of such diseases as syphilis or gonorrhea receded into the background. The syphilis spirochete that once could destroy the mind and career of Lord Randolph Churchill now just called for a shot in the rear. The physicians, when they revised their Code of Ethics, left out the pestilence provision; perhaps it seemed that the entire notion of pestilence was outmoded in the confident new age of antibiotic medicine. AIDS was a rude awakening.

The problem surfaced anew when polls began to show that physicians, nurses, and other health care workers in training were stating that they did not want to care for HIV+ individuals when they entered practice. Other studies suggested that a large number of licensed practitioners were refusing their services on one ground or another. Finally, authentic voices of the profession, such as the *Southern Medical Journal*, were raising questions whether, since seropositivity was "self-inflicted," there should be any ethical obligation to care for AIDS patients. Let the sinners die![44]

Health care workers have argued their right to refuse care on three grounds: (1) that they are facing an unacceptable hazard; (2) that they have a personal need for and a right to job satisfaction; (3) that the caregiving relationship is a free and contractual one. All three sets of arguments have been officially and emphatically rejected by the leading professional organizations. Both the American Medical Association and the American College of Physicians have restated the classical position that "the denial of care to patients for any reason is unethical. . . . Refusal of a physician to care for a specific category of patients—for example, patients who have AIDS or who are HIV+, for any reason is morally and ethically indefensible."[45] This is clear enough and comports with the 1846 Code of Ethics. Further, the American Medical Association now provides an ethics forum in both the Journal of the association as well as its newspaper, *American Medical News*.[46] But there can be a great deal of slippage between the official position of any professional association and practice in the field; if you are a patient, it is the attitude of practicing physicians that is crucial, not the policy position of a medico-political elite. Consequently I think it important to treat the objections to caring for AIDS patients as serious reservations by serious people.

THE HAZARDS OF AIDS CARE

Undeniably there are significant risks involved in caring for AIDS patients, particularly in a surgical, emergency, or intensive-care setting. How great these risk are is extremely difficult, perhaps impossible, to state with any assurance. Research published in the *Journal of the American Medical Association (JAMA)* calculated that the risk of seroconversion to a surgeon was on the order of 1:130,000 to 1:4,500. Any estimate with this much spread is at once suspect, and certainly not very useful to a person trying to assess his or her occupational risk. What it really says is, "We don't know."[47] On the other hand, merging mathematical models and experience, a San Francisco surgeon with a substantial AIDS clientele calculates that each time he suffers a needle-stick injury he has a 1:2,000 chance of seroconverting, and since he incurs at least ten needle-sticks per year his yearly seroconversion odds are 1:200. He purchased a large disability policy as a result of his calculations.[48]

A review of the literature on the matter simply underscores that no one has a good grasp on the actual odds. There are too many variables to allow calculations that produce clear, defensible guidelines. Significant variables involve, for example, the kind of service rendered, the condition of the patient, the stage or progress of his infection, the care facilities available and the proficiency of those using them, and the attitudes and training of those rendering care. Only one thing is clear, that the risk is too substantial to be ignored or minimized by official policy statements.[49]

Nonetheless, the simplistic answer seems to be the only one: risk comes with the territory. Admitting that this formula seriously oversimplifies a complex situation involving almost infinite gradations of risk among various types of health care providers, it seems to be the only appropriate place to take a stand on the ethical issues.[50] The annals of medicine are filled with names of those who rendered care at great personal sacrifice and risk. Men like Benjamin Rush, one of the founding fathers of American medicine, cared for Yellow Fever victims in Philadelphia's 1793 epidemic in the same selfless way many other caregivers have done in countless epidemics down through history. They followed a professional instinct definitively stated by William Boghurst, a London apothecary who lived during the Plague of 1666:

> Every man that undertakes to bee of a profession or takes upon him any office must take all parts of it, the good and the evil, the pleasure and the pain, the profit and the inconvenience altogether, and not pick and chuse;

for ministers must preach, Captains must fight, Physicians attend upon the Sick.[51]

No one has said it any better; there is little more to say.

JOB SATISFACTION

Another argument supporting the right of the caregiver to withhold service relates to the expectations and satisfactions that motivate the practice of medicine. It is argued that direct service health care providers see themselves primarily as healers whose job it is to get the sick out of bed and back on the job. Consistently failing to do so leads to burn-out, loss of morale, lowered efficiency, and professional depression, all to the detriment of their patients. The practice of medicine is already a high-stress occupation without the additional problem of a no-win illness like AIDS. Of course, if a caregiver wishes to undertake this additional stress that is all right, but it ought not to be required ethically or legally.

A sense of professional failure that accompanies the death of a patient is a very real emotion, not to be treated lightly. No one likes to lose, least of all highly skilled professionals whose self-image and professional reputation are at stake in the mortality rate. The language we use to describe the situation describes how we all feel about it. The doctor "loses" his patient; that is, in a battle of wits with death, the caregiver has lost. Heroic efforts notwithstanding, eath gets the prize. Incurable AIDS demotes the physician and his supporting personnel from healers to maintenance staff. This is not the satisfying role that a young intern, nurse, or paramedic had in mind to play and, indeed, it must be seriously frustrating and destructive of morale.[52] The problem of burnout in AIDS care is very real and well documented.

This rationale for withholding professional services must be taken seriously and confronted in health care administration. We need to call upon our experience with battlefield medicine to develop programs of support for the caregiver's morale. At the same time, however, it constitutes a reasonable position only from those who have already assumed a significant AIDS caseload, *not from those who anticipate* that their morale might suffer if and when they decide to service AIDS patients. The issue is serious, but it is hard to take seriously those in the second group who express it. All caregivers must accept the loss of patients; like risk, this also comes with the territory.

THE DOCTOR-PATIENT "CONTRACT"

By far the most significant and far-reaching argument advanced—the argument most emphatically rejected by the AMA—was that (1) physicians were "just like" the members of any other professional group, and (2) physicians should have the right to contract their services for reasons and fees they feel appropriate, as well as to a clientele of their choice, that is, the physician ought to have the legal right to allocate his time and service on the basis of any criteria he thinks applicable, whether they are medical or nonmedical. The architect can decline to design your home, the contractor can refuse to build it, the interior designer can decline to decorate it, and the physician can withhold services to those who live within it. Those who start from this premise insist that there is nothing morally or legally wrong with a caregiver refusing service to an alcoholic, a drug user, a Black, a Jew, a homosexual, a communist, or an AIDS victim, not because the caregiver lacks competence (which everyone admits is a compelling reason), but merely because the caregiver dislikes or disapproves of the client as a person.

The first prong of the argument states that physicians are just like other professionals and should be treated as such. But the facts are otherwise. Whether they be Indian shamans, African witch doctors, Mexican curanderos, or American R.N.s or M.D.s, the populace has always placed caregivers in a special category and accorded them status, deference, and perquisites commensurate with their importance to society. Caregivers, especially physicians and nurses, are not just plain folk! In contemporary America their professional associations are given quasi-governmental status with significant regulatory and policing powers. Their importance is signaled by our willingness to heavily subsidize their education in order to guarantee an adequate supply. The individual physician pays dearly in time, dedication, hard work, and money for his license; but the truth is that, regardless of whether he graduates from a public or a private university, the lion's share of the cost of training the physician is borne by either the taxpayers or private endowments or a combination of both. The cost of a modern medical education is such that, if society said "Pay your own way!" we would have neither doctors nor nurses. By the time practice begins, the American physician is probably the most heavily subsidized product of our graduate education.

No, healers are not ordinary businesspeople. That is their pride and their burden. Their training is not ordinary, their arts and skills are not ordinary, there is an altruistic and moral aspect to their proper professional motivation, and our reliance upon them is extraordinary. The physicians and their immediate support staffs are special. We think so, and, in truth, so do they. Many of their professional associations are currently arguing before state legislatures in support of special limits on malpractice liability, and their arguments always commence with the assertion that their services are essential to society. Health caregivers demand, deserve, and receive a special place in our social economy; I would argue that, as a consequence, society has the right to place them under obligations not shared by other professionals and, at minimum, insist that they stand fast and do their job in a time of epidemic.

The second prong of the argument asserting that caregivers should have the same liberty of contract to grant or withhold services as other professionals is superficially appealing; it does tie-in with the powerful American tradition of free enterprise capitalism which insists that state restraint on liberty of contract needs strong and special justification. However, in the face of this basic tenet of our national political faith, various groups have successfully argued a compelling case in many areas. Statutory and case law expressions of policy are sharply limiting individual contractual choice for the greater good of society. Within the past fifty years the U.S. Supreme Court and the Congress have ruled that services in the following areas may not ordinarily be granted or withheld on the basis of racial, ethnic, or sex considerations: education; employment; public facilities, from buses and planes to golf courses; private facilities like restaurants, motels, hotels, or theaters which cater to the public; rentals or sales of homes by owners or realtors; and admission to private, but business-oriented clubs. It takes no great leap of imagination to frame an argument, if one is really needed, that health care must not be denied to the sick regardless of who the sick are. I can think of no better way for the caregiving profession to encourage the development of a completely nationalized system than to insist on a contractual right of discrimination when the political and legal trends are clearly in the opposite direction.

It is unlikely, however, that constitutional and/or occupational scruples motivate the objections to treating HIV+ individuals. Much more likely is an understandable but unacceptable fear and completely intolerable bigotry.[53] Church defined and transmitted hatred of homosexuals, and a cultural disdain and fear of IDUs (especially Black and Hispanic ones) are the headwaters of much policy and behavior in America's reaction to this epidemic. The patent fact that the groups earliest affected in the United States were and are male homosexuals and IDUs allowed underlying hatreds to surface in many forms including that of withholding health care.[54]

No caregiver has suggested that for reasons of occupational safety, job satisfaction, or constitutional law, pediatric cases be left untreated, that children be refused care. On the contrary, the care of pediatric AIDS victims is well funded and staffed. Children are the "innocent victims!" The rest are sinners and deserve to die. No more than 13 percent of the federal health budgets prior to 1990, which ran into the billions, were earmarked for direct care for teens and adults. The Ryan White Act of September 1990 hopefully may change that (see chapter 6).

History offers many examples of caregivers refusing or corrupting their services for ideological, political, religious, or other personal, nonmedical reasons, but none seem to offer much support in the current American context. Nazi physicians refused treatment to Jews, Southern Whites turned away

Blacks, and Soviet psychiatrists placed themselves at the service of state security by certifying political dissidents as insane. However, no one suggests that these are models that should be emulated in America. The Jews, the Blacks, and the dissidents had one thing in common: they were outcasts in their own societies—just as the homosexual and the IDUs are today.

Over six hundred years ago a surgeon advised his students, "If you are asked to treat a patient with no chance of recovery [because of infection with bubonic plague], say that you will be leaving town."[55] It seems at times that we have progressed too little a distance. There are 600,000 physicians and 180,000 dentists in the United States, but a shortage of those who will take AIDS cases. Five percent of the nation's hospitals care for one half of the cases. Private physicians are not counseling their patients on AIDS, and former Surgeon General Antonia Novello's call for help goes unheeded.[56] A 1990 survey revealed that 50 percent of the physician-respondents would not treat an HIV+ patient if given the choice. In 1994 the AMA sent a twenty-five-page guide, "AMA Guidelines on Early HIV Intervention," in an attempt to overcome reluctance at the primary care level to deal with HIV patients. Altogether too many of our doctors and dentists, it seems, have left or are "leaving town" to escape the political and personal impact of the AIDS epidemic.

VIRUS TESTING: HOW AND WHO?

Mandatory testing for everyone for evidence of a spreading, fatal disease would seem, at first glance, to be an unremarkable and sensible action for governments to undertake. School children used to be routinely checked for exposure to TB (and may have to be again if the current rise in TB continues), and voluntary breast and prostate cancer screenings have been used for a number of years. Similarly, there is widespread testing for HIV administered by ASOs, blood banks, hospitals, military, prison, and other government programs. Public agencies are now administering more than two million HIV tests annually. There is nothing new or startling about general population testing as a public health measure.

There are differences, however, and those differences make HIV testing, especially involuntary or "routine" testing, a matter of heated debate. In the case of breast and prostate cancers, screening is justified as a means of instituting effective treatment. With TB, screening serves not only to commence treatment but also as the function of protecting others until medication annuls the bacterium's ability to infect. Unfortunately, such compelling justifications are lacking for HIV screening. There is no known way to stop the progress of the disease in an individual, nor any medical way, such as a vaccine, to protect others from transmission. The main arguments for mass HIV testing, voluntary or involuntary, relate to the information that it would provide both the testee and the government. Hopefully, it would serve to induce the testee, if positive, to avoid further risk behavior and begin health monitoring; for governments, better data could lead to more effective safer sex campaigns as well as more intelligent allocation of research and intervention resources.

Part of the debate over HIV testing stems from the technology itself. This book is not the place to delve into the intricacies of testing technology,[57] but I want at least to indicate some of the individual, social, and political problems that arise directly out of that technology.

There are many tests that can be used to determine whether someone has been infected by HIV, but only two are used widely—the Elisa and the Western Blot blood tests.[58] Neither tests directly for the virus but rather for antibodies the immune system has created, after infection, to fight the virus. The Elisa is our main screening test, while the Western Blot is our principal means of double-checking an HIV+ reading by Elisa. The American Medical Association recommends that three tests on the same serum sample be administered before certifying someone as HIV+.[59] In both the Elisa and Western Blot, the result in any given test administration represents a *prediction* that the virus is (+) or is not (-) in the blood sample presented; that is to say, both tests make a statement like this: "If you wish to isolate or detect virus particles from this sample of blood, the likelihood that you will be (or will not be) successful is 98.5%."

Needless to say, a great deal rides on this prediction—a prediction that, like all predictions, can be wrong. Error can creep into biologic testing due to inadequately sensitive or selective testing; but this is not the case with the HIV tests, they score very high in both respects. Errors can also result from careless lab work, but while this happens, it does not happen enough to affect national figures. However, there are several sources of significant error. First, a person's immune system must have had sufficient time to generate antibodies against HIV before an antibody test can be effective. Generally the body requires from six weeks to three months after infection, although, in rare cases, the period can be much longer. In viral terms, "the viral population must rise to around 10^9, which would take about 30 (viral) generations" before it is detectable.[60] In any case, if there are no antibodies, then a test will read negative even though the testee is, in fact, positive. At the outset of infection, the person may well test negative even though he or she may have a large quantity of virus in the blood and be very infectious.[61] This "window" period makes it possible, for example, for infected blood to get into the national blood supply in spite of screening and for people unwittingly to transmit the infection in sexual relations. It is also one of the reasons why one test is ineffective as a premarital check. Parties planning marriage, to be really sure, would have to be strictly monogamous or abstemious and undergo two tests about three months apart.

Another source of error, one with larger sociopolitical implications, stems from the fact that the predictive accuracy of the tests is contingent not only upon their sensitivity and specificity but also upon the proportion of the population being tested that, in fact, has been infected and developed the antibody. As a general rule, *the smaller* the proportion of those in the tested population who are infected, *the higher* a test's positive error rate will be; conversely, the higher the proportion of those in the sampled population who are HIV+, the more reliable a positive prediction will be. To put this another way, a prediction by Elisa that you are positive is very reliable *if* you are a member of a group in which there is much HIV infection, a high risk group. On the other hand, if you are a not a member of such group, then the test result is less reliable, more prone to error. This shortcoming of the Elisa and Western Blot is common to all such biological tests. Why not test for the virus directly? The answer is cost. The polymerase chain reaction assay will accurately test for the presence of the virus (not the antibody), but the cost is approximately $200.00, and it takes about two weeks to get results— clearly too costly and too slow for general population or blood screening uses. The overwhelming majority of the American population is not in a high risk group and is not infected; the overall seroprevalence is estimated at .004 (1 million HIV+ over 250 million population). If the nation were to be tested with the Elisa alone, the number of false positives would be staggering, in fact, they would greatly outnumber the true positives. The consequences of such a result are incomprehensible—morale, suicide rates, marriage, productivity, insurance, politics, everything would be shaken as if by a giant hand. If the Elisa positives were checked by the Western Blot, then the number of false positives would be greatly curtailed, since it is 99.9 percent selective for blood samples that have no trace of HIV. But the costs would be staggering. Elisa tests cost about $10; Western Blots cost around $55 and take more time to process. Given the great number of false Elisa positives, assume three fourths of the population would require at least the first two, then reasonably accurate testing would cost over $10 billion—not to mention the cost of getting our laboratory capacity to the level of such a nationwide test. This is at least one reason that demands are no longer heard from politicians for mass mandatory screenings. Perhaps, enough has been said to indicate that what seems, at first glance, to be a sensible thing to do— test everyone—is individually and politically like walking into a whirlwind.

TESTING POLITICS

In September 1991 a weak, emaciated Kimberly Bergalis testified for just a few seconds before a subcommittee of the Committee on Energy and

Commerce, U.S. House of Representatives. She asked Congress to pass legislation to help ensure that no other person—patient or caregiver—be infected as she was, in the very health care setting itself. In 1987 she had kept a dental appointment with AIDS, and since diagnosis, she, her family, and other patient advocates have campaigned for a program of mandatory HIV screening of both caregiver and patient. Kimberly Bergalis died a few months after her congressional appearance, at age twenty-three. As of March 1992, five more of her dentist's patients have been found to be similarly infected; Dr. David Acer has died.[62] Sherry Johnson (age eighteen), another infected Acer patient, announced in 1993 that she would try to continue the campaign for mandatory testing and disclosure.

This first *recorded* "doctor to patient infection" case did not start the debates over HIV testing in the health care setting, but it did give them emotional dimension and focus. Ms. Bergalis's activism forced people to confront that they were not arguing merely technical points relating to the Elisa or Western Blot HIV tests, or about what groups should be tested under what conditions; she made everyone realize that they were disputing issues involving life and death, something easily lost sight of in the forest of statistics, arguments and counterarguments. In this way she gave meaning to the remainder of her life, and she presented the nation's Congress with a challenge it still has not met, the challenge of forging a coherent national policy on HIV testing.

It is fair to say that, on the multiple issues involved in HIV testing, we are in a state of confusion and disarray. The issues involve professional pride as well as prejudice and discrimination; the character and/or limitations of our testing techniques; the expenditure of billions, and, as always, the related matter of "who pays?"; which level of our government system should be responsible for what, and at what political costs? Hovering above all the technical, political, and economic arguments is a blanketing fear, a fear that AIDS so readily—and rightly—inspires in all of us.

The Medical Perspective. The health care community* wants all patients requiring invasive procedures (from simple tissue removal for biopsy to orthopedic surgery) to be tested for HIV, preferably with consent, but without if need be. This includes all patients admitted to hospitals and many seen in the office.[63] The position of dentists is less clear; at this juncture, they seem more concerned to avoid mandatory testing for themselves than insisting upon it for patients.

The health care workers (hereafter HCWs) justify this position on two grounds: (1) that various studies[64] indicate that HCWs are at some measurable risk of HIV infection in many procedures and that knowledge of the

---

*By "medical care community" I refer to those in direct caregiving contact with people, such as physicians, RNs, LVNs, therapists, dentists, hygienists, and so on (not pharmacists, dieticians, etc.) —about 4 million people.

patient's status, if positive, would signal them to scrupulously observe all infection control rules thus reducing their risk; and (2) that testing would enable attending physicians to produce faster and more accurate diagnoses in cases of emergency admissions.

With respect to the risks of transmission, The Centers for Disease Control Cooperative Needlestick Surveillance Group announced an infection rate of from 0.42 percent to 1 percent following a single hollow-bore needlestick contaminated with HIV+ blood. The usual odds cited are 1:300 for each incident.[65] Such injuries constitute about 80 percent of the reported HCW exposures to infectious blood, and, of course, they occur largely to (60%–75%) the nursing staff and lab technicians handling blood rather than physicians or housekeeping staff.[66] Another 12 percent of the exposures involve open wound or mucous-membrane exposures, which carry significantly less risk of transmission because contaminated blood is not injected into the body. From 1983 to June 30, 1991, for example, HIV tests were given to 1,548 HCWs six months after exposure. Of the 1,366 with needlestick exposures, four tested positive; of the 182 whose exposure was through mucous-membrane or open wound, none tested positive. To put the HIV risk in some perspective, exposure to Hepatitis B under the same circumstances carries a 6 to 30 percent risk of an infection that kills 250 HCWs annually.

Through March 31, 1992 there were 8,088 cases of AIDS in HCWs (it is important to keep in mind that this figure represent only those with CDC-reported AIDS, not all those who may be seropositive or have unreported AIDS).[67] Included in this figure, there were 227 dental workers, 841 physicians, 56 surgeons, 1,745 nurses, 1,448 health aides, 151 paramedics, 1,140 lab technicians, and 421 therapists. As of January 1, 1993, 71 percent of the HCWs with AIDS had died. Approximately 5 to 6 percent of these AIDS cases have been documented to be occupationally related infections and thus become relevant to an assessment of occupational risk. The remainder were either lifestyle-related (sex/drug = 78.2%) or undetermined. In September 1992 the Centers for Disease Control released updated figures registering 111 new seroconversions. Thirty-two were determined to be the result of occupational exposure in a specific, known incident; sixty-nine others were classified as "possibly occupational."[68] However they might have been infected, these approximately eighty two hundred individuals represent a tiny fraction of the some 4 million individuals working in patient-contact health care.

As regards the contention that diagnostic efficiency would be enhanced, it can best be cast as a scenario: A patient presents himself to the emergency staff running a high temperature and various other diagnostic markers of some form of pneumonia. The working assumption is a standard community-derived pneumonia and an antibacterial treatment is commenced while various tests are ordered. Blood is drawn, vital signs read; the patient is clearly sick and is admitted. Several days later the first tests come back but do not indicate a usual pneumonia, so spinal taps and lung X-rays are ordered. More time is spent, and the patient is not responding to the usual treatment. Five days later the correct diagnosis of *pneumocystis carinii* pneumonia is made. Once diagnosed, the treatment is well known and effective. Had the admitting physicians known of the patients seropositivity, the correct course of treatment would have been started immediately for this common and dangerous HIV related opportunistic infection.

My scenario is, in fact, based on a scene commonly played out in hospitals throughout the land. At San Francisco General Hospital, which has much AIDS experience, the signs would have been recognized, but this is not necessarily the case elsewhere. A young counselee of mine was in San Antonio's Medical Center for a week before the correct diagnosis was made.

These data and considerations seem sufficient to the medical community to warrant a call for mandatory patient testing. Their spokespersons and resolutions prefer not to use the word "mandatory," using the term "routine" instead. This is disingenuous at best, deceitful at worst. To classify the HIV test, over which hangs a sentence of death, as though it were the same kind of "routine" test as that for blood type, is meant to defuse opposition by misleading the public mind. The American Medical Association and other industry unions want mandatory patient screening; a rose, by any other name, is still a rose.[69]

On the other hand, the medical industry sees no reason for routine/mandatory screening of HCWs, particularly physicians. Their unions insist that there has never been a completely documented case of physician/nurse to patient transmission, and this is true. The Acer/Bergalis case involved a doctor of dentistry. Further, they exclude from their area of responsibility the thousands of infections resulting from surgical organ transplants and transfusions. These infections raise a difficult point bearing upon the ethics of responsibility: Should an attending physician or surgeon, like the captain of a battleship, be held ultimately responsible for what transpires under his command, even though he personally is not at fault? Finally, they dismiss the Centers for Disease Control's statistical estimates (see below) of patient infections as ill-founded and unwarranted speculation.

In December 1991, the AMA's House of Delegates adopted resolutions that probably represent the majority of medical opinion. The resolutions called upon physicians to observe infection control precautions, to determine their own HIV status, and to establish local monitoring boards to oversee and guide the practice of HIV+ members. However, determining one's status, reporting to a monitoring board, and submitting to its guidance would be entirely voluntary. The local boards, moreover, should be immunized from all legal accountability for their guidance. Physicians who voluntarily submitted to, but repeatedly ignored guidance, should be reported to state licensing boards by the local boards. Resolutions also encouraged HIV+ physicians to refrain from invasive procedures wherein the patient might be presented with risk of infection. The Association also reaffirmed its opposition to routine/mandatory testing for physicians, and its support for the reporting of all individuals (patients) who test positive to state health boards.[70] On behalf of its membership, the Association also authorized a million dollar public relations campaign to improve the public image of physicians.

The Patient Perspective. Those like Kimberly Bergalis, who advanced the interest of patients, generally call for mandatory testing of both HCWs and patients, coupled with disclosure of the HCWs serostatus to the patient. This is needed, it is argued, to allow the patient to make a reasonable judgment as to the degree of risk he/she wishes to take. Patient advocates point out that physicians, surgeons especially, are very careful to advise patients of all possible risks involved in major medical interventions as a way of minimizing their malpractice liability if things should not go well and as a way of allowing the patient to make intelligent choices about his or her life. Before surgery, the patient is asked to sign forms stating that he/she has been advised and accepts those risks. Why should the possibility of transmitting a fatal infection from health care provider to patient, or transmission from infected to uninfected patients via medical procedures, be treated any differently than the possibility of fatal transplant rejection?

To that salient question, the HCW usually responds, "Because there is no data indicating that there is any risk of transmission." What is the patient's risk? The answer is that there are no clear answers, such as more or less do exist for HCW risk. There are several reasons for the uncertainty. First, researchers within the medical establishment who have studied risk to health care providers have not been as interested in studying patient risk; thus, the results are few studies. Second, it is difficult to track patients in our highly mobile society, especially if they have been infected with a virus whose effect may not appear for ten years. Third, if you accept the position of the AMA and exclude infection from HIV contaminated organ transplants, surgical transfusions, and infections incurred in dental procedures, then prior to 1989 there were no cases of transmission from doctor directly to patient, or indirectly from patient to patient via procedures under the control of doctors. Since 1989 three patients undergoing nuclear medicine procedures in the United States received HIV contaminated blood.[71] In 1993 an Australian physician transmitted an HIV infection to four patients from a fifth by ignoring prescribed instrument sterilization procedures.[72] Although the American and Australian case prove that patients can get infected in the health care setting from physicians, the results of American "look-back" studies (studies tracing patients of an infected HCW) indicate, again, that the risk is small.

CDC studies involving over 19,036 patients treated by 57 HIV+ health care workers have not located any instances of patient seroconversion (other than those mentioned), directly attributable to infected HCWs passing on their infection.[73]

Granting all this, there are data which bear upon judgment. The Centers for Disease Control, not accepting that the Acer/Bergalis case represents the sole example of doctor to patient infection, did create a mathematical model that predicted that since 1981 from three to twenty-eight patients had been infected during surgery, and from ten to one hundred had been infected during dental work. Neither the American College of Surgeons nor the American Dental Academy accept this study. However, even if you assume its validity, the results do not point to a significant risk.

Another bit of relevant information would relate to the number of HIV+ health care workers the patient is likely to encounter in any given year. Only a general professional testing would establish the figure with precision, but there are some indications of the extent of infection. In 1993 the National Commission on AIDS estimated that there were 5,000 physicians, 1,200 dentists, 360 surgeons, and 35,000 others in various other health care roles infected with the virus. These estimates roughly comport with extrapolations from the number of CDC-reported AIDS cases of HCWs (see "The Medical Perspective"), to the number of HIV+ in the health care community. The ratio between AIDS diagnoses and HIV+ status is stated variously between 1:5 and 1:8.2 by different authorities. Applying this (probably conservative ratio) to HCWs, and using the CDC-reported AIDS diagnoses as the base, then there would be about 41,000 to 67,000 infected HCWs. So what can you say? Not much, except there seems to be little evidence that the patient is at much risk of even meeting an infected health care worker (remember there are over 4 million), much less getting infected by him or her.

Patient advocates also would require disclosure of serostatus. Mandatory disclosure, the shearing away of privacy, is troublesome from the standpoints of both patient and HCW. Probably an HIV+ doctor would have few patients if they knew. There is little question but that the entire weight of discrimination, employment loss, cancellation of insurance, and so on, now generally felt only by HIV+ patients, could also fall upon health care workers who disclosed their status. On the other hand, Pennsylvania and New Jersey courts have ruled that the HCWs interest in employment does not weigh heavily in a scale the other tray of which contains the patient's interest in survival.[74]

Viewed from either perspective, that of the patient or of the health care worker, there is really no case in the currently available risk data warranting mandatory testing of anyone.[75] One spokesman for the medical viewpoint

rejected the patients' position with the comment that it was more likely that
the patient would get hurt in an accident while riding to the hospital in an
ambulance than that he would get infected once there. But exactly the same
holds for the doctor; it is much more likely that he will have an accident on
the expressway than a patient will infect him once he arrives on duty.

Actually there is no evidence that AIDS has changed the risk that has
always been part of the medical/dental context, it has just publicized it.
Patients have always taken a basically blind chance on the health, competence, and caring of their health care providers (both the ones they hire and
those hired by the ones they hire), and health care workers have always
faced the risk of infection from their patients. As far as HCWs are concerned,
many recent studies in *The Journal of the American Medical Association* and
other professional sources indicate that what little occupational risk there is
could be cut further by safer procedures. If hospitals insisted upon and
HCWs were retrained in better, safer techniques (especially surgical and IV-
line), most dangerous exposures to blood could be avoided.[76] If Congress
feels the need to "mandate" something, let it mandate the development of
compulsory, professional, infection control seminars. In the context of the
mandatory testing debate, both sides should acknowledge that there is no
such thing as "zero risk," and both should admit that the current data do not
indicate any significant risk one to the other.

With respect to the contention that mandatory or "routine" testing would
enable the physician to serve the patient better, the response is obvious: If
this is true, then simply explain the benefits to the patient and obtain his/her
informed consent. It is not honest to bury an HIV consent clause in a general admission consent form—which can run seven pages—and expect the
patient to read and digest it all while the admitting nurse is standing there
tapping her pencil. Indeed, the expectation of this approach is that the
patient will not read the fine print or at least will not raise a fuss about one
phrase among many. The response of the physicians' unions to the issue of
HIV testing in the health care setting has been narrowly and obviously self-
serving and, for that reason, unconvincing. If a responsible testing program
is not in place upon the occasion of the next Acer/Bergalis case—and
inevitably there will be another—then political forces outside the profession
will impose one. Perhaps the program will be sensible, perhaps it will not
be; my guess is that it will simply echo the old adage: "What is good for the
goose, is good for the gander."

There is one aspect of both perspectives that deserves special comment.
Acknowledging the serious negative consequences that can flow from
knowledge of positive test results, both sides insist that the results of HIV
tests would be or should be handled with "sensitivity and confidentiality."
Under current law and practice, this assurance is worth next to nothing.

Once a person, whether medical or lay, has a positive test entered on the records, the information is shared by a wide assortment of people from the office secretary/receptionist who types and routes records, to all the nurses, LVNs, aides, orderlies, administrators, and clinical or surgical physicians associated with the case. It would be more honest to replace the word "confidential" with the phrase "not public domain," indicating thereby that there might be some adverse legal consequences to printing the test results in the hospital newsletter. I asked three physician-friends the same question: "Assume you are admitting a patient to the hospital, how many people would have easy access to the patient's records?" They answered variously, but all agreed on a minimum one dozen, and one thought that in a surgical admission it could run much higher. The *only* secure test result is the one obtained in an *anonymous*, not confidential, testing procedure where the testee is known only by number or pseudonym. "Confidentiality" in the health care setting means little more than that visitors and patients cannot easily get personal health information.

The Government Perspective. Government agencies from the Centers for Disease Control to the Congress have been caught in the heated cross-fire between these contending interests. In 1991 the CDC, in conjunction with the AMA, recommended that physicians get tested and voluntarily refrain from procedures that carried a risk of infecting patients if they were HIV+. Hardly a daring proposal! Then in mid-year the CDC went further and proposed a four-part plan designed to limit the presumed infection potential of HCWs: (1) a listing of all "exposure-prone" procedures, such lists to be developed by the various medical and dental specialty unions; (2) a vigorously encouraged program of in-house HIV testing; (3) the establishment of local peer-group committees of physicians and dentists, using the "exposure-prone" lists, to monitor and guide the practice of those HCWs who were identified as HIV+; and (4) finally, that before an HIV+ physician engages in an exposure-prone procedure, the patient be informed, counseled, and give specific consent.

The release of the CDC plan in July 1991 started a major battle between the agency and the professional associations, which the CDC lost by December. Of all the major associations, only the AMA gave limited support to the CDC, while the others (some forty associations) flatly refused to cooperate in drawing up the "exposure-prone" lists, the necessary first step. Uniformly they complained that there were no data indicating doctor to patient risk, that there was no "scientific basis" for creating "exposure-prone" lists, and that the CDC was just running scared before a tide of public hysteria caused by the Acer/Bergalis case.[77] The CDC attempted to mollify the doctors by recommending in September that all acute care hospitals commence "routine" testing for HIV and by setting up committees of CDC-specialty consultants to see if compromise positions could be evolved. However, the agency did insist on the lists and set November as the deadline for receiving them. Implied was the threat that it might write its own lists if the associations refused to act. The only effect of these later actions was to rouse the opposition of the American Hospital Association, which complained that the CDC had not told them how they were going to fund the estimated $1.65 billion annual cost of all the new testing and counseling, while the consultants merely reiterated the stands of their associations—that the CDC was letting hysteria drive public policy. November came and went without the lists. In December the CDC capitulated, backed away from its July proposals, and began talking about "invasive procedures" rather than "exposure-prone" ones.[78]

Meanwhile Congress picked up on the hysteria. Senator Helms and Representative Dannemeyer proposed stronger medicine—mandatory testing of doctors and patients, backed by criminal penalties of ten years' imprisonment plus $10,000 fines for HIV+ physicians convicted of treating patients without obtaining informed consent. The Senate adopted the Helms proposal but then abandoned it the House-Senate conference committee trying to write a jointly acceptable bill. Congress ended its efforts in September 1991 by passing a bill requiring the states to adopt the CDC program or its "equivalent" or face loss of federal health care grants.[79] The one agency that responded to public health concerns in a unified fashion was the Occupational Safety and Health Administration which, in December, issued a new set of job safety rules applying to 5.6 million workers in hospitals, nursing homes, medical and dental offices, correctional facilities, emergency response fire and police agencies, and funeral homes. The ten pages of new rules require employers to provide masks, gowns, gloves, special waste receptacles, and the like, in an effort to cut both hepatitis and HIV transmission. President Bush's contribution to our thinking about AIDS in 1991 was to state that he was not in favor of a plan to distribute condoms in high schools.

States and local health agencies reacted variously. In October 1991, Illinois began a massive search of all records in the offices of the 208 state health care workers who had AIDS. The search was for evidence of "invasive procedures," a term the law failed to define, that might have put clients at risk. The clients, if any, would then be notified by mail of possible exposure, and testing would be advised—but not at state clinics because there was inadequate budget and personnel for the task. All this was without one known case of HCW to patient transmission in the state! In November Texas became the first state to adopt the CDC proposal in its entirety— even though by that time the CDC was abandoning it.[80] New York and Michigan announced that they were writing their own laws, the San Francisco Department of Health denounced the CDC proposals, and the South Carolina Medical Association initiated one that, in some respects, went further than the original CDC plan by authorizing "certificates of compliance" to be issued for people to hang on their walls—a thinly disguised form of coercion.[81] By the end of the 1991, eleven states had some program in place, and another eighteen states were debating.

Meanwhile, back on the farm, a large Atlanta, Georgia, dental firm began advertising, "AIDS-FREE DENTISTRY," and the AMA's House of Delegates, speaking on behalf of three hundred thousand members, concluded its deliberations with a suggestion that Congress should consider a tobacco-package warning to be flashed as a caption on TV depictions of sex—something like, I suppose, "Warning! The Surgeon General has determined that unsafe sex can be hazardous to your health." In the war against AIDS, 1991 will not be remembered as our finest hour.

Since then, however, various national and state agencies have issued revised infection control procedures to minimize risk of transmission. Anyone who has visited a dentist's office in the past year can personally attest to the impact of the Acer/Bergalis case; the hygienist who cleans my teeth looks as if she is clothed for chemical warfare, mumbling directions from behind a clear plastic full-face shield modeled on an arc welder's helmet. Still, in spite of all the attention to infection control, glaring examples of bad judgment and carelessness crop up now and then as, for example, the 1993 case of a physician using the same hypodermic for multiple flu injections in the Washington, D.C., bureau of *Time* magazine.[82]

HIV TESTING: PROPOSALS FOR A NATIONAL PROGRAM

The government of the United States has never confronted the AIDS epidemic with a unified program. President Reagan ignored it as much as he dared; his successor followed in his footsteps. The low-profile presidential stance seemed to flow partly from personal belief and partly from the need to conciliate right-wing politics and religion. The result during the Republican administrations was a piecemeal approach, programs with no overriding coherence. The Congress was mainly concerned with the development of medical research programs in and through the National Institutes of Health, with some funds, channeled through the states, designated for AIDS education and care. The Department of Health, Education, and Welfare, through components like the CDC, and the Food and Drug Administration concentrated on defining the epidemic and overseeing drug development. As for HIV testing, the national government has restricted its programs to limited groups like penitentiary inmates, military personnel, Job Corps applicants, Foreign Service officers, and immigrants; for all of these groups testing is mandatory and for none of them is there a clear and convincing rationale. Congressional legislation encouraged states to develop their own testing and counseling programs with predictably variable results—California insists on anonymous testing and Colorado insists on names, though it lets people sign, "Ronald Reagan."

The direction in which the nation is moving is what I call "creeping coercion." First came the mandatory federal programs, then mandatory (if you need the job) employment testing permitted by forty-one states, then mandatory testing for insurance (if you need the policy), then state sponsored hospital and health care programs, and on and on, without planning, unified design, or adequate protection for the individual. We are in a mess now, as the debate inspired by the infection of Kimberly Bergalis illustrates. It is likely to get much worse unless President Clinton provides the leadership the system needs. My own feeling is that everyone (whether they wanted to admit it or not) was waiting for the miracle cure that would bail us out, the "magic bullet" that would shoot down the Human Immunodeficiency Virus. Unfortunately, it did not arrive, nor is it likely to in the foreseeable future. We either craft a rational response, or sink into a deadly virus infected swamp of contradictory, ineffective, and damaging policies.

An integrated national policy would have to have four dimensions: testing, education, medicine/care, and protection. The necessary foundation and beginning point is a voluntary, vigorously encouraged, presidentially led national testing program.[83] The testing program would have to be far more elaborate and costly than those which are today mounted by the states. HIV testing of the entire population would confront the need for multiple tests to combat the problem of false results that inevitably occur in larger, heterogeneous populations. Further, testing would have to include the more expensive testing involved in CD4 blood counts in order to accommodate the 1993 revised definition of AIDS.

A national testing program would not run counter to public opinion—a 1987 Gallup Poll indicated that a majority of the public thought everyone should get tested—and we do have applicable experience in the war bond and polio vaccine campaigns. However, the single most important factor in the success of a national voluntary program would be the high-profile, vigorous support of the president. As a way of launching a program, I would hope that President and Mrs. Clinton, Secretary of Health and Human Services Shalala, and the White House AIDS Policy Coordinator Gebbie would publicly support and encourage such an effort by being tested. Such action by our head of state could be coordinated with other celebrity support to create a public climate favoring HIV testing. Research published in the *New England Journal of Medicine* demonstrated that celebrity action had a profound and immediate effect in increasing the demand for tests.[84] All results, of course, would be private to the testee, citizen and president alike. Nothing could diminish the fear and stigma associated with the HIV test more readily and successfully; nothing would underscore its seriousness or its importance to the nation more dramatically. It would be an example of leadership worthy of enshrinement in our national history.

Why not extend existing programs of mandatory testing to everyone and be done with it? Those who favor this approach point to the success of the U.S. military in their testing program, but they forget that America is still a civilian society with a very wise civil Constitution. Although the courts generally have been sympathetic to claims of public health, it is still not possible to line up the civilian population for inspection and testing as though it were an oversized regiment. We would be sacrificing our Constitution, the world's oldest and finest, to the fear of AIDS.

The government should be direct and honest in seeking help from the general public. It needs better information, and should admit it, with respect to the parameters of the epidemic. Such information can only come from a national testing. Even now, thirteen years into the epidemic, we do not have accurate data mapping the extent or characteristics of our national infection. This is like going into battle without knowing the number or disposition of enemy troops, and if that is not stupid, then nothing is. Of course, no voluntary system can be perfect, but if properly promoted, it would produce information far superior to anything we have now.

What should be done with the information gathered? If a national voluntary testing program were operated on an anonymous basis, then its benefits would be limited to providing much better epidemiological data. This, in turn, would allow more rationale design of safer sex campaigns and regional allocations of money and facilities. If the program were confidential rather than anonymous, that is, a program that would identify HIV+ individuals, then it would allow public health authorities to consider the application of classic techniques such as reporting, counseling, and contact tracing. The old techniques would have to be modified in terms of the AIDS context, but all might have useful functions. AIDS counseling is a more elaborate, time consuming, and, therefore, costly process, than previous STD counseling, but it certainly is an absolutely necessary adjunct of testing and reporting. Contact tracing for any disease confronts the facts that today, as compared to, say, 1935, our population is much more mobile and has greater opportunities for anonymous sex. Still it could be useful as a method of reaching the reasonably constant sexual partners of someone who is seropositive. If the partner is still negative, then warning could help preserve that condition; if positive, then the partner could be counseled. Recent studies indicate that it is unlikely that the seropositive partner will warn his or her sexual partner(s).[85] A modified quarantine in the form, perhaps, of electronic house confinement as now used in probation, might be applicable to positive individuals who refuse to desist from activities likely to transmit the virus.[86] These traditional methods have largely been rejected because they do present difficult civil rights problems. However, as the epidemic worsens, they might be reconsidered for their utility in slowing the spread of disease as well as getting help to people who need it.

The other side of the coin of public cooperation must be the assumption by the national government of responsibility for the medical care of individuals testing positive, before and after progression to AIDS. There are a number of funding possibilities from AIDS-specific funding on the model of existing kidney programs through expanded Medicaid access to inclusion in a genuine national health program such as President Clinton is urging. Every method has its strengths and drawbacks, but almost any national approach would be preferable to the continuance of the state-grant-in-aid technique, with its cost-ineffective and variable results. In any case, with a national commitment to care, testing would both identify and support the seropositive individual. Further, there are an increasing number of drugs, like pentamidine, bactrin/septra, foscavir, acyclovir, and ganciclovir, which are effective in treating infections that just a few years ago were cripplers. In this new context, identification and tracing make sense, just as the existence of antibiotics justifies contact tracing for tuberculosis or syphilis.

In addition to rethinking approaches, there should be consideration for those whose seropositivity threatens their ability to continue in their work, for example, an HIV+ surgeon.[87] Programs, perhaps jointly operated by government and professional associations, could offer retraining so that the physician could contribute in the health care setting but without presenting risk or the perception of risk. For example, Dr. G. Edward Rozar Jr. voluntarily ceased performing cardiac surgery when he discovered his infection and became, with the support of his hospital, the director of the peripheral vascular laboratory, a position of importance in supporting active surgeons.[88] I have focused on HCWs, but others might benefit from retraining as well. In addition, joint governmental and professional relocation programs could match training and need. An HIV+ health care worker might be helped to locate and move to a position that specialized in HIV+ patients. Such a program could alleviate the shortage of personnel in high impact areas such as San Francisco, Houston, or Miami.

Both the identification and care elements must be present and linked. All who submit to an HIV test today are sticking their necks out in many ways; it must be made more worthwhile and less hazardous. A voluntary, confidential program must address the question "What's in it for me?"

An effective national testing program must partly answer that question with "better protection against breaches of confidentiality." Even though what is proposed is a program of mass involvement, still the results are not and should never be in the "public domain." Admitting that a "confidential" system always has the potential to leak, it does not have to leak like a sieve. There must be incentives for testing, as well as protection for those tested. Congress must enact strong, uniform laws supporting the privacy of personal medical information to displace, through federal preemption, the crazy-quilt of state laws now more or less in force. If someone in legitimate possession of your personal information, such as a lab technician, divulges test results to an unauthorized party, then there should be serious civil consequences. Once the fact of disclosure is established, the disclosing party should be placed under a rebuttable presumption of intention to harm; it would be his job to justify why he told his friend, who then told another friend, who turned out to be your boss's secretary. If Congress wanted to go further, it could establish treble damage awards on the model of our antitrust law, or it could reach back to England's seventeenth-century habeas corpus law and make those who fail in their duty removable from position or office. It might be possible, also, to extend the concept underlying the Americans with Disability Act so as to cover discriminatory harm that flows from unauthorized divulgence or receipt of personal medical information. There are many possibilities. If OSHA can tighten occupational safety rules for workers, surely the Congress can tighten privacy and confidentiality standards for our nation.

Any national program would necessarily be complex and costly. We should have an intelligent debate on any such program's components and implications; it should not be left to the self-interested design of medical associations, politicians running for office, public health officials, or, for that matter, organizations of people already infected. However, I think all would agree that any coherent and complete national program would have to rest upon the testing program. Without national testing our data is necessarily faulty. With faulty data our educational campaigns suffer. Without identification we cannot mount an effective program of medical and personal care. And without protection too few will participate in the testing program.

Kimberly Bergalis begged Congress for a national program reflecting her own experience. It was too narrow a focus. Congress should have responded with a national program based on broader perspectives and all that we now know of the virus. In fact, Congress did little more than suggest that the states do something. That's not good enough. The great medical and dental associations limited themselves to protecting their members from what they called "public hysteria." That's not good enough either. The president and legislators we elect, as well as those in the associations to whom we look for enlightened care, have a duty to respond more effectively and for all of us. And they must respond soon. There are three hundred and fifty thousand and counting.

UNCONVENTIONAL THERAPIES

There is an old saying that fits the situation in AIDS perfectly: "When there is no cure, there will be a Thousand Remedies." Mainline allopathic medicine has produced a significant number of new or newly applied drugs to deal with the principal infections associated with AIDS. These have undeniably alleviated many opportunistic infections, improved the quality of life of the PWA, and been responsible for the gradual lengthening of life-span after AIDS diagnosis. However, the failure of science to develop a cure, a vaccine, or an effective long-term management has generated a profusion of allopathic, nonallopathic, and nonmedical therapies that hold out a promise of accomplishing what mainline medicine so far cannot.

The range of these therapies is great—from Zimbabwe witch doctors applying herbs and traditional rituals to promising, but unproven, drugs from Western research institutes.[89] "Alternative or unconventional therapies," as I am using the term, denotes any therapy that has *not* been subject to the elaborate and controlled testing required for government approval or is not in the process of such testing. From whatever source they come, using whatever techniques, these share one thing in common—they are *not* approved by the U.S. Food and Drug Administration, the Federal Centers for Disease Control, or other official regulatory bodies for use as therapeutic agents or protocols in the treatment of AIDS.[90]

This lack of approval does not mean that a PWA cannot resort to them; indeed, many do. A 1993 study in the *New England Journal of Medicine* reported that one third of all PWAs rely completely on some form of alternative therapy. In addition, one quarter of all those who see physicians supplement that care with alternative therapy. The $13.7 billion spent each year on alternative therapies is over one third the amount spent on all conventional medicine ($36 billion).[91] However, lack of approval does mean that licensed health care workers (medical and osteopathic physicians, dentists, nurses, and so on) take risks in using them for treatment and cannot prescribe the remedies. Practioners who do may run afoul of state and national occupational licensing rules as well as laws punishing medical fraud or malpractice with civil and/or criminal penalties.

Besides lack of approval, the alternative therapies characteristically rely for their legitimation on what is called "anecdotal evidence," rather than data collected in laboratories or drug administrations as part of a clinical trial. The anecdote is just what its name implies, it is a "story," usually a very personal story that relates the speaker's state of mind. The HCW asks, "How do you feel today. Any pains? Where are they and what are they like?" I answer with an anecdote, that is, a personal and individual version of my bodily, mental, and emotional state. It may or may not match the story told by my lab tests, or a previous patient who, it turns out, suffers the same illness. Anecdotal evidence is perfectly legitimate and useful so long as its basic limitation is understood; it is not generalizable and, thus, not reliable when applied to someone other than the original storyteller. In fact, it is not all that reliable as an accurate statement of the storyteller's condition. In any case, it is *my* felt-symptoms, my aches, my pains, and my fears that I speak of, not yours. Yours are yours.

Gathering information that applies reasonably well to large groups of similarly afflicted people is a very difficult, arduous, and controlled process precisely because it is necessary to eliminate the personal, the individual, the subjective, the idiosyncratic to arrive at generally applicable formulae of care. As any student of the effort to find cures for cancer, rheumatoid arthritis, and AIDS can tell you, it is easy for promoters to gather reams of testimonials praising the efficacy of this or that nostrum. People giving testimonials are not lying; they do believe, and believe fiercely, in the efficacy of the frequently useless treatments they are undergoing. Recent studies have shown that the placebo effect is much stronger than generally acknowledged,[92] but most important, patients *want and need* to believe, and that is, of course, the key.[93]

For convenience, I will divide this brief examination of alternative therapies into two segments. The first, "allopathic experiments" describes examples of unapproved (for AIDS) therapeutic drugs or protocols that have emerged out of the search for cures within the conventional research and/or medical setting. This group of remedies relies upon classical intervention techniques such as drugs, surgery, blood treatment, and transfusions. It is conventional, but unproven medicine. The second category, "nonallopathic experiments," deals with therapies that evolved outside the conventional setting and, in their very existence, frequently challenge the foundations of modern medicine. In this category are found remedies ranging from herbal through ritualistic and the medical approaches that are not allopathic in their theoretical foundation. Typically there is no reliance on a pharmacopeia of drugs or surgery.

Allopathic Experiments

Many alternative therapies emerge out of the biomedical research process, but for one reason or other do not enter or complete the toxicity, dosage, and efficacy trials required for approval. Literally hundreds of drugs and/or protocols fall into this category of "risky and unapproved" treatments. They are tried in spite of their lack of approval (meaning that people take their own chances), most accumulate testimonials on their behalf, but none have been shown to halt or slow the course of the disease; most fall by the wayside.

Three experimental initiatives will illustrate the category: DNCB, hyperoxygenation therapy, and hyperthermia therapy. DNCB, dinitrichlorobenzene, is a photochemical that has long been used in industry. Its enthusiasts claim that it has the ability, when used as a topically applied ointment on humans, to trigger an immune response that boosts the production of killer T cells, the cells that patrol the blood system and destroy blood cells infected by HIV or other pathogens. Thus, it is argued, it can and does enhance the "search and destroy" capability of the immune system. A major proponent is Charles Caulfield of the *San Francisco Sentinel*, who is himself a long-term survivor (twelve years since diagnosis). He credits DNCB, among other things, for his survival. Those who approach the DNCB data from a clinical trial perspective feel that the evidence marshalled by its proponents is too anecdotal and insufficient to warrant a recommendation beyond "Try it if you want to. It probably won't do any harm if you are careful."[94] Another approach is called hyperoxygenation therapy. This therapy starts from the accurate observation that HIV cannot survive in an oxygen atmosphere. If, so the theory goes, it were possible to flood the blood system with high concentrations of oxygen, it might be possible to kill billions of virus. How might this be done? Several procedures, some taken from other fields of medicine, have been suggested and/or tried: (1) infusion of water with ozone (a corrosive gas) and then use of the water as an enema, (2) pressurizing the patient in a compression chamber with a high concentration of oxygen such as used for divers, (3) sipping 35 percent concentrations of hydrogen-peroxide (the standard drugstore variety is 3 percent). All of these are potentially very dangerous treatments (the FDA has condemned the first, and deaths have been attributed to the third), and none have been proven efficacious. Detractors point to the fact that HIV has the ability to reside in internal systems not reached by the usual circulation of plasma and is thus insulated from contact from the high-oxygen concentrations. Finally, a team of oncologists attempted to apply a protocol that showed some promise in cancer, namely, hyperthermia.[95] This involves removing the patient's blood, heating it to a temperature fatal to the virus (or cancer cell), and then, after cooling, reinfusing it. Despite the elaborate equipment and obvious expense involved, it was appealing in its theoretic simplicity—if the right temperature is used, anything can be killed. Press releases from Atlanta Hospital were so encouraging that the NIH sent a special team of investigators to check the claims; the team's conclusion was that there was no objective reason to continue the experimental treatments.

All these initiatives, and hundreds more that are proposed, tried, and reviewed yearly, share some features in common. First, they are mostly proposed by intelligent, sincere people looking for an effective weapon against HIV. These are neither scams nor remedies handed to grateful earthlings by galactic aliens on the space deck of their saucer. Second, all have a foundation in Western science, and their advocates can advance plausible arguments on their behalf. Third, none have undergone rigorous, controlled clinical trials, though all have been "monitored" by professional health care workers and have considerable testimonial support. Finally, none of them have become part of mainline medicine's arsenal of weapons against AIDS.

A legitimate question arises when one reviews the many initiatives that have fallen by the wayside, "How could so many people, and so many plausible approaches, have missed the mark?" Those given to conspiracy theory are apt to say, "Ah, but they did not miss! Big drug companies, or a government dominated by homophobes, or an international racist conspiracy, or something else, is holding known cures off the market." But there is little need to resort to comic book explanations. There are many considerations that bear upon an answer—which of them applies to specific cases, of course, changes with the cases. First, most physicians are not trained researchers—it just seems that way to people with no science background whatever. Clinical physicians are generally not schooled in, and have no need for, the rigorous tools and concepts of experimental bench science. They are trained as healers, not as biochemists, microbiologists, and virologists. Like anyone else, they can be misled by their own hope, their own enthusiasm for an idea, their compassion for their patients, and their own lack of research experience. This is a nice way of saying that, as researchers, most physicians are good clinicians. The pressures generated by AIDS have led even world-class research scientists, like Jonas Salk, for example, to be overly optimistic about possible progress. Another consideration, and one that relates to the previous one, is that HIV infection is a notoriously uneven disease in its development or progression. A friend of mine registered T cell counts of only 200 per milliliter of blood (not good) in June 1993, but by December they were up to 600 (much better)—with absolutely no change in treatment or lifestyle to explain it. Because of uneven progression, an observer could quite easily attribute an improvement to new treatment, when, in fact, there was no relation between treatment and condition at all. This is apparently what fooled the oncologists experimenting with hyperthermia. The accurate documentation of cause and effect is what controlled drug trials are all about. Finally, there is no agreement within the professional research community as to what signs or markers should be used to assess whether a patient is, in fact, getting better or worse. Obviously if a patient dies, then he has gotten "worse," but between initial infection and death there are infinite shadings that appear over a long period of time, and there is no agreed method of measuring or describing these stages. Without such measures, how can the efficacy of new drugs or protocols be assessed? This is a problem that plagues both the professional and the amateur AIDS researcher.

One thing is clear. The gradually revealed complexity of both pure and applied HIV viral research has humbled everyone. I no longer read, in serious journals, news about "major medical breakthroughs" coupled with predictions, such as that made by President Bush's secretary of Health and Human Services, that a vaccine was just around the corner. In the 1990s researchers have become much more careful in their public statements and predictions; the weight of many optimistic, but inaccurate, projections, much false hope, and many abandoned "cures-of-the-week" has induced a new reticence and caution in statement.

However, it is important to note that unsuccessful or, at least, unproved initiatives have their own importance. They may not be successful as remedies, but they indicate areas where the answers do not reside. Science progresses via unsuccessful as well as successful discovery; in that sense, there are no "failures" in scientific research. In a universe of infinite variety and choice, to know where the answer is not likely to be found, is to have valuable information.

Nonallopathic Therapies

This classification covers an enormous range of therapeutic possibilities from forms of nonallopathic medicine like homeopathy or chiropractic to the herbal/ritual practices of shamans, witch doctors, curanderos, and faith healers.[96] At the outset it should be noted that the term "unconventional" in this context is very culture- and class-bound. In Zimbabwe traditional witch doctors number in the thousands, have their own union (the twenty-thousand-member Zimbabwe National Traditional Healers Association), and represent the conventional form of health care. The government of that nation is trying to ensure that their methods are, at minimum, not spreading HIV—forget curing it. In southwestern United States the curandero is a very important traditional healer for Hispanics in both rural and urban areas, as is the faith healer in America's Bible Belt.

Advertisements and articles in a monthly periodical devoted to these approaches, *Healing AIDS*,[97] reveal a rich array of methods including homeopathy; chiropractic; massage; acupuncture/acupressure; Chinese herbal medicine; psychoimmunity; vegetarianism; macrobiotics; spiritualist channeling; crystal healing; art and music therapy; "Energetics"; various body "detoxification" regimes; diets using garlic, blue-green algae, Echinacea, Shitake mushrooms, or wheat grass, and many forms of Yoga, stress reduction, breath control, meditation; or "positive thinking or visualizing" including the currently popular *Course in Miracles*[98] or Louise Hay's *You Can Heal Your Life.*[99]

There is little new in all this. Dietary, pseudoscientific, and mystical modes of healing are as old as sickness. Various forms of faith healing are prominent features of America's fundamentalist, born-again evangelical, and New

Age movements. Homeopathy is almost two hundred years old and was widespread in nineteenth-century rural America; my farm relatives from Wisconsin used homeopathic manuals and materials. Some forms of traditional Chinese medicine express a thousand years of therapeutic experience with a vast array of herbs and other natural materials. Yoga's ability to achieve stress reduction, which is important to PWAs, has been refined over centuries. The ancient Romans believed strongly in the curative properties of certain gemstones, a belief that has resurfaced in New Age literature on "crystal power." Americans and Europeans have long enjoyed "detoxifying" their bodies with mud baths, sulfur springs, and other "curative" spas. Since the mid-nineteenth-century cereal and graham cracker craze, Americans have taken up one "health food" or dietary enthusiasm after another. The use of certain vegetables and/or herbs is also ancient. In 1664 the London College of Physicians recommended the following for those afflicted by the plague:

> [T]ake a great onion, hollow it, put into it a fig, rue cut small, and a dram of Venice treacle; put it close stopt in a wet paper, and roast it in the embers; then apply it to the tumor.

In addition fat people were advised to stay out of the sun, and garlic was to be eaten raw as well as kept in one's shoes.[100]

The alternative approaches have some elements in common, even if their particular methods vary greatly. Generally they reject conventional Western medicine's reliance on the germ theory of illness, that is, the position that illnesses are usually traceable to an invading bacterium, fungus, or, as in the case of AIDS, virus; they also reject reliance upon Western scientific methods of inquiry. Chinese herbal and acupuncture therapies are examples of alternate theory as well as alternate therapy. Chinese theory conceptualizes illness as a product of disrupted, unbalanced, or blocked "flows" of energy within the body; energy channels or "flows" within each person are considered to be part of the energy-flow within the universe itself. These channels are neither objective nor measurable and do not relate to human skeletal, muscular, or neural anatomy—you cannot see them, feel them, or X-ray them. Treatment by herbal potion or acupuncture is designed to bring the flow back into balance.

Another common element is that evidence of treatment efficacy is generally anecdotal, circumstantial. After drinking the prescribed herbal potion or undergoing acupuncture, the patient says "I feel better, more energetic, happier, the pain is relieved." The Chinese see no reason to collect and systematize such data as would convince the skeptical Western analytic tradition. There are now some attempts to scrutinize Chinese methods with Western scientific techniques—using modern chemistry to isolate and purify the active compounds in various herbs, for example.[101] Generally speaking, however, Western science cannot easily prove or disprove the claims put forward on behalf of unconventional treatments because the practioners, not believers in Western scientific method, have not framed their knowledge in such a way as to make it testable. "Evidence" in these traditions equals anecdotes, sometimes a millennia of them.

A further common element is that the alternative approaches tend to stress the mind/body connection and the influence of the mental or spiritual state upon the body's well-being. For Christian Scientists this connection is all-important; physical illness is conceptualized as a delusion, the product of spiritually imperfect mind. The function of the Christian Science Reader is to help the person work through patterns of incorrect thought using Mary Baker Eddy's *Science and Health with Key to the Scriptures* as a guide. The Native-American shaman uses ancient rituals and prayers to bring the patient's spirit into harmony with the natural order of the universe so that his herbs and potions will have the desired effect.

Finally, there is much common agreement that effective treatment must be holistic; it must deal with the whole person, and often the whole family or tribe, not just an affected limb or an invading bacterium. The validity and importance of some of the attitudes, approaches, and insights commonly found in unconventional nonallopathic approaches are just now being acknowledged in mainline Western medicine—the central importance of nutrition, for example. Partly, at least, the willingness to look anew at these approaches is due to AIDS, or rather the failure of conventional medicine to solve AIDS. Certainly this was behind the congressional mandate, in the 1992 Budget Act, that the National Institutes of Health establish a new office specifically to fund research on alternative, unconventional treatments. The NIH has reluctantly obeyed by creating an Office of Alternative Medicine (OAF) with a staff of four, and funded with $2 million from the $10 billion NIH budget.[102]

Overall, what can be said of the range of unconventional, nonallopathic remedies? No cure has emerged from this avenue either. Nor have the alternative remedies proven (in clinical trials) effective against such opportunistic infections as *Mycobacterium avium complex, Pneumocystis carinii, Cytomegalovirus retinitis*, or the many other opportunistic infections associated with advanced HIV infection. Some, such as aloe vera and acupuncture, have demonstrated palliative value, especially in the alleviation of pain and dermatologic discomfort. My own belief is that, when cures, vaccines, or major new treatments develop, they will be the product of time-consuming, meticulous, and imaginative scientific research in the world's laboratories of virology, microbiology, biochemistry, and pharmacology—the birthplaces of all our effective medical remedies. They will not be the byproduct of spirit communion, spinal adjustments, Ayurvedic diet, aura manipulations, or endless mantras, no matter how well meaning.

However, that is not the same thing as saying that these approaches are valueless. They have their place. To some extent they harness the intangible, but awesome, power of faith. It is undeniable that faith and will power can heal some maladies, can make even more at least tolerable, and finally can help in the treatment of all of them. Any physician can attest to the importance of the patient's mental and emotional outlook. Insofar as these various approaches and their remedies serve as a means of triggering the curative powers of mind, then they should be encouraged. If a practice reduces stress, then it is beneficial since HIV, like many other pathogens, thrives when a person is highly stressed. Insofar as an apparently effective alternative therapy combines ritual with herbal potion, then biochemists must purify the active ingredients involved (as, for example, Acemannan has been extracted from aloe vera), and pharmacologists and clinicians must determine, in controlled trials, whether the chemical is helpful or harmful in HIV therapy.[103] Certainly there is a place for the alternative approaches, but the place is as a supplement to, not a replacement for, mainline allopathic medical treatment.

FRAUDS AND PHONIES

It is unfortunately true that wherever there is sickness and suffering, a certain vulturelike subgroup of our species will descend from the skies to feed. Like many illnesses before it, AIDS has become the focal point of a high-dollar industry and has thus attracted such vulturelike people. There is money to be made. A September 20, 1993 article in the *Detroit Free Press* alleged that only 4 percent of the $450,000 collected by a group pretending to support children with AIDS was used for actual services for them. The group has now disbanded; but another will take its place as sure as the sun sets.[104]

Fraudulent charities and fake healers have always been part of the American scene. Before donating any money or signing on for treatment, it is wise to check with the local AIDS service organizations first because they generally know who is in town raising money or offering therapy. All the devices familiar to fraud investigators have reappeared, retrofitted for AIDS, from magnetized bracelets or shoe inserts to "draw out the virus," to elaborate machines which have no effect other than enriching the seller. My favorite in this latter class is a hi-tech adaptation of eighteenth-century phrenology. This "science" asserted that ailments could be diagnosed by "reading" the forms and indentations of the human skull, a sort of palmistry of the head. The contemporary machine adaptation resembles a Star Trek helmet of clear plastic fitted with many sliding needlelike probes. These probes (replacing the phrenologist's fingers) are fitted to the skull and, through electronic circuitry, "read" a diagnosis. Then, with a mere flip of the switch, imaginatively named electric charges are directed to the appropriate portions of the skull to effect a "treatment."[105] It is easy to laugh at some of this stuff—until you are dying, that is.

There are, of course, criminals and charlatans in both conventional and nonconventional healing, but the varied nonconventional alternative therapies have an especially difficult problem in weeding them out. As far as I know, no unconventional therapy sponsors a national hotline (1-800-776-CERT), such as is provided by the American Board of Medical Specialties through which the consumer can check upon the training and credentials of a physician before employing him or her as a healer.[106] In some states, Chinese herbal, acupuncture, and the nonallopathic medical practicioners are developing some standardization of training and licensing,[107] necessary steps toward effective professional policing. However, it is still easy for anyone to hand out a shingle as an AIDS counselor, a "vitamin and nutrition specialist," or an Ayurvedic or faith healer. Even in states like California, which have serious fraud detection and prosecution agencies, the enforcement cannot cope with the numbers of imaginative con artists.

When the afflicted leave the domain of mainline medicine, they are mostly on their own in sorting out frauds and fantasies. The protection of the law is weak, but there are some useful rules to guide the process. The following are based upon those that appeared in San Francisco's Project Inform bulletin, *PI Perspective*, April 1992:[108]

BEWARE OF

1. Products claimed to be a "cure" or said to render patients "HIV negative."
2. Promotion as a "miraculous," "foolproof," "secret," or "suppressed."
3. Non-specific, vague claims to "boost the immune system."
4. Products coming from little known doctors or "researchers" from distant countries (whose credibility can't be verified).
5. Claims of support from obscure foreign universities, laboratories, or journals.
6. Claims that a product also works for other diseases such as cancer.
7. High unexplained, unwarranted costs.
8. Promotion based solely on personal testimonials and second-hand reports, while clinical trials that will happen "any day now" never materialize.
9. A promoter who claims suppression because of unconventional views, which threaten "big business" medicine.
10. A promoter who claims to have solved what everyone else has missed.

11. A promoter who claims he's too busy saving patients to collect checkable data.
12. A promoter who claims that the medical establishment is out to get him.
13. A promoter who attacks the integrity of all those who question him.
14. A promoter offering treatment outside the territorial reach of the American legal system.

Individuals seeking help in the world of alternative therapies, be they allopathic or nonallopathic, have an incredible range of choice, but they are also pretty much on their own. Both the honest and dishonest promoters of alternative therapies will continue to flourish in the field of AIDS and discerning the difference between them frequently boils down to guessing at motives—is a promoter after your welfare or your wallet? Only major breakthroughs in conventional medicine will divert promoters of unconventional treatments to other human tragedies. Whatever can be said about the efficacy of their elixirs, they offer hope and, with or without AIDS, a world without hope is a dismal place to be.

Notes

1. The full list of periodicals covering AIDS exclusively is available from the AIDS Info BBS, San Francisco, CA, 1-415-626-1246, compiled by Ben Gardiner, 1993.
2. Largely as a result of AZT and pentamidine, the survival prospects have increased from about nine months (after diagnosis) to nearly two years. See for example editorial, *JAMA* (November 25, 1988); Centers for Disease Control, *Draft Proposals for Early Intervention*, Fifth International Conference on AIDS, Montreal, Canada, June 1989. A. E. Glatt et al., "Treatment of Infections Associated with Human Immunodeficiency Virus," *Medical Intelligence* 318, no. 2 (May 1989), 1349–1448. Probably the most dramatic therapeutic improvement has been the use of Pentamidine or Bactrin as a prophylactic against *pneumocystis carinii*, which in the early years of the epidemic (and still in the third world) was the most deadly and common form of opportunistic infection. See also Roger Rickleps, "Thanks to New Drugs, Patients are Surviving and Working Longer," *New York Times*, September 2, 1988, 1.
3. "Editorial: Improving Survival in Acquired Immunodeficiency Syndrome: Is Experience Everything?" *JAMA* (May 26, 1989), 3016. Also see "Editorial: The Rocky Road to Effective Treatment of Human Immunodeficiency Virus (HIV) Infection," *Annals of Internal Medicine* 110, no. 1 (January 1989), 1; "Editorial: Controlled Trial Methodology and Progress in Treatment of the Acquired Immunodeficiency Syndrome (AIDS)," *Annals of Internal Medicine* 110, no. 6 (1989), 417.
4. Less than 6 percent of AIDS patients live more than five years beyond diagnosis. However, there are some who remain relatively healthy for a decade or more. See "Group of Long-Term Symptom-Free HIV-Infected Patients May Hold Key

to the Development of an AIDS Vaccine," *Internal Medicine World Report*, November 1–14, 1992, 1; Dave Gilden, "Berlin: Long-Term Survival Studies Suggest New Treatment Strategies," *AIDS Treatment News*, July 9, 1993, 3.

5. Quoted in "Advance in AIDS Treatment," *New York Times*, November 14, 1990, A1.

6. For a moving portrayal of a young physician and the impact of AIDS care on his maturation as doctor, see William A. Check, "Growing up Fast: A New Generation of AIDS Physicians," *Observer* (American College of Physicians) 9, no. 10 (November 1989), 1.

7. See the story of Dr. Stephen Herman, director of Research at Stephens Pharmaceutical in Joyce Niles, "AIDS Researcher Arrested," *Internal Medicine World Report*, March 1, 1990, 12.

8. *Health InfoCom Network News* 2, no. 31 (1989), 16 (distributed electronically on the InterUniversity BITNET system), News Release date, July 18; issue date, August 28. The network is called "The AIDS Clinical Trial Information Service"

9. The announcement of Anthony Fauci, M.D., director of NIAID and the accompanying article in *American Medical News*, December 9, 1988, 3. There is a good discussion in *AIDS Treatment News*, nos. 84, 85, August 1989. A current description of the outlines of this development can be found in Albert R. Jonesen and Jeff Stryker (eds.), *The Social Impact of AIDS in the United States* (Washington, D.C.: The National Academy Press, 1993), chapters 4 and 6. A description of one of the more active community groups can be found in Cheryl Clark, "Private Groups Helping Test AIDS Drugs," *The San Diego Union-Tribune*, July 11, 1993, A1.

10. Peter S. Arno and Karyn L. Feiden, *Against the Odds: The Story of AIDS Drug Development, Politics, and Profit* (New York: Harper Collins, 1992).

11. In this connection it is worth noting that every university in the United States must have a special committee to review all research proposals that involve humans. This is to guarantee that humans not be used inhumanely.

12. Gina Kolata, "News of Advance in AIDS Treatment Delayed 5 Months," *New York Times*, November 14, 1990, A1. See also the follow-up response from NIAID in *New York Times*, November 16, 1990, A13, and the analysis in *AIDS Treatment Issues, The GMHC Newsletter of Experimental AIDS Therapies* 4, no. 8 (November 30, 1990). The charges and answers are well summarized in *Internal Medicine World Report*, December 1990, 4, and January 15, 1991.

13. A case in point was the controversy that developed around unorthodox, semi-underground clinical "tests" in 1989 of Compound Q, a promising antiviral drug. See Gina Kolata, "Critics Fault Secret Effort to Test Aids Drug," *New York Times*, September 17, 1989, 21, and *New York Times*, September 20, 1989, 10.

14. John Schwartz and David Brown, "A Deadly Medical Gamble. Test of Promising Drug Turns into Calamity," *The Washington Post*, July 8, 1993.

15. The standard·drug development and approval process breaks down approximately like this: *Preclinical Testing* (Years 1 & 2)—the phase during which the safety and biological activity of the new drug is tested, frequently on animals. *Phase I Testing*: Testing to determine safety, dosage, toxicity on humans using small groups of *healthy* volunteers (under one hundred). Seventy percent of the Investigational New Drugs (INDs) will pass this stage. *Phase II Testing* (Years 4 & 5): The drug is tested on from one hundred to two hundred *patient* volunteers to evaluate effectiveness, possibly dangerous side effects, and so on. Thirty-three percent of INDs will pass this stage. *Phase III Testing*: Tests on from one

thousand to three thousand *patient* volunteers to verify Phase II and monitor for long-terms effects. Under new "Expedited Review" procedures these two phases can be combined to shorten the approval process for new medicines addressing life-threatening diseases like AIDS. Twenty-seven percent of INDs will pass Phase III. *Food and Drug Administration Approval* (Years 9–11): This phase involves FDA review of all the documentation (test results, lab findings) that accumulate. About 20 percent of all INDs will survive the process and gain FDA approval. After approval there is still elaborate safety monitoring as the drug goes into manufacturing, distribution, and use.

16. An interesting discussion of the problem by John S. James, "The Drug Treatment Debacle, parts 1 & 2," *AIDS Treatment News*, nos. 77–78, 81–82 (1989).

17. A good brief introduction to the problem of differing perspectives was written by Natalie Angier, "Cultures in Conflict, M.D.'s and Ph.D.'s," *New York Times*, April 24, 1990, B5.

18. John James, *AIDS Treatment News*, no. 77, 4. James points out that in an exponential progression, such as applies roughly to this epidemic, the last doubling of case numbers before a medical advance or cure is found will account for about one half of the cumulative total of AIDS deaths throughout the entire epidemic.

19. In the 1830s Alexis de Tocqueville observed that the single-minded drive for profit was one of the characteristics that set apart the American from other cultures of the West. See his classic *Democracy in America*, Vol. 2, Phillip Bradley, ed. (New York: Knopf, 1945), 247–48.

20. *New York Times*, Medical Sciences Section, April 18, 1989; *Business Week*, April 24, 1989; *AIDS Treatment News*, April 21, 1989.

21. *AIDS Treatment News*, April 21, 1989, 5.

22. John S. James, "Needed: Compulsory Licensing of Pharmaceutical?" *AIDS Treatment News*, May 19, 1989, 4.

23. As an example of the problems, see "Correspondence: The Pressure to Keep Prices High at a Walk-in Clinic," *New England Journal of Medicine*, January 19, 1989, 183.

24. "AIDS, Drugs, Need and Greed," (Editorial) *New York Times*, September 29, 1989, 24. *Australian AIDS News* (distributed electronically on the InterUniversity BITNET system), October 28, 1989, reported a major debate in that country about the importation of AZT as a result of such reported profits.

25. *San Antonio Express-News*, November 10, 1990, 4G.

26. Gina Kolata, "AIDS Group Plans to Buy Drug for Less in Europe," *New York Times*, September 25, 1989, 11. The American manufacturer is Lyphomed of Rosemont, Illinois. The firms was granted "orphan status" for its product by the Federal Food and Drug Administration even though the drug is not even patented. "Orphan status" means that the firm has a seven-year legal monopoly on manufacture and distribution protected by federal law. There is no market competition restraining the price. Therefore Lyphomed charges whatever the traffic will bear. The same is true of Burroughs Wellcome's AZT.

27. Warren E. Leary, "Companies Accused of Overcharging for Drugs Developed with U.S. Aid," *New York Times*, January 26, 1993, B9.

28. Centers for Disease Control, *AIDS Daily Summary*, October 5, 1993, quoting *Boston Globe*, "AIDS-Drug Maker Plays Hardball Over Price," October 3, 1993.

29. C. Everett Koop, "The Health Care Mess," *Newsweek*, August 28, 1989, 10. See also *San Antonio Express-News* coverage of a San Antonio address given by

Koop on June 4, 1989.

30. Associated Press Release, *San Antonio Express-News*, February 13, 1993.

31. National Directory. See note 33.

32. For a highly personal history of the New York group, see Larry Kramer, *Reports from the Holocaust: The Making of an AIDS Activist* (New York: St. Martin's Press, 1989). Kramer, an author and playwright, was one of the founders of the Gay Men's Health Crisis. But the organization quickly became too "establishment" for his tastes, and he became a vocal opponent and gadfly. He later organized ACT UP, a confrontational advocacy group. Both are active groups.

33. For a complete listing, see The U.S. Conference of Mayors, *Local AIDS Services, The National Directory, January 1990* (available for $15 from the Conference of Mayors, 1620 Eye St. NW, Washington, D.C. 20008). For a study of the upstate New York experience, see Donald B. Rosenthal, "The Institutionalization of AIDS Service Organization: The Upstate New York Experience," paper prepared for delivery at the 1989 Annual Meeting of the American Political Science Association, Atlanta. Dr. Rosenthal is at the State University of New York at Buffalo.

34. Peter Nully, "Where All That AIDS Money Is Going," *Fortune* (February 7, 1994), 139.

35. See Charles Perrow and Mauro F. Guillen, *The AIDS Disaster: The Failure of Organization in New York and the Nation* (New Haven: Yale University Press, 1990). The authors conclude that the inability of various public and private organizations to confront the problems presented by the epidemic was probably inevitable. HIV was too new and involved too many emotionally charged issues.

36. For a description of similar problems in New York City's famous Gay Men's Health Crisis organization, see "An AIDS Service Agency Struggles to Meet Needs of Competing Groups," *New York Times*, May 28, 1993, A18.

37. Jonathan Kwitny, *Acceptable Risks* (New York: Poseidon, 1992).

38. "The AIDS Crisis: Learning from Mistakes," *Financial World*, March 2, 1993.

39. The four counties of the state reporting area–Bexar (San Antonio), Comal, Guadalupe, and Wilson—have registered 1,701 cases of AIDS since 1981. Using the customary extrapolation ratios of 1:5 or 1:8.2 (used by CDC), then the area would have approximately the number of seropositives mentioned.

40. Some of the larger ASOs are now receiving grants from drug manufacturers and the national government to underwrite costs of various programs such as community clinical drug trials. There are perfectly legitimate reasons for both offering and accepting such grants. But, undeniably, they raise conflict-of-interest problems for ASOs whose organizational roots include care-delivery and PWA advocacy. The problem for the ASOs is how to take the money they need for programs (that ultimately benefit PWAs) while still using tough pressure tactics to force manufacturers to lower prices (also for the benefit of PWAs).

41. For a disturbing overview, read Marc A. Rodwin, *Medicine, Money, and Morals— Physicians' Conflicts of Interest* (New York: Oxford University Press, 1993). Other analyses: David E. Rogers and Eli Ginzberg (eds.), *Public and Professional Attitudes Toward AIDS Patients, A National Dilemma*, Cornell University Medical College 5th Conference on Health Policy (San Francisco: Westview Press, 1989), and Christine Pierce and Donald Van DeVeer (eds.), *AIDS, Ethics and Public Policy* (New York: Wadsworth, 1988).

42. There is a good summary of the arguments in the *New England Journal of Medicine* 321, no. 19 (1990), 1334–36.

43. As quoted in A. Zuger and H. M. Stevens, "Physicians, AIDS, and Occupational

Risk, Historic Traditions and Ethical Obligations," *JAMA* (October 9, 1987), 1926.

44. See, for example, Richard Goldstein, "AIDS and the Social Contract," *The Weekly Newspaper of New York*, December 29, 1987.

45. Statement adopted by the ACP in 1987. See *New York Times*, March 13, 1987, A21; July 10, 1987, D18, and November 13, 1987, A14 for reactions and official statements of the medical associations. And see the "Interim Report on the Prevention and Control of AIDS" adopted by the AMA's House of Delegates at the 1987 Annual Meeting at Chicago, June 21–25, 1987.

46. *American Medical News*, February 16, 1990, 49 for the current position of the AMA and its new programs.

47. M. O. Hagen et al., "HIV Occupational Risk," *JAMA* 259 (1988), 1375. And see M. Brown et al., "The Third International Conference on AIDS: Risk of AIDS in Healthcare Workers," *Nursing Management* (March 1988), 33–36.

48. Sari Staver, "One in 250 HIV-Infected Sticks Transmits Virus–Studies," *American Medical News*, January 13, 1989, p.3, 19.

49. See "Commentary: Why Fear Persists, Health Care Professionals and AIDS," *JAMA* (December 16, 1988), 3481; Theodore Hammett and Walter Bond, "Risk of Infection with the AIDS Virus through Exposures to Blood," *AIDS Bulletin* (U.S. Department of Justice, National Institute of Justice) October 1987; Richard Ratzan and Henry Schneiderman, "AIDS, Autopsies, and Abandonment," *JAMA* (December 16, 1988), 3466.

50. Special report: "Fearful Healers," *New York Times*, November 11, 1990, A1.

51. Quoted in Zuger and Stevens, "Physicians, AIDS, and Occupational Risk." This is an excellent preliminary exploration of the subject.

52. "Commentary: Supporting the Health Care Team in Caring for Patients with AIDS," *JAMA* (February 3, 1989), 747.

53. See the analysis of Dr. Molly Cook, "HIV Fear Tied to Homophobia and Racial Bias," *Internal Medicine News*, February 15–28, 1990, 1 et seq.

54. One of the many ironies of the epidemic's course in America is that the homophobia that underlies a claim to deny care is easily traceable to the "Judeo" part of the Judeo-Christian tradition and the Pauline theological foundation. But the same Jewish culture produces a firm legal and ethical mandate commanding physicians to heal all patients without regard to their age, sex, race, creed, disease, or lifestyle. See "Jewish Law and the Obligation of the Physician to Heal Patients with AIDS," *JAMA* (April 21, 1989), 2199.

55. Quoted in Zuger and Stevens, "Physicians," 1925.

56. Bruce Lambert, "AIDS War Shunned by Many Doctors," *New York Times*, April 23, 1990, A1.

57. I would refer the reader to the discussions and references found in Christine Pierce and Donald VanDeVeer (eds.), *AIDS: Ethics and Public Policy*, Part III, especially the article by Kenneth R. Howe, "Why Mandatory Screening for AIDS Is a Very Bad Idea" (Belmont, Calif.: Wadsworth Publishing Co., 1988); Gerald J. Stine, *Acquired Immune Deficiency Syndrome* (Englewood Cliffs, N.J.: Prentice Hall, 1993), chap. 10.

58. There are two types of tests used to detect infection. One type is antibody tests which detect the presence of antibody to the virus. If the antibody is present, it is reasonable to infer that the virus is also. They are Elisa (enzyme-linked immunosorbent assay); Western Blot; immunofluorescence; radio-immuno-precipitation; hemagglutination. Although generally very sensitive and selective, these tests can react to agents other than HIV and give false positive or

indeterminate results. For example, at the San Antonio AIDS Foundation we found that pregnant women frequently tested positive when, in fact, they were not. Apparently the Elisa was reacting to hormone increases. The other type is used in cases where there are serious doubts as to the accuracy of positive results from the above tests. The client then can use the second type of test which reacts to the presence of the virus directly. These are the polymerase chain reaction assay, the P24 assay, and the HIV culture/co-culture tests. Why not use these to begin with? Because they are too expensive, require too much special equipment and training, and too much time to be used as a broad screening test.

59. The AMA recommends using the Elisa as the preliminary screening test, and if it is positive, confirming it with the Western Blot and one of the other available tests.

60. Manfred Eigen, "Viral Quasispecies," *Scientific American* (July 1993), 45.

61. Ironically, an infected individual may also test negative at the very end of his life—during the terminal stage of AIDS. By that time, the immune system has collapsed and can no longer generate antibodies against anything.

62. Centers for Disease Control, "Possible Transmission of Human Immunodeficiency Virus to a Patient during an Invasive Dental Procedure," *Morbidity and Mortality Weekly Report*, 39 (1990), 489–93. CDC, "Update: Transmission of Human Immunodeficiency Virus Infection during an Invasive Dental Procedure— Florida," *Morbidity and Mortality Weekly Report* 40 (1991), 21–27. Note that the CDC dropped the term "possible" from the title of its Update.

63. "AMA for HIV Tests with No Patient Consent," *Medical Tribune*, December 26, 1991, 1.

64. See, for example, Adelisa L. Panlilio, et al., "Blood Contacts during Surgical Procedures," *JAMA* (March 27, 1991), 1533–1547; David K. Henderson, et al., "Risk for Occupational Transmission of Human Immunodeficiency Virus Type 1 (HIV-1) Associated with Clinical Exposures," *Annals of Internal Medicine* (November 15, 1990), 740–45; Editorial, "Transmission of Human Immunodeficiency Virus Type 1 (HIV-1) by Exposure to Blood: Defining the Risk," *Annals of Internal Medicine* (November 15, 1990), 729–30; Keith Henry and Joseph Thurn, "HIV Infection in Healthcare Workers," *Postgraduate Medicine* (February 15, 1991), 30–38.

65. "HIV Risk in Exposed Health Workers '1 in 300'," *Internal Medicine News*, December 1, 1991, 20; Keith Henry and Joseph Thurn, "HIV infection in Healthcare Workers," *Postgraduate Medicine* (February 15, 1991), 30.

66. *CDC HIV/AIDS Surveillance Report, First Quarter 1993*, Table II: "Health-care Workers with Documented and Possible Occupationally Acquired AIDS/HIV Infection, by Occupation," reported through March 1993, United States.

67. Michael Howe (ed.), *AIDS Information Newsletter*, AIDS Information Center, V.A. Medical Center, San Francisco, January 1, 1993, "HIV/AIDS in the Health Care Environment, Part I."

68. Centers for Disease Control, *Morbidity and Mortality Weekly Report*, 1992M, 41:823–45.

69. States vary in their existing policy. California prohibits testing without informed consent. New York's highest court recently ruled that physicians cannot dispense consent procedures, particularly ones that might trigger contact tracing of sexual partners. See "N.Y. Court Rejects Move to Require Testing," *American Medical News*, May 20, 1991, p.4.

70. "AMA Votes to Allow HIV Testing of Patients without Specific Consent," *American Medical News*, December 23, 1991, 1.

71. "HIV Exposure during Nuclear Medicine Procedures," *JAMA* (September 9, 1992), 1253.

72. "4 Australians Infected with HIV in Surgery," *New York Times*, December 16, 1993.

73. The Centers for Disease Control, "Update: Investigations of Persons Treated by HIV-infected Health-Care Workers—United States," *Morbidity and Mortality Weekly Report*, May 7, 1993. As of the date of the report, ninety-two HIV+ patients were identified, but eighty-six of those seroconversions could plausibly be explained by their involvement in other risk activities; five had no identifiable risk factors other than contact with an HIV+ worker and therefore could have been infected in the health care arena. However, genetic sequencing analysis does not support a finding that the virus in the HCWs and the five patients are the same. "Search for Patients of HIV Infected M.D.'s Costly, with Unlikely HIV-positive findings," *Internal Medicine World Report* (December 12, 1991), 1.

74. State courts in Pennsylvania and New Jersey have already ruled in favor of the patient's right to know about the positive status of his or her physician. See Julius Landwirth, "Courts Look at Disclosure of Physicians' HIV Status," *Infectious Disease News*, January 1992, 13; "Medical Society of New Jersey Calls for Routine HIV Testing," *Internal Medicine World Report* (June 1, 1991), 1.

75. Bernie Ankney, "HIV Risk Seen Identical for Patients," *U.S. Medicine* (November 1991), 1.

76. Letter: "HIV Infected Surgeons" (describing with diagrams safer surgical techniques), *JAMA* (February 12, 1992), 803. Adelisa L. Panlilio, et al., "Blood Contacts during Surgical Procedures," *JAMA* (March 27, 1991), 1533. The article states that the most important single variable relating to the probability of surgical needlestick injury is the amount of time the surgeon has been working. After one hour the surgeon is more likely to puncture is glove and finger while working on the patient. Simply stated, he gets tired just like the rest of us.

77. "Opposition Mounting against CDC Plan for 'Exposure-prone' List," *American Medical News* (October 28, 1991), 1.

78. "CDC Abandons Risky Procedures List for Doctors with HIV," *Infectious Disease News*, February 1992, 2.

79. "States' Interpretation of 'Equivalent' Key to Congress' Mandate on HIV Guidelines," *American College of Physicians' Observer* (November 1991), 1.

80. "Texas Law Restricts Infected M.D.'s," *Internal Medicine News*, November 1, 1991, 1.

81. "Medical Society Launches Controversial Testing Program," *American Medical News*, February 10, 1992, 16.

82. "Needle Scare at *Time* Magazine," *Washington Post*, November 5, 1993, G1; summarized, CDC, *AIDS Daily Summary*, November 5, 1993. The physician's practice ignored CDC guidelines long in place. The magazine's staffers will now have to undergo hepatitis and HIV testing.

83. Proposals of Marcia Angell, executive editor of the *New England Journal of Medicine*, in "A Dual Approach to the AIDS Epidemic," May 23, 1991, as well as various responses to her proposals in the September 12 issue.

84. Amy Fairchild et al., "More Disclosure of AIDS in Celebrities," *New England Journal of Medicine* (February 1993).

85. Research from the University of North Carolina at Chapel Hill on the issue of

partner notification found that when it was left up to the HIV+ individual, only 7 percent of the partners were told of the infection. Fifty percent of the partners were notified when the program's counselors undertook the task. See *Medical Tribune*, January 30, 1992, 13.

86. See the case of Ed Savitz of Philadelphia in the *San Antonio Express-News* (Associated Press), March 28, 1992, 9a and March 31, 1992, 2a.

87. Sari Staver, "A Life of Work Unravels," *American Medical News*, February 3, 1992, 36.

88. G. Edward Rozar Jr., M.D., "I'm HIV-Positive, but I Won't Give Up Being a Doctor," *Medical Economics* (December 2, 1991), 43–45.

89. An informative review of many alternative therapies, from shark cartilage to vitamins, was published in the *Gay Men's Health Crisis Newsletter*, "GMHC Treatment Issues," Special Winter Issue, 1993–94.

90. Information on unconventional treatments can be obtained from Healing Alternative Foundation, 1746 Market Street, San Francisco, CA 94114.

91. David M. Eisenberg et al., "Unconventional Medicine in the United States," *New England Journal of Medicine* (January 28, 1993), 247. Ruth M. Greenblatt et al., "Polypharmacy Among Patients Attending an AIDS Clinic: Utilization of Prescribed, Unorthodox, and Investigational Treatments," *Journal of Acquired Immune Deficiency Syndrome* (March 1991), 136–43.

92. See the excellent survey article, Daniel Goleman, "Placebo Effect Is Shown to Be Twice as Powerful as Expected," *New York Times*, August 17, 1993, B6.

93. Larry Tate and Martin Delaney, "Hope, Folly, or Fraud," *PI Perspective* (newsletter of Project Inform, San Francisco), April 1992, 11.

94. Project Inform in San Francisco published a statement of its findings on DNCB in August 1993. The bottom line "is that any claims of efficacy should thus far be taken with considerable skepticism."

95. Dr. William D. Logan and Dr. Kenneth Alonso, Foundation for Virology and Oncology, reported impressive results in inhibiting HIV replication in a Kaposi's sarcoma patient, press release of May 31, 1990, issued at Atlanta Hospital. Dr. Alonso's last treatments were reported from Mexico City.

96. A 1989 survey showed that one fourth of all patients were trying treatments that had neither the approval of the FDA nor that of their physician. These included megadose vitamins, fetal sheep blood injections, and unapproved drugs. *American Medical News*, December 22–29, 1989, 21. See also William J. Kassler, et al., "The Use of Medicinal Herbs by Human Immunodeficiency Virus-Infected Patients," *Archives of Internal Medicine*, November 1991, 2281–88.

97. *Healing AIDS, A Magazine of Healing Tools, Resources and Aids* (3835 20th St., San Francisco, CA 94114).

98. Published by The Foundation for Inner Peace, Tiburon, California (nd).

99. Louise Hay, *You Can Heal Your Life* (Santa Monica, Calif.: Hay House, n.d.).

100. AIDS patients are also advised to stay out of the sun, or use a high-protection sun block. It has been demonstrated that ultraviolet radiation has a significant impact on activating HIV. And one of the nation's longest surviving PWAs (now dead) credited his longevity to a daily diet of raw garlic. And see Ryan Ver Berhmoes, "Hucksters, Healers, and Heroes," *American Medical News*, January 27, 1992, 29–34.

101. See Carles R. Caulfield and Billi Goldberg, "Chinese Herbs for HIV: A Critical Review (in two parts)," *San Francisco Sentinel*, August 20 and September 22, 1992. The articles can be accessed on Internet, sci.med.aids newsgroup, same

dates, archive 11,142.

102. Dave Gilden, "Alternative Medicine Advocates Divided over New NIH Research Program," *AIDS Treatment News*, April 2, 1993.

103. People generally assume that herbal remedies lack the possibly harmful toxicities of manufactured drugs because they are "natural." This is not the case. CDC's *Morbidity and Mortality Weekly Report* (July 16, 1993) contains a case report on lead poisonings of forty children of Mexican descent resulting from their mothers' administration of traditional ethnic herbal laxatives. Similarly, Colorado health authorities traced some life-threatening illnesses to the use of a traditional Chinese herbal product known as Jin Bu Huan tablets, available at health food stores. David Dodell, M.D. (ed.), *Health Info-Com Network, Medical Newsletter*, vol. 26, issue 53, December 5, 1993, Internet.

104. CDC, *AIDS Daily Summary*, November 5, 1993.

105. *American Medical News*, April 1, 1988.

106. The Hotline is published in two thousand Yellow Pages directories and can access information on about two thirds of the nation's eight hundred thousand physicians who have ABMS board certification in some specialty.

107. For example, practitioners of traditional Chinese medicine are licensed by the California State Board of Medical Quality Assurance, carry the title of licensed acupuncturist, and are regarded as primary care physicians. San Francisco has several professional institutes for training and delivering care: The Quan Yin Healing Arts Center, The American College of Traditional Chinese Medicine, and the Immune Enhancement Project. All of these institutes receive some government funds to subsidize their care programs and have strong connections with traditional allopathic medical programs.

108. The Project Inform guidelines are, in turn, based upon those issued by the California AIDS Fraud Task Force.

5

Avoiding Aids:
The Problem of Behavior

THE HAZARDS OF LIVING

We live surrounded by risk that, for the sake of our emotional balance, we ignore as much as possible. The law requires us to strap on seat belts in an effort to cut the more than fifty thousand deaths per year. Former Surgeon General Koop's #1 priority was not AIDS, but the elimination of smoking, which is implicated each year in over one hundred fifty thousand deaths—three times the number killed in the Vietnam War. Swimming, motorcycle, electrical, and handgun accidents account for another forty thousand deaths. Truly, living is dangerous to your health. Torts, a major field of the law, flowers in the dangerous but beautiful garden of our collective lives. A major risk of living has always been that of encountering in some fashion or the other one of the organisms that prey upon us, be it a shark or a bacterium. The HIV has added another danger to an already long list. Accompanying every form of risk there are avoidance possibilities which flow from the nature of the predator itself. Thus it is unlikely that a shark will bite you on land though any ocean fisherman can tell that it can and has happened. Similarly risk of infection with HIV can be diminished to tolerable levels by simply paying proper respect to the modes of transmission by which the virus is transferred from one host to another.

As an introduction to the topic of avoiding AIDS, here is an approximate rank ordering of standard risk activities as I read the data. The intervals between each category are not equal. The rank ordering from greatest to least is based upon the possibility that you will be infected if you are involved, willingly or otherwise, in this activity, and there is HIV contamination:[1]

1. Transfusion of HIV contaminated blood or blood products—the direct introduction of the virus into the bloodstream.

2. The use of shared, unsterile apparatus for injecting drugs, in or out of health care settings.
3. Being the recipient partner in anal intercourse during which no condom is used.
4. Industrial-medical negligence and/or accident.
5. Being the recipient partner in vaginal intercourse during which no condom is used.
6. Being the insertive partner in vaginal intercourse during which no condom is used.
7. Being the insertive partner in anal intercourse, during which no condom is used.
8. Oral sex (receptive fellatio).
9. Anal intercourse with condom protection.
10. Vaginal intercourse with condom protection.
11. Transfusion of screened blood or blood products.

Other than being born to an infected mother (25 percent chance of transmission) there are *NO* other standard routes than the above and their variations.[2] A survey of fourteen separate American and African studies seeking to document various modes of transmission concluded that there was no credible evidence of seroconversion other than through the above routes.[3] There are no documented instances of seroconversion due to human or insect bites, sitting on toilet seats, donating blood, sharing foods, glasses, straws, or cooking or eating utensils, shaking hands, and hugging. There are no documented cases of seroconversion as a result of exposure to infected individuals in the occupational pursuits of firefighting, law enforcement, emergency response technicians, or general office or educational work. This is not to say that transmission can never occur in such environments; there have been and will continue to be a small number of freak transmissions, transmissions that occur outside the normal pattern. The absolute number of nonstandard transmissions will grow as the epidemic encompasses more and more people, but the percentage will always be small.[4] About the only good thing that I can say about the present form of the virus is that it is not easy to get; if it were, the world be in much bigger trouble.

However, there are innumerable variations on the risky behaviors that create nuances and shadings that, in real life, affect the relative placement of risk. For example, the insertive partner's risk (6, 7) is seriously heightened if he is uncircumcised, has genital ulcers, or has or receives another venereal disease at the time the virus is transmitted.[5] Similarly it makes a huge difference if a user patronizes a "shooting gallery" or uses his own "works" at home. Further, it is impossible to disentangle some behaviors, like kissing and intercourse, so that attribution of seroconversion to the intercourse alone is certain.

A final complication stems from the fact that there are many interrelated physical variables, but no one can precisely state what the interrelationships are. Still, a useful way to think about risk is in terms of variables (apart from your or your partner's behaviors) that are involved in a possible transmission. Ranked from high to low risk, those variables include (1) the fluid type that is exchanged: blood, semen, vaginal/cervical secretions, breastmilk, saliva, tears, urine, sweat, and excrement;[6] (2) the route of absorption or transmission into the body: direct injection, rectum, vagina, placenta, break in skin, penis, mouth, newly inflicted wound, eyes, nose, intact skin; (3) the inoculum: large volume, repeated exposures, occasional exposures, small volume, one exposure, no exposure; (4) the health status of the party to whom a possible infection might have been transmitted: sick at time of transmission, infected with other STDs, malnourished, drug user, alcohol and tobacco user, highly stressed, pregnant, healthy. The Colorado Department of Health uses a 4x4 matrix with the above variables as a rough-and-ready tool to estimate the potential for transmission.[7] Clearly, however, neither this method, nor my opening list, nor anyone else's chart can provide precise answers.

Finally, I should mention that the difficulties in getting precise statements are partly reflections of the three other factors: (1) the paucity of data on sexual behavior in general; (2) the newness of the entire field of retroviral research; (3) the highly conditional nature of statistical statements.

LIES, DAMNED LIES, AND STATISTICS

AIDS has not made dangerous behavior that was all that safe before. But it does force us to reassess risk and adjust our attitudes and behavior. We need to think about how to evaluate, in personal terms, the various statements that bombard us daily. For example, people read in the newspapers that the odds against an American heterosexual contracting AIDS are astronomical. They believe that they are safe; they are wrong. Probability statements can establish parameters of time and action within which a certain result is likely to occur. *If* you always flip a coin *exactly* the same way, *then* it is probable that "x" times it will come up heads, and "y" times it will be tails. However, probability statements cannot tell you when the specific occasion of a head or tail may occur. You may get a run of twenty-five heads, followed by a run of ten tails, or the two sides might alternate. The point is that no one can know whether the next flip will produce a head or a tail. Nor can anyone tell you whether the next sexual or drug encounter will be safe or not. Further, in real life there is much slippage in that word "exactly." These truths apply to the problem of describing how to avoid AIDS, just as they apply to flipping coins. The only honest response to the "Me worry?" reaction is to point out that people are dying within the odds. If it is sexual transmission, the very first encounter may be infectious,[8] or it may be the five thousandth, or never. There is no way to predict the safety of the individual event. If we could extrapolate from general odds to the specific occasion, no one would lose at Las Vegas.

Furthermore, probability statements are accurate only within strictly defined limits. Statisticians who project from existing data to future probabilities can only do so after assuring that their base data are accurate and timely, and after prescribing certain constants or assumptions. The figure often seen in the press that 1–1.5 million Americans are infected with the virus is a figure which is very suspect.[9] The original estimate was projected from two sources: (1) an extrapolation from 1986 existing case data of about 30,000 cases, and, (2) a "guesstimate" based on Kinsey's 1940s estimate that about 10 percent of the American male population was dominantly or exclusively homosexual. If this remained the case in the 1980s, then it could be projected that about 10 percent of them would contract AIDS. The final figure was, in other words, an estimate based on the current reported cases, plus an estimate based on 1940 data, and assumed a certain course of infection. It is no exaggeration to call it "guesstimate."[10] In 1989 the California Medical Association estimated that there may be as many as 2.1 million seropositives in that state alone.[11]

A 1989 article in *Science* argued that the Centers for Disease Control estimates of seroprevalence levels among whites relative to ethnic minorities, and Midwesterners relative to Easterners was much too low. The CDC answered that methodology of the authors was flawed. The *Science* authors then countered with the projections of the Government Accounting Office which suggested that they had, in fact, been gentle in their criticism of the CDC studies.[12] The CDC's estimates of the seropositives within the population has ranged from a low of 650,000 to a high of 1,500,000. The most recent CDC estimate settled on 1,000,000 by calculating backward from the number of reported AIDS cases to the number of supposed seropositives; it remains to be seen whether the estimate of seropositivity will jump as a result of the increase in AIDS reports under the 1993 revision.[13] A further complication stems from the fact that, regardless of whether domestic or international reported figures are being discussed, the AIDS cases reflect the incursion of HIV into the population approximately ten years previous. AIDS data reported in 1994 reflect 1984 behavior and infection; what the actual infection rate is now (as you read these words) is anybody's guess. Global estimates of the World Health Organization and other groups run from 14 to 30 million infected. The estimates will vary with the particular studies used, the data comparisons, and the political climate. In the Reagan-Bush administrations there was a tendency to downplay the epidemic, especially the extent of its intrusion into the middle-class heterosexual community.[14] If several possible figures are possible, announce the most optimistic one, and one that fit the Reagan-Bush view of the epidemic as a gay problem. Obviously, this eased the pressure on government to do something. Indeed, one of the most serious casualties of the epidemic's politicization has been the CDC's reputation for political impartiality and scientific objectivity.[15] However, the numbers game is played by all sides. Stephen Joseph, formerly commissioner of Public Health for New York City, ran into a whirlwind of criticism and opposition when he cut the estimate of seropositives in the city by half, from 400,000 to 200,000.[16] He thought the gay community would be happy with the new lower estimates; instead it was outraged. For both sides, the figures connect immediately to budget and funding.

Part of the problem in getting a firm figure stems from the definition of AIDs. When you read that "X% of HIV+s will progress to AIDS within 5 years of primary infection," it is important to keep in mind that the statement does not say that you will get "sick" in five years, but that you will have developed the collection or syndrome of symptoms which the Federal Centers for Disease Control has defined as constituting certifiable AIDS. This definition is very complex,[17] and its periodic revisions have an immediate impact on the figures delimiting the epidemic. The August 1987 revision produced a 20 percent increase in reported cases, both here and abroad.[18] The 1993 CDC redefinition, adopted in January 1993, increased the total reported cases 111 percent for that year. Using the 1987 definition, there would have been approximately 48,063 cases, but the 1993 definition added 55,432 to the total (see Figure 3.6). An additional 20 percent is expected for 1994.[19] Furthermore, it is quite possible to get sick and die of infections stemming from an HIV infection without, by definition, dying of AIDS. As a matter of fact, a study published in 1993 indicated that our counting of AIDS cases was inaccurate by fully one half prior to 1986 for the simple reason that HIV/AIDS had not yet been added to the international code book for certifying cause of death; after 1987, certifications jumped by 81 percent.[20] Consequently, physicians and coroners used traditional categories like "pneumonia" or "cell-mediated immune deficiency." Epidemiologists estimate that there are from five to eight times as many individuals whose health is impaired by HIV infection as there are those who have certifiable AIDS. Such individuals make up the large group of asymptomatics or ARCs (people with Aids Related Conditions), who are sick and sometimes dying of "Almost AIDS."[21] It is very likely that the official statistics on the epidemic, although grim, are not half grim enough.

Furthermore, many of the critical definitions that provide the foundation for projections and recommendations are themselves skewed and suspect.

For example, our official reporting system for the spread of AIDS is based on questionable delineations of the groups involved. The drug user category is reasonably clear (although its ranking in the hierarchy of groups has the effect of making the heterosexual category look smaller). The straight and gay classes are entirely self-defined (that is, people self-identify). I suppose that is the best that can be done because, though it may seem extraordinary, it is nonetheless a fact that we do not have an acceptable definition of "straight" or "gay." There is good reason. Forty years ago Kinsey stated flatly that the population did not fall into these simple-minded categories:

> Males do not represent two discrete populations, heterosexual and homosexual. The world is not to be divided into sheep and goats. . . . It is a fundamental of taxonomy that nature rarely deals with discrete categories. Only the human mind invents categories and tries to force facts into separate pigeon-holes. The living world is a continuum in each and every one of its aspects. The sooner we learn this concerning human sexual behavior the sooner we shall reach a sound understanding of the realities of sex.[22]

Regardless of Kinsey's warning, the Centers for Disease Control uses such pigeonhole categories to report all data on the epidemic. Its *Morbidity and Mortality Weekly Reports (MMWR)* uses such categories as "homosexual," "bisexual," "heterosexual," to organize and present figures on reported AIDS cases to the nation. All other discussion in the newspapers, the TV, and the lecture hall relies upon them.[23]

But who is "gay" and who is "straight"? The CDC classifies as heterosexuals only men who state that they have had no same-sex sexual encounters. A person is classified as homosexual or bisexual if he admits to any same-sex sexual activity. In all cases, the reliability of the data depends upon candor, selective memory, and, above all, culturally determined perceptions of sex.[24] According to Kinsey 30 percent of the sexually active male population has had at least "incidental" homosexual experiences. The results, then, are that the CDC's heterosexual category applies to about 70 percent of the male sexually active age group.[25] But it is a shifting or dynamic division, not a static one. As Kinsey put it, "It is true that there are persons in the population whose histories are exclusively heterosexual. . . . And there are individuals . . . whose histories are exclusively homosexual. . . . But the record also shows that there is a considerable portion of the population whose members have combined . . . both homosexual and heterosexual experience and/or psychic response. There are some whose heterosexual experiences predominate, there are some whose homosexual experiences predominate, there are some who have had quite equal amounts of both types of experience."[26] Can all the nuances that one finds in real life usefully be lumped into gross categories? Why, for example, should the "bisexual" be combined with the "homosexual" category: "Homosexual and Bisexual Males"? Why not use the equally logical "Heterosexual and Bisexual Males"? It is not at all clear whether the bisexual male is a homosexual who occasionally has sex with females, or a heterosexual who occasionally has sex with males.

It is all categorical nonsense. Being Haitian, "straight," or "gay," cannot be "risky" as such. HIV is spread by specific behaviors found to a greater or lesser extent in all groups; why not report in terms of known risky behaviors by whomever performed, such as anal sex?[27] The answer is that the current thirteen categories—one half of which are "heterosexual"—have become partly political rather than purely epidemiological. In the early days of the epidemic the official risk classification system reflected the perception of the epidemic as the "Gay Plague." However, various projections of the American epidemic into the twenty-first century agree that it will become predominantly a heterosexual infection, just as it is already in Africa and the Caribbean.[28] Then the heterosexual category will contain the chilling numbers. Will it then become a "Straight Plague"? It is long past time to clean up the classification system so that sexually active people are given neither a false sense of security nor an equally false sense of despair, but they are given full warning and guidance on what behavior to avoid.

HIV infection is clearly capable of being transmitted in several ways, but the virus itself is indifferent to the lifestyle preferences of the host. Reporting data in terms of the CDC classification encourages and perpetuates a misidentification of the essential problem. It focus attention on other more or less defined groups of people, like gays or hemophiliacs. However, what is really important to us, as it is to the virus, is human behaviors, for some are much more apt to spread HIV than others. In discussing IV drug use and/or safer sex, it *is* important to know the kinds of behaviors to avoid; more often than not it is impossible to know what individuals to avoid.

Avoidance assumes that you have the necessary information to classify that person and that the classification embodies a valid relationship. Ordinarily you do not. First, most of America's carriers are unaware of their condition. Second, a number of studies indicate that those who are aware are not eager to reveal their status. Lies not infrequently accompany the search for sex.[29] And, finally, no one displays any outward sign of seropositivity until late in the course of the infection. If you have more money than good sense, you can join a club that supplies a "Certified AIDS Free" membership card for use on dates. However, good sense requires that we discuss risk behaviors, not presumptively risky people.[30]

In other words, statistics and definitions have limitations, even when they come from authoritative sources like university research centers or the CDC.

Many of the arguments in health and public policy stem from professional differences with regard to definitions and statistical methods. The sex researchers Masters, Johnson, and Kolodny challenge many of the figures, projections, and conclusions of the AIDS "establishment" in their book *Crisis: Heterosexual Behavior in the Age of AIDS*. They argue that the official estimate of the infection's prevalence in the population is underestimated by about one half and that many public health conclusions (for example, that kissing is safe) were based on inadequate data.[31]

In addition, there are caveats that stem from the very nature of science itself and the business of data collection. The nonscientist must try to remember that the word NEVER does not exist in the vocabulary of laboratory science. The sun *might not* rise tomorrow, and you *might* get AIDS from the bananas packed for you by an infected grocery clerk, but these things have not, in fact, ever been recorded. I remember the head of the San Antonio AIDS Foundation losing his temper at a strategy meeting with physicians on just this point. The Foundation counselors were trying to determine what they should and should not say to people who called on the AIDS Hotline for practical advice on how to avoid HIV infection. The scientists in attendance were hemming and hawing in their usual professional way when the Foundation president blew up and shouted, "How many centuries did it take for you guys to admit that people couldn't get syphilis from a toilet seat?" Silence reigned until someone sheepishly answered, "Oh, just one." Be that as it may, both the training and the philosophy underlying modern science absolutely rule out the "absolutely never."

Finally, there is a big difference between "hard" and "soft" data, and this difference frequently becomes critical in sensible discussions about AIDS related behavior. Hard data are obtained when an observation embodies and reflects the use of commonly accepted and invariant standards—for example, when I state that this brick weighs ten pounds. Others can check it out, weigh it themselves, and validate my data against a commonly accepted standard. This is "hard" data. There is precious little of it in the world of AIDS. What we generally have is indirect evidence, "soft" data, that is, data which may embody a person's judgment, cultural definitions, memory, or candor, or data that just seems to support the probability of a hypothesis. For example, one of the arguments for locating the geographic origin of HIV in Central Africa is the very high rates of AIDS measured there. It seems a reasonable proposition that HIV must have been spreading a long time to establish such high rates of infection, and it had the time because it started there. Another example of soft data are the statements made by interviewees in polls. Let us say that you want to know how many of HIV+ males in Mexico City have seroconverted as a result of male to male sex. You conduct a poll, ask whether the interviewee is homosexual, and discover that 50 percent of the HIV+s will honestly answer "no." You conclude that there must be a high rate of heterosexual seroconversion. But the conclusion may be wrong because Latin males who are the active or insertive partners in male intercourse or oral sex do not consider themselves and are not considered by their culture to be homosexuals.[32] Epidemiologists, statisticians, and others go to great lengths to establish the reliability of their data, but inevitably their data gains authority through weight of numbers rather than conforming to a strict logical or standardized format as in the case of hard data. Soft data are generally less precise and subject to more interpretation than is the case with hard data. How important this can be will be seen in the discussion below on the risks of oral sex.

Practicing physicians have their own set of professional limitations. A sense of limits flows from the fact that all competent physicians are painfully aware of how imprecise an art medicine really is and equally aware of how much many patients emotionally need the assurance of a certain diagnosis. Thus, with one eye on medicine's limitations and the other on a possible malpractice suit, the physician prefers to say as little as possible and state that little in very conditional terms.

It may seem that I have muddied the waters of risk-assessment, but I really haven't—they are already muddy. As a former counselor I am acutely aware of what it is that everyone wants—clear, absolute, unambiguous guidance about what behaviors they could safely undertake. But as a counselor, I know that no one is going to get them from honest sources. Like it or not, all that knowledgeable people can endorse is behavior that will, with a little luck and in the greatest number of cases, enhance the chances of *avoiding* AIDS. What it comes down to in the end is that each individual must read the arguments, look at the data, and make up his or her own mind as to what chances to take and with whom.

AIDS AND DRUG USE

Obviously the most direct road to infection is direct injection of the virus into the bloodstream, the natural home of HIV. Devices from acupuncture needles, through blood transfusion needles, to hypodermic syringes and needles used to inject everything from antibiotics to heroin will accomplish this.[33] All that is required is that the needle be contaminated with the invisible virus. In the United States, the likelihood of infection through a contaminated transfusion or the use of unsterile needles in a legitimate health care operation is very low. Accidents can and will happen that gravely concern the individuals involved, and there will be more accidents as the size of the epidemic increases, but, still, they will be too few to constitute a public health hazard.

Such is not the case with transmission of HIV through drug use, by direct injection or indirectly through use of stimulants such as crystal and crack.[34] The practices of 1.5 million injecting drug users (IDUs) in the United States do pose a major hazard both to themselves and to the general community. The drug user subgroup has become a living storage reservoir for the virus, a source from which it is being transmitted to the greater community. IV drug users now account for about 30 percent of the total cases, and they are the major source of heterosexual and perinatal transmission.[35] The bridges are prostitution and the sale of blood to commercial plasma collection centers (*not* blood banks) by the addict.[36] There can be no battle to keep HIV out of the drug community; it is already well established, the virus having been introduced into the New York area drug community in the 1970s. Further, sometime in late 1987 data began to indicate that the rate of HIV infection in the groups practicing intravenous drug injection was increasing relative to those practicing anal intercourse. To put it another way, many of those practicing anal intercourse were getting the message about AIDS avoidance, but the drug user was not. The surgeon general began warning that the control of·AIDS in the future would be tied to the containment of drug use, and his warning was later echoed by Admiral Watkins, chairman of the Presidential AIDS Commission.[37] Unfortunately these warnings did not register on the Reagan-Bush White House. The National Commission on AIDS (the congressionally established successor to the Presidential AIDS Commission), in its December 1989 report, urged the president to take notice of this dangerous connection and revise the allocation of resources in its "War on Drugs" to account for the AIDS/drugs connection.[38]

Illustrative seroprevalencies within various IDU subgroups are: San Franciscans enrolled in a community drug treatment program, 55 percent;[39] Chicago, west side, 30 percent, south side, 15.6 percent, and north side, 19.1 percent;[40] Manhattan clients of detox and methadone programs, 60 percent;[41] Atlanta clients of an STD center, 10 percent;[42] clients of a Puerto Rican drug treatment center, 45 to 59 percent;[43] and a small sample of Manhattan prostitutes, 50 percent.[44] The overall number of infected IDU in the United States is estimated to be two hundred thirty-five thousand people or 16 percent of the total. Most epidemiologists expect these figures, which are already on par with those found in urban Central Africa, to go up unless some way can be found to change patterns of drug use. Clearly, AIDS containment within the IDU community is necessarily part of the larger "war on drugs" being waged by the federal government.

After Teddy Roosevelt left the White House, he went on an African safari and wrote a book on his prowess as a Great White Hunter. Illustrations showed Teddy standing on the carcass of an elephant, a dead rhinoceros, and other luckless animals that got in the way of his gunsights. With his usual flair and showmanship, he managed to convey the idea that the "Dark Continent" was forever illuminated by his brief sojourn there. But except for a few less animals, he left it as he found it. Somehow the Reagan-Bush "war on drugs" reminds me of Teddy's conquest of Africa. Newspapers showed Reagan's Attorney General Meese proudly standing in front of a pile of confiscated heroin. Nancy Reagan composed the administration's battle cry—"Just Say No!"—sweetly oblivious to the fact that the very nature of addiction is that you cannot say "Just say No." President Bush, in an inspiring address on August 7, 1989, mobilized the Boy Scouts of America for the "war on drugs." Lots of showmanship, but nothing really changes. The domestic and international drug industry continues to grow, increase its profits, and spawns ever more violence and destruction.

The interconnected wars to contain both the virus and drug use have many elements in common.[45] Winning them will be very expensive, although not as expensive in the long run as not winning them. Neither will be won without radical departures from currently acceptable approaches, nor will they be won without principled and courageous presidential leadership—the kind we associate with Abraham Lincoln. There is no likelihood, for example, that we will make a dent in the unbelievably lucrative drug traffic until the profit is taken from it. Americans should understand the power of the profit motive. That cannot be done by episodic, media-event drug raids or pious admonitions to middle-school students.

The national government could become the only legal supplier to those already addicted, combine free or low-cost supply with treatment programs both for addiction and AIDS if need be, and gradually (over the course of several generations) wean the commonwealth from its dangerous dependencies. However, the consternation, in and out of the Clinton's White House, that greeted Surgeon General Joycelyn Elders's modest proposal in 1993 that perhaps we ought to study the matter, indicates that the nation is not ready for real medicine.[46] On a less sweeping level, it could encourage shooting gallery "house doctors" to promote the use of sterile needles. The cooperation of the "house doctors" (who are the shooting gallery experts at helping addicts find a usable vein) would have more effect on stemming the spread of AIDS via contaminated needles than all the press releases of the national government. Or the president could help sell the public on the notion that needle exchange programs are not designed to encourage drugs but to discourage the spread of AIDS. If the president needs a national model to follow, he need look no farther than the Netherlands, Vancouver, British Columbia, and some forty American state programs, including one in New York City.[47] All of these programs treat the distribution of clean needles and condoms as equally important aspects of the fight to contain AIDS.[48] Further, they are showing some impressive positive results in decreasing HIV transmissions attributable to injecting drug use.[49] Moreover, if all of this is considered too radical for a national politician, a good deal of progress could be made simply by congressional funding of existing drug treatment programs at the level called for by the population of drug users. Our programs can currently accommodate about 10 percent of the addicted population.[50]

SAFETY AND SEX

The necessary starting point for any discussion of safe sex is that there isn't any. There never has been. Sex and love have always been high-risk enterprises as perhaps befits their centrality to the human experience. It has always been one of the main functions of both church and state to exert some controls lest our hot pursuit damage the very community that our drives serve to perpetuate. From the days of Helen, whose face launched a thousand ships for the Siege of Troy, to the somewhat more mundane current possibility of contracting one of about twenty-four sexually transmitted diseases,[51] sex and love have been a problem—but one, I hasten to add, the burdens of which we have gladly assumed. Omar Khayyam, the great twelfth-century Persian poet, immortalized our fantasies in his *Rubaiyat*:

> Here with a Loaf of Bread beneath the bough,
> A Flask of Wine, A Book of Verse—and Thou
> Beside me singing in the Wilderness—
> And Wilderness is Paradise enow.

The Persian word for garden (pardis) is the source of our word *paradise*, a place of fulfillment, beauty, peace, a place to share with your beloved. Gaining access to, retaining, and leaving a loved partner—one's microcosmic paradise—has always had fatal potential. Indeed most literature, poetry, and drama (as well as current TV soaps) revolve around the heady game. But always we have felt that the ultimate moment of passion and possession made the risks worthwhile. Now AIDS has dramatically upped the ante, and we are desperately searching for safer forms of sex.

What are the forms of safer sex in the context of AIDS, and what do I mean by "safer sex"? Safer sex practices are those for which there is no scientifically documented instance of seroconversion from negative to positive or where the evidence indicates a very low risk; by "documented" I mean findings corroborated by accepted scientific procedures sufficiently controlled to warrant being published in such reputable journals such as the *New England Journal of Medicine* and *The Journal of the American Medical Association*. There are now well over three hundred and five thousand cases of clinically recorded AIDS in the United States alone. These case records, as supplemented by an impressive body of epidemiological evidence, enable public health authorities to make recommendations that they would have hesitated to offer only a few years ago.

KISSING AND PETTING

As far as AIDS is concerned, kissing is safe—light or deep, on the cheek, on the hand, on the stomach, or wherever the spirit moves you. There are no documented cases of seroconversion attributable to kissing.[52] It is interesting to compare the U.S. government's brochures on avoiding AIDS in 1987 and 1988. The earlier cautioned against deep or "French" kissing, while the latter—mailed to the entire nation—stated flatly, "You won't get AIDS from a kiss."[53] Kissing is safe for several reasons. First, the virus apparently cannot penetrate unbroken outer skin layers (inner cervical or rectal membranes are another matter). Second, enzymes occurring naturally in saliva present the virus with a hostile environment, and stomach acids are fatal. Third, the infectivity of the virus is partially dependent upon its concentration in the fluid involved, and only very low quantities have been isolated from the saliva of even very advanced cases of AIDS.[54] Of course, there are always those who for reasons of private profit or fear will create theoretically dangerous scenarios—IF you have an open sore on your lip or tongue, and IF you let someone who is HIV+ chew on it for awhile, THEN seroconversion might possibly result. True. Anything is possible in this world; it is even possible that such people will grow up. But that possibility is probably much less than the chance of infection due to kissing. Unlike smoking, the surgeon general has certified that kissing is *not* hazardous to your health.

On the other hand, kissing presents us with an excellent example of the difficulties in making unqualified recommendations when HIV is involved. Although you will not be infected by the virus from kissing, you might get tuberculosis. People with HIV damaged immune systems are susceptible to two forms of TB, one of which is transmissible by oral contact, coughs, and sneezes. It is not clear whether the increasing incidence of TB is the result of the activation of earlier infections or is the result of wholly news ones. Whichever, it is now recommended that all HIV+ individuals undergo annual TB skin tests, and, if positive for TB, determine whether he or she is currently infectious. Fortunately, there is effective treatment; unfortunately, persistent coughing must now be regarded as a warning to affectionate friends and/or partners.

Other sexual expressions are without risk—hugging, cuddling, suppers by candlelight, the entire gambit of more exotic erotic fetishes (foot, clothing, pictures, etc.), pornography, cross-dressing, drag, massage and/or mutual masturbation, dancing, and hot tubs. The extraordinarily rich and imaginative array of behavior this side of intercourse is all still available as means of pleasuring your partner and yourself, of saying, "I love you, but am not willing to die for you." Once we get over being frightened by AIDS, we may find that it compels us to search our imagination for ways, other than ultimate ways, to express affection. We may even rediscover some past ways. A smart manufacturer could reproduce the colonial bundle-bed and bring old-fashioned country bundling back into vogue.

ORAL SEX

We have taken care of the lighter play. What about oral sex, sex involving contact between the mouth, the genitalia, the breasts, and other erotic zones? The signals from the research community are mixed on oral sex. The earliest studies found no evidence whatever that HIV is transmitted through oral sex regardless of by whom performed, how performed, and on whom performed. Indeed, these findings so surprised researchers reporting in the British medical journal, *The Lancet*, that they made a point of mentioning what they had *not* found:

> The absence of detectable risk for seroconversion due to receptive oral-genital intercourse is striking. That there were no seroconversions detected among 147 men engaging in receptive oral intercourse with at least 1 partner . . . accords with other data suggesting a low risk of infection from oral-genital (receptive semen) exposure.[55]

No researcher has totally discounted the possibility, but it is fair to say that all the early American and English studies heavily discounted the probability of seroconversion through oral sex.

The team of Masters, Johnson, and Kolodny dispute these findings as, indeed, they dispute many current understandings relating to the transmission of HIV. With regard to fellatio, they argue that "there is no known viral or bacterial sexually transmitted disease that is not spread—at least at times—by oral-genital contact." Their point has a certain common-sense persuasiveness.[56] But they do not present data that sustains their position.[57]

However, in October 1989, San Francisco's health director, Dr. David Werdegar, announced that his researchers were "absolutely sure" that they had recorded two cases of seroconversion through oral sex. The evidence consisted of interview testimony.[58] This was followed a year later, in October 1990, by an announcement by Dr. Warren Windelstein, professor of epidemiology at the University of California's School of Public Health, that results of a study of eighty-two men in the Bay Area indicated that 17 percent seroconverted as a result of participating receptively in oral sex. The men in question denied that they had been involved in any other risk behaviors, such as anal intercourse or IV drug use.[59] If such data are ultimately found to be persuasive by the scientific community, the early understandings will have to be altered.[60] I want to underline that most of the studies and observations have related to male-with-male oral sex, not male-with-female, or female-with-female. There is some very incomplete evidence that oral sex between men and women and between women can transmit the virus. The best that one can say is that, if it occurs, it is very unusual.[61] My own sense of the data is that with respect to all possible oral infections, transmission of the virus does happen, but it is rare.

At this point it is important to recall previous comments with regard to hard and soft data. The new findings suggesting that oral sex presents a higher risk than previously believed necessarily rest upon the accuracy of statements made by interviewees as to the character of their sexual behavior. More specifically it turns upon their denial of acting as the passive or receptive partner in anal intercourse.

My experience at the San Antonio AIDS Foundation and my understanding of Western intellectual history lead me to advise great caution in accepting such denials. At the San Antonio AIDS Foundation, counselors have often seen initial denials retracted as the clients gained confidence in the discretion and caring of the counselors. Why should a man fervently deny being the passive partner in intercourse? Because an unbroken intellectual tradition, stretching back to Aristotle, condemns it as contrary to the "nature" of man. This view asserts that the male was designed to be the dominant, active sex; passivity or receptiveness would be, therefore, a perversion of the proper order of nature. Early Christian thinkers such as St. Paul and St. Augustine embellished Aristotle with assertions of a divinely ordained "natural" male superiority. It was pointed out that Adam was, after all, first, and was made in the image of God. Both of them denounced men who allowed themselves to be used "as a woman" because it "lowers" a man, the original creation of God, to the lesser status of a woman. These ideas became part of early church law and the general Western moral code. They remain powerful today and can easily control verbal, if not always physical, behavior. The Aristotelian-Pauline-Augustinian assumptions and arguments should no longer be considered persuasive, but they are. Even on cursory examination they trip over one major and conclusive error—women are not, in fact, inferior to men. The premise is wrong. Still, it is not at all uncommon to encounter gay men, to say nothing of men who consider themselves straight, who cannot admit they participate in anal sex. To do so, they believe, would lower themselves to the status of women; they are hostages to a very wrong-headed Western tradition. It is easy for the scientist to overlook the awful, compelling power of our taboos because they are not readily measurable. Given the strength of data correlating receptive anal intercourse with HIV infection, given the paucity of data correlating receptive fellatio with infection, and given the power of the operating taboos, I would view statements denying anal sex with skepticism. Any study that finds an enhanced risk for oral sex on the basis of such denials must be examined with the greatest care. Each year thousands die of AIDS without being able to acknowledge the cause of their death even to relatives and friends. Similarly, I would wager, thousands become HIV+ without being able to admit to the behavioral source for their infection.[62]

Is oral sex risky or not? What is the answer? The answer is that, in the context of AIDS, the jury has returned a verdict of "possibly risky." However, it has long since rendered firm verdict with respect to other sexually transmitted diseases. Syphilis, gonorrhea, herpes, hepatitis B, various enteric diseases, and others are all transmitted through this practice, and there is ample evidence that the microbes involved in these diseases can be co-factors in the transmission and/or activation of HIV. The United States is experiencing epidemic levels of these STDs as well as AIDS.[63] The bottom line is that, to be on the safer side, barrier protection from condoms or dams is indicated.[64]

SEXUAL INTERCOURSE

Last, but hardly least, is sexual intercourse, vaginal or anal. Sexually speaking, these practices are the high road to HIV infection, especially for the receiving or (badly mislabeled) "passive" partner. Both forms of intercourse have strong potential for transmission of HIV particularly for the recipient partner; either infected seminal fluid is ejaculated into the partner's body, or the penis is put in contact with infected anal or vaginal tissues and fluids. In either situation, the virus can then make its way from its point of origin into the recipient's bloodstream either through ruptures in the interior linings or by direct interaction with mucosal cells.[65] The only access more direct to the bloodstream would be direct injection or transfusion with contaminated blood. The two modes of sexual intercourse do involve different public perceptions, resulting policies, and levels of risk.

Anal Intercourse. If there is any subject that has ranked high on the list of America's nondiscussable subjects, it is heterosexual or homosexual anal intercourse. In schools, Latin and Greek texts referring to this ancient sexual practice were left untranslated, mistranslated, or kept under lock in rare book rooms.[66] The fact that anal intercourse is one of the world's oldest and most widespread method of birth control is largely ignored in America. The general American public attitude toward it is revealed by opinion polls indicating that many believe you can get AIDS through anal intercourse even though neither partner is infected with the virus![67] Only very recently (and as a result of the examination of our behavior forced by AIDS) is explicit American evidence surfacing. A letter published in the July 24/31, 1987, issue of the *Journal of the American Medical Association* indicates that as many as 25 percent of American women engage in some anal intercourse, and about 10 percent do so regularly. The conclusion was that

> the number of women at risk through anal sex appears to equal the entire homosexual population of this country and exceed the number of homosexual men practicing receptive anal intercourse.

An ongoing study by Dr. David R. Bolling, M.D., director of Woman's Health Center of San Antonio, Texas, indicated that 728 of the 1,000 patients of the Center had tried anal intercourse, and 238 of those (33 percent) were frequent participants.[68] One of the principal works on heterosexual transmission lists heterosexual anal intercourse as a major vector.[69] In many Latin countries the possibility of exposure through anal intercourse is even more striking. The power of the Catholic tradition is such as to make condoms illegal or difficult to obtain, even if people wished to use them. In addition, the feudal-based traditions of "machismo" dictate that a woman be virginal upon marriage.[70] Both the requirements of premarital birth control and the maintenance of a technical virginity are met through anal intercourse. In addition to heterosexual anal intercourse, there is, of course, homosexual anal intercourse. There is no accurate measure of how many homosexuals participate in anal intercourse both as active and passive partners, but it is probably a sizeable majority. In any case, the number of sexually active people involved is large, and all are participating in risky sex.

Wherever practiced and for whatever reason, the fact is that of the myriad sexual modes, anal intercourse carries the highest risk of infection for the receptive partner, regardless of that partner's sex. In the British study on this subject the investigators stated that "receptive anal intercourse was the only sexual practice shown to be independently associated with an increased risk of seroconversion to HIV in this study, and could account for nearly all new infections."[71] Similarly, an American study concluded that "The data . . . confirm that receptive anal/genital contact is the major mode of transmission of HIV infection."[72] A recent study from the University of California at Berkeley reported that the men of a large cohort who were not receptive intercourse partners had an infection rate of 8.6 percent, whereas the men who were receptive partners had a rate that ran from 17 to 56 percent, depending upon the number of partners.[73] However, the risk for the active or insertive partner is less clearly established; none of the studies I have seen have been able to establish that the insertive partner was at enhanced risk for seroconversion, that is, a risk greater than would usually be associated with condomless intercourse.[74] In other words, the risk of transmission through anal intercourse is very asymmetric, and the receptive female or male bears most of the risk.[75]

Vaginal Intercourse. The dominant practice of the dominant majority carries the third highest risk of seroconversion; only direct transfusion and anal sex outrank it. What are the odds? The answer is that there is no clear answer. Most studies that have dealt with vaginal-intercourse transmission from one partner to another have used as their original or "index" HIV+ partner someone who was infected by surgical or blood product transfusion. The results indicate that the rate of transmission is extremely variable, from 10 to 61 percent. This variability is reflected also in the data relating to the relative risk of the male and female partners; some studies suggest that the risk is approximately equal or symmetrical, others that the female's risk is some seventeen times higher than that of her partner.[76] The variabilities can be explained partly by differing methodologies and parameters, and significantly different target groups from "non-drug using partners of IV users" to "wives of patients in Zaire." There are just not enough data in hand to be clear about the relative risks. A very theoretical study that received public attention in April 1988 stated that the chances of seroconverting as a result of one heterosexual encounter with someone who had tested free of the virus and during which a condom was used was 1 in 5 billion.[77] Other results from the same study indicated that the odds of seroconverting on the first encounter are 1 in 500 after engaging in condomless sex with an HIV+ partner and 2 out of 3 on or about the 500th.

Such findings are theoretically defensible, but no more useful than the statement: "It is highly improbable that you will be hit by a car while walking on an ice floe in the Antarctic." The authors of one of the studies mentioned above asserted that it was far more important that people chose partners carefully than that they avoid anal intercourse, use condoms, or limit their number of partners. More specifically they advised that heterosexuals should protect themselves by having sexual relations only with partners they know to be in "low risk" groups, even though they acknowledge that this is difficult to know. Advice that cannot really be implemented is of questionable value. An individual can refuse receptive anal intercourse, insist on using condoms, and limit sexual partners, but just how does a person determine that the attractive someone is neither directly nor indirectly (through past or other partners) involved in a high-risk category?[78] The authors have fallen into the trap of which Kinsey warned. The world is not divided into sheep and goats; on the contrary, sexually it is a world where frequently one cannot tell the sheep from the goats.

SAFER SEX AND PUBLIC POLICY

Properly considered, the risk statistics should give little comfort to anyone. *Sex has become an all-or-nothing game, that is, EACH TIME you play you are in a win/no-win situation.* It is totally unlike playing the odds elsewhere. If you lose betting on the races or buying a Lotto ticket you can, with luck, recoup another day; *if you lose playing the AIDS odds, the loss is irreversible and irremediable and your luck has completely run out.*

This harsh fact of life has many important implications for personal behavior as well as for government policy. For every individual it should rule out being the receptive partner in anal intercourse; all studies pinpoint this as the most dangerous sexual behavior. Regardless of one's sex, a personal policy of "Just saying NO!" can, in fact, save your life.

On the public level we must learn to discuss the "unmentionables." One of the most extraordinary revelations brought about by AIDS is the depth of ignorance about the possibilities, functions, and dangers of sex. When I was a boy, a well-meaning adult sat me down and gravely informed me that my sanity would be endangered if I masturbated. He was wrong, but that was sex education in the early 1940s. The recently published *Kinsey Institute New Report on Sex* leaves the impression that the level of general understanding has not changed much since.[79] Alan Wabrek, president of the World Association for Sexology, lamented, "There is probably no other field of knowledge where, as a society, we even suggest that keeping people ignorant is the best policy."[80]

In San Antonio, the Metropolitan Health District has made little headway in persuading the local school districts to implement meaningful AIDS avoidance education programs, and everywhere in the nation efforts at realistic sex education is met with determined opposition.[81] Except in the states most heavily affected by AIDS, colleges are not noticeably more enlightened. Some are now adding sexually transmitted diseases (STD) courses in recognition of the abysmal ignorance of the average first-year student. This is not to say that an eighteen year-old does not know how to have sex; he or she most certainly does! Not a great deal of "education" is needed there. It means only that the entering student is blissfully ignorant of the implications and dangers that lurk in sex. Nonetheless, progress is slow; it is an uphill battle to get open and honest courses in the first or second year college curriculum. School superintendents and college presidents alike dread sparking religious controversies and are wary of the public relations impact on parents who, being parents (I do not exempt myself), prefer to think of their children as serious students, rather than horny adults. The danger of these attitudes lies in the patent fact that the only thing more deadly than the virus itself is ignorance about it.

For its part, Congress continues to refuse funding for the national studies we need to get accurate information on American sexual behavior and will only support the blandest of anti-AIDS public education campaigns. The distaste and denial associated with anal intercourse and its incorrectly exclusive association with homosexual behavior is so strong that it is difficult to have any dialogue. Public education campaigns that honestly and directly confront the real world dangers are apt to be denounced by politicians and church leaders as pandering to "queers" and "sin," with predictably devastating results for funding. Even at the primary advising and care level, our taboos get in the way; it is often difficult to get AIDS counselors to raise the matter with clients, and the clients frequently do not want to hear it.[82] Nonetheless, pious and ambiguous generalities are not strong enough to help contain an epidemic.

In addition to avoiding anal intercourse, the number of sexual partners must be decreased, preferably to one. A point made strongly by most studies is that the risk of seroconversion is positively related to the number of different sexual partners. The subgroups within the San Francisco Men's Health Study displayed a range of seropositivity from 17.6 to 70.8 percent, depending upon the raw number of partners.[83] The results of the General Social Survey indicated that there were about eight hundred thousand men in the United States, ages eighteen to forty-four, who admitted to ten or more partners in the preceding twelve months.[84] As in the case of receptive anal sex, the figures clearly point to sensible personal policy.

However, the public policy implications stemming from multiple-partners data are more complex and difficult. Should government promote the formation of loyal, monogamous relations and discourage incidental, transitory relationships? If so, how? Should it, for example, make possible homosexual marriage so as to introduce some legally backed stability into those relations? Homosexuals are frequently criticized for being "unstable" and promiscuous, but currently no state provides legal recognition for a stable homosexual union. Should government make divorce more difficult, or exert tighter controls on sexually explicit, fast-track advertising and programming? Currently our media glorifies a lifestyle that is anything but an exemplar of stability, monogamy, and loyalty.

Any discussion of the multiple-partner problem must inevitably acknowledge the fact the fact that America supports an enormous, varied, and thriving sex industry from old-fashioned whorehouses, porno theaters, and sex shops, to so-called massage parlors, photo salons, dating clubs, baths, and singles bars, all of which promote transient contact and multiple exposures. Americans like sex; they just do not like to think about it. Different areas of the industry relate to the problem of containing AIDS in different ways. For example, if unbiased studies indicate that pornography is frequently used as a substitute for physical sex, and does not lead to interpersonal violence, then it would make sense for the national, state, and local governments to stop harassing the industry. On the other hand, a good argument can be made for closing or seriously regulating sex shops (as Nevada regulates prostitution) that provide the location and facilities for anonymous, fleeting homosexual or heterosexual sex. The impact on the sustainability of the epidemic that results from the activities of a superactive subgroup who regularly patronize these businesses is substantial. James R. Thompson, professor of statistics at Rice University, calculated that

> if only 10 percent, say, of the gay community frequented bathhouses, *even if the less active members of the gay community decreased their contact rate in order that the same total number of contacts in the gay community was maintained*, it could have the same practical effect as would have been obtained if the entire gay community doubled their contact rate.[85]

Thompson argues that had the bathhouses been closed early in the epidemic, HIV's spread might have been significantly curtailed. For a time fear accomplished what public health authorities were reluctant to do, but this time has passed—new sex emporiums are opening in New York City, San Francisco, and other places.[86] In any case, public fear never went so far as to demand closure of the heterosexual side of the sex business, though its role in sustaining other STDs like herpes is well documented.

A final point of agreement among the studies examining transmission is that the "proper use" of barrier latex condoms lessens risk.[87] By how much? The large statistical study referred to earlier assumed a 10 percent failure rate for condoms, a figure that manufacturers insist is too high. The Federal Drug Administration's inspection tolerance level is 4 defective (leaky) condoms per 1,000, a standard that resulted in the rejection of many manufactured lots in 1987–88. Condoms have been twisted, stretched, filled with water, blown-up like balloons, and pumped in machines—all in an effort to establish their reliability. They were even the subject of a major rating and testing article by *Consumer Reports* in March 1989.[88] All the data are necessarily inconclusive because none of the studies really field-tests the device. What happens in the course of anal and vaginal intercourse is what is really important, not what happens in laboratory simulations of what happens in bed. Still, lab simulations, anecdotal review by users, and commonsense are the best we are likely to get in this area.

No one can argue that condoms provide complete protection; they do fail for various reasons, and people have seroconverted in spite of consistent use.[89] The clearest evidence of efficacy comes from studies of so-called discordant couples, couples where one party is seropositive and this is known by the other. In those cases, consistent and careful condom use reduced risk of HIV transmission by 69 percent (87 percent effective in preventing pregnancy).[90] In addition, rates of all sexually transmitted diseases, including HIV, have dramatically decreased since 1982 within the San Francisco white, heterosexual and homosexual population, and this decrease is attributed by researchers to sharply increased use of condoms.[91] In sharp contrast to the

Reagan-Bush policy, the Clinton administration is clearly in favor of their use; in 1993 the Centers for Disease Control, the Food and Drug Administration, and the National Institutes of Health jointly issued a report on condom effectiveness and joined in urging their use.[92]

Data on adequacy aside, condoms are the only significant protection against the transmission of HIV during sex presently available. They are not only reasonably effective, they are an existing, cheap, and available means of prevention on the individual and the public level. Critics of them should be asked what they offer that provides protection while, at the same time, permitting sexual relations. I think the answer will usually reveal that it is not condoms they are opposed to, it is sex.

AVOIDING AIDS

So, how does one avoid being infected with the Human Immunodeficiency Virus? From the viewpoint of both drugs and sex, the basic answer is, "Don't let it into your body!"

If you shoot up the virus, you have committed suicide. Group use of syringes and needles is double dumb. Drugs are dumb to begin with; add HIV and unsterile works, and it totals double dumb. If multiple use of hypodermic syringes is practiced, then at least thoroughly cleanse and sterilize the works with a wash of household bleach.

What is "safe" sex? The answer is that it is a wonderful, romantic myth. What is "safer" sex? Safer sex is first and foremost an attitude. It is the belief that you can give and receive love without endangering yourself or your partner, that there are emotionally satisfying exchanges short of sexual intercourse. The attitude that people have to "go all the way" to prove their masculinity, femininity, or commitment always was juvenile and risky, but it is now potentially fatal. Unless there is a change of our basic attitudes relating to sexual relations, the educational campaigns urging safer behavior are not apt to have much sustained effect.

As a behavioral matter, the answer to what is safer sex involves a combination of proscriptions and recommendations, and *they are the same regardless of one's sex or sexual disposition—straight, gay, bisexual, or whatever.*

But first I must make one exception. I do not believe that the concept of safer sex can apply to sexual relations between individuals—one of whom is known to be HIV+ and the other not—unless sexual intercourse and receptive oral sex are absolutely excluded. Omitting these sexual responses, there still remains a rich assortment of oral, visual, and tactile stimuli, including massage and masturbation. So the exclusion does not mean that one cannot have a loving, sexual relationship with an HIV+ partner; it means solely that any penetrative sexual relationship is risky. There is nothing to

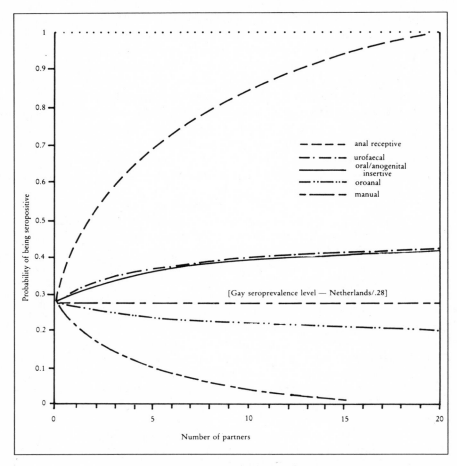

FIGURE 5.1 Sex Practices and Risk

Source: G. J. Van Greinfen, R. A. P. Tielman, and J. Goldsmit, "Prevalence of HIV/HTLV III Antibodies in Relation to Lifestyle Characteristics in Homosexual Men in the Netherlands" (paper presented at the International Conference on AIDS, Paris, June 1986), as reproduced in Tony Coxon, "The Numbers Game—Gay Lifestyles, Epidemiology of AIDS and Social Science," in Peter Aggleton and Hilary Thomas (eds.), *Social Aspects of AIDS* (London: Falmer Press, 1988).

be gained, and much to be lost, by ignoring the fact that penetrative sex with someone known to be HIV+ is a form of Russian roulette. The use of condoms does not change this perspective. First, in neither vaginal nor anal intercourse does the receptive partner have a reliable way of insuring that a condom, or an effective condom is, in fact, being used. Second, it may well be that even consistent use of condoms does no more than delay the inevitable; condoms can leak and can fail.[93] There is evidence that many established couples (especially in hemophiliac families) make a conscious decision to continue sexual intercourse even after one has seroconverted (so-called discordant couples); they make a judgment that the maintenance of their sexual bonding and love is more important than the possibility of transmission. That is their right, and we can only wish them well. However, I cannot label it safer sex. It is dangerous—but then, love and sex have always been dangerous.

The reality, however, is that in most cases, a person entering into intimate relations with another will ordinarily not have reliable information about the partner's HIV status. The partner may be genuinely HIV negative, may not know one way or the other, may be misinformed (as when he or she has tested negative, but falsely), or may lie. Under these circumstances the only reasonable course is to assume that the partner is a potential carrier and protect yourself either by abstention from the most intimate forms of sexual relations or by using such protection as has been demonstrated to offer good protection.

No form of sexual expression other than unprotected, condomless intercourse has been shown to present a major risk for the transmission of HIV. Barrier protection with condoms or dams, especially if lubricated with products containing 65mg nonoxynol-9, a spermicide toxic to HIV, reduce risk to acceptable levels.[94] By "acceptable levels" I mean levels of risk lower than we assume in our daily lives without much thinking about it—the risk of a fatal auto accident, of sport and gun accidents, and active and/or passive smoking, for example. Anal intercourse is extremely dangerous for the "passive" partner even with a condom, since condom failure is more likely in this mode.[95] Until a preventive vaccine is developed, receptive anal intercourse should be unequivocally excluded from everyone's portfolio of sexual expression. Vaginal intercourse is safer in that it is a less efficient mode of viral transmission and is less likely to produce condom failure. The risks involved in both forms become unacceptable if one partner has a sexually transmitted disease of any kind but especially one that produces genital sores or lesions. If you see a sore or a rash, go no further. What evidence we do have indicates that oral sex is not an efficient means of transmitting HIV, but remember, it works just fine for everything else. So condom use is indicated here also. Finally, multiple partners and/or using any substance, like alcohol or drugs, to the point where your sense of self-preservation is dulled, enhances all risk, perhaps fatally.

The U.S. Public Health service estimates that by the end of 1993 millions of Americans will prove to be infected by the Human Immunodeficiency Virus. The AIDS syndrome that terminates this infection will have killed more than two hundred thousand of us. It has also killed a game that millions once enjoyed, a game called "Casual Sex."

Notes

1. Except for the anchor categories, the ranking is approximate and suggestive only. Clearly the transfusion of contaminated blood (#1) presents an almost 1:1 (95 percent) chance of infection. The chance of infection from blood bank supplies would depend upon the seroprevalence within the population of donors. In Zambia the chance would be high, in the United States low. For #11: The American Association of Blood Banks stated in 1989 that the chance of being infected by screened blood in the United States was between 1:100,000 and 1:200,000. Estimates as to the possibility of infection through unprotected anal intercourse (for the recipient partner) and medical accident like a needlestick from an HIV+ patient are both about 1:200.
2. Some of the variations, however, would not easily occur to someone not reading the literature. For example, a major concern has been the transmission of AIDS through the use of sperm, frozen or otherwise, dispensed from Sperm Banks. In October 1989 New York passed stringent new regulations requiring that sperm banks test donors twice in a six-month interval before their sperm was used in artificial insemination.
3. Robyn R. M. Gershon, David Vlahov, and Kenrad E. Nelson, "The Risk of Transmission of HIV-1 through Non-percutaneous, Non-sexual Modes: A Review," from the Department of Environmental Health Sciences, and the Department of Epidemiology, The Johns Hopkins University School of Hygiene and Public Health, distributed by the Gay Men's Health Crisis, *AIDS Clinical Update*, October 1, 1990.
4. For example, in 1993 there was transmission between brothers, one an HIV+ hemophiliac. Apparently they were using the same razor. Another involved a transmission between two small children, one of whom was subject to frequent nosebleeds. See *AIDS News Service*, VA Medical Center, San Francisco, December 10, 1993.
5. Uncircumcised men may be five to eight times more likely to seroconvert from heterosexual intercourse than circumcised men; genital ulcers increase one's chances of seroconversion four to five times. See "Circumcision May Protect against AIDS Virus," *Science* (August 4, 1989), 470. Research released at the IX International Conference on AIDS document that having syphilis, gonorrhea, or other STDs can increase the chance of successful HIV transmission "a hundred fold." Similarly a simultaneous transmission of HIV and another STD is a guarantee of both infections. See Lawrence K. Altman, *New York Times*, June 11, 1993, A6.
6. Others fluids can also be infectious but are not likely to be encountered, such as cerebrospinal, synovial, pleural, pericardial, peritoneal, and amniotic.
7. "Transmission Risk-Estimate Matrix," developed by The Center for AIDS and Substance Abuse Training, Falls Church, Virginia—a group sponsored by NIAID, and the Colorado Department of Health. Disseminated by the sci.med.aids newsgroup, *Internet*, December 4, 1993.
8. There is a documented case of "first encounter" transmission in the story of

Slidon Gertz who was exposed in her first sexual encounter at age 16. See *USA Today*, August 10, 1992, A2.

9. For a good summary of the problems in accurate projections, see "Projecting the Incidence of AIDS," *JAMA* (March 16, 1990), 1538 et seq. On the original estimate of the Coolfont Planning Conference, see M. I. Macdonald, "Coolfont Report: A PHS plan for Prevention and Control of AIDS and the AIDS Virus," *Public Health Reports* 101 (1986), 341–48; and D. J. Bergman et al., "Future Trends," same issue.

10. For a brief but very good discussion of the data reliability and projection problems, see Peter Aggleton and Hilary Thomas, *Social Aspect of AIDS* (London: Falmer Press, 1988). Chapter 7, "The Numbers Game," deals specifically with the difficulties of getting reliable responses for statistical data on matters involving sex. The authors are generally, to be put it mildly, very skeptical of the American data in general and the CDC reports in particular.

11. *Health InfoCom Network News*, October 16, 1989.

12. E. O. Laumann et al., "Monitoring the AIDS Epidemic in the United States," *Science* (June 9, 1989). CDC's answers and the authors' counterreplies are in September 1, 1989 of *Science*. The General Accounting Office, in a backhanded swipe at the CDC estimates, suggested that perhaps the CDC needed a larger budget to expand its surveillance staff. See *National Journal* (July 1, 1989), 1715.

13. The CDC uses a method that assumes an incubation period of ten years before an AIDS diagnosis. Using the number of AIDS cases *reported*, and given a ten-year period, the number of seropositives needed to produce that number of AIDS cases can be estimated. There are many problems with the system. Most nongovernmental epidemiologists come up with higher seroprevalence figures than does the CDC—it is a conservative estimate.

14. For a good review of the statistical problems and the understatements, see William B. Johnston and Kevin R. Hopkins, *The Catastrophe Ahead* (New York: Praeger 1990) chap. 3.

15. Criticism of the CDC's catering to White House political directives has come from many sources and perspectives. See *Journal of the American Medical Association* (September 16, 1992), where the CDC was flatly accused of "public health malpractice" as it strived to be politically rather than medically correct in its presentation of data and recommendations. One glaring example from the early history of the epidemic comes from the disclosure that the CDC did possess data relating to the intrusion of HIV into the injecting drug community but did not use it because it would confuse the presentation of the epidemic as strictly a gay problem. Another example can be found in the CDC's adoption, in 1992, of very conservative "obscenity" tests for screening AIDS education and prevention programs submitted for funding. The CDC, in allocating its $350 million educational support funds, insisted, in line with Reagan-Bush policy, that AIDS control messages stress abstinence and be cleared by local panels as not "obscene" or "offensive." Also see Elizabeth Etheridge, *Sentinels for Health, A History of the CDC* (Berkeley: University of California Press, 1992).

16. Stephen C. Joseph, *Dragon within the Gates: The Once and Future AIDS Epidemic* (New York: Carroll and Graf, 1992), chap. 6.

17. The definition used by U.S. Social Security System and by the various state rehabilitation commissions in determining whether someone is eligible for AIDS disability financial assistance runs six, double-columned, single-spaced pages of small print. More than one person living with AIDS has died before the bureaucrats could

determine whether the individual was "sick" within the definition.
18. See various reports in *JAMA* 260, no. 15, 2213.
19. I should note that, to confuse things further, some states, like Texas for example, commenced using the definition adopted by the federal government in 1993 almost a year earlier. Furthermore, both the national government and the states recalculate their annual reported totals as cases are more accurately attributed to the year of diagnosis. Thus a case reported in 1994 may actually have been first diagnosed in 1990. It will eventually end up back in the 1990 total, although it will first appear as a 1994 report. This makes for historical epidemiological accuracy, but a great deal of confusion as well, because the figures take a long time to stabilize.
20. P. Chu et al., "Cause of Death Among Persons Reported with AIDS," *American Journal of Public Health* (October 1993), 1429. The manual involved is the World Health Organization's *Manual of the International Statistical Certification of Diseases, Injuries, and Causes of Death* (Geneva, 1977, updated 1987).
21. The "ARC" designation is now considered obsolete. Earlier it was thought that there might be a syndrome of conditions which would not necessarily progress to AIDS, and which could, therefore, be properly thought of as a separate set ailments. It is now clear that this is not so.
22. Kinsey, Pomeroy, and Martin, *Sexual Behavior in the Human Male* (New York: Saunders, 1948), 19. And see Kinsey et al., *Human Behavior in the Human Female* (New York: Saunders, 1953).
23. The CDC uses these criteria to classify: (1) "Homosexual or Bisexual" equals anyone who reports same-sex sexual contact. (2) "Heterosexual" equals [a.] anyone who reports specific opposite-sex contact with someone in a high-risk groups, e.g., IDU, or [b.] anyone who does not report same-sex or risk-group contact but was born in a Pattern II nation as defined by the World Health Organization. A Pattern II country is one in which the dominant form of transmission is heterosexual.
24. For example, if you tell a Latin American, Caribbean, Mediterranean, Middle Eastern, or Azerbaijani male that he is "gay" because he has a male lover, you may provoke a dangerously violent reaction in defense of his machismo or honor. Those cultures limit the idea of homosexuality to the so-called passive partner. AIDS workers quickly discovered this in San Antonio, where a HIV+ Puerto Rican emigre may have both male and female sex partners and be considered absolutely straight—so long as he is the dominant or active partner.
25. Kinsey, Pomeroy, and Martin, *Sexual Behavior in the Human Male*, 25.
26. Ibid., 19.
27. The model for projecting AIDS cases developed by mathematician Yakov Fuxman takes this approach. His model reflects individual risk factors, rather than categorized groups. For that reason it projects farther into the future and more accurately. See Rebecca Voelker, *American Medical News*, December 22, 1989, 4.
28. For example, see the scenarios portrayed in Johnston and Hopkins, *The Catastrophe Ahead*, 137–46. The World Health Organization projects that by the year 2000, 80 percent of all HIV infections will have resulted from heterosexual contact, up from 60 percent at present. See *HIC Medical News*, December 9, 1990.
29. Susan D. Cochran and Vickie Mays reported on their studies on this matter in the Correspondence section of the *New England Journal of Medicine* (March

15, 1990), 774. Their general conclusion was that a sizeable percentage of college-age, sexually active students (more men than women) do not tell the truth about their sex lives to their partners.

30. Across the United States and the World there is a significant variation in population seroprevalence. The New York-Washington-Boston population corridor has the highest seroprevalence rate in the nation, with the South Bronx the highest within that area. On the other hand, North Dakota is, so far, relatively untouched by the epidemic. The entire picture, then, relates both to what you do and where you do it.

31. Masters, Johnson, and Kolodny, *Crisis: Heterosexual Behavior in the Age of AIDS* (New York: Grove Press, 1988), chaps. 1 and 2.

32. See the story filed by Nancy Nusser from Mexico City, Cox News Service, "AIDS on Increase; Gays Ignore Risks," *San Antonio Express-News*, September 16, 1990, 2G. "Study of Behavior—Non-identifying Gay Men," *CDC HIV/AIDS Prevention*, August 1993, 6.

33. An acupuncture case was reported from France. See *New England Journal of Medicine* (January 26, 1989), 250.

34. The use of crystal and crack contribute greatly to unsafe sexual practices. A person, especially a female, on these drugs is twice as likely to contract AIDS in a sexual setting then one who is not.

35. See the study and its citations Jordan B. Glaser and J. Strange, "Heterosexual Human Immunodeficiency Virus Transmission Among the Middle Class," *Archives of Internal Medicine* 149 (March 1989): 645–49.

36. "Drug Abusers with AIDS Virus Are Selling Plasma, Study Finds," *New York Times*, April 25, 1990, A10, reporting on a Johns Hopkins School of Hygiene and Public Health study that documented that 23 percent of the 2,921 IV drug users surveyed in the Baltimore area in 1988 and 1989 said that they had sold plasma or donated blood after they began IV drug use.

37. See *Wall Street Journal*, February 28, 1988, 24E.

38. The National Commission was so disturbed that it took the unusual step of issuing a preliminary report eight months earlier than mandated by the Congressional Act creating it.

39. Heterosexual IV drug users enrolled in a San Francisco Drug Treatment Program. Richard Chaisson et al., "Cocaine Use and HIV Infection in Intravenous Drug Users in San Francisco," *JAMA* (January 27, 1989), 561–65.

40. See "Study of IV Drug Users and AIDS Finds Differing Infections Rate, Risk Behaviors," *JAMA* (December 2, 1988), 3105. "Links between Cocaine and Retroviral Infection (Editorial)," *JAMA* (January 27, 1989), 607–8.

41. Don C. Des Jarlais et al., "HIV-1 Infection among Intravenous Drug Users in Manhattan, New York City, from 1977 through 1987," *JAMA* (February 17, 1989), 1008–1012.

42. Robert A. Hahn et al., "Prevalence of HIV Infection among Intravenous Drug Users in the United States," *JAMA* (May 12, 1989), 2677–2684.

43. Ibid., 2679.

44. Ibid., 2679.

45. See D. C. DesJarlais and S. R. Friedman, "AIDS and IV Drug Use," *Science* (August 11, 1989), 578. The authors point out that the drug problem is really not one problem; there is considerable variation to be found within the total group that uses intravenous injection. In Sweden, for example, 50 percent of the heroin users are HIV+, while only 5 percent of the amphetamine injectors

are. Why? Similarly, the seroprevalence rate among IV users in New York City is 50 percent, in San Francisco 15 percent, and in Los Angeles 5 percent. Again, why the differences?

46. Stephen Labaton, "Surgeon General Suggests Study of Legalizing Drugs," *New York Times*, December 8, 1993, A11.

47. Stephen Joseph, former New York City Commissioner of Health, tells an interesting story of how his proposals for needle exchange got caught up in the Koch versus Dinkin mayoralty campaign. To the delight of Black and White ministers, Dinkin, the challenger, spoke earnestly of the immorality of Koch's exchange program, and Koch's support of needle exchange was one of the factors that beat him. After Dinkin took over as mayor, he cancelled the program, but later he reinstituted and took credit for it. Stephen Joseph, *Dragon within the Gates: The Once and Future AIDS Epidemic* (New York: Carrol & Graf, 1992), chap. 8.

48. Michael Gray, "Fighting AIDS with Needle Exchanges," *American Medical News*, February 16, 1990, 33 et seq. On the Vancouver program, see *New York Times*, April 17, 1990, A7.

49. See Don C. DesJarlais and Samuel R. Friedman, "AIDS and the Use of Injected Drugs," *Scientific American*, February 1994, 82–88; and "Two Studies Back Idea That Addicts Will Trade in Their Drug Needles," *New York Times*, January 17, 1994, A12.

50. See the testimony of Dr. Evridiki J. Hatziandreu, Congressional Office of Technological Assessment, *New York Times*, September 19, 1990, A12.

51. Alan R. Hinman, M.D., Director of the Division of Sexually Transmitted Diseases, Centers for Disease Control, *Sexually Transmitted Diseases Treatment Guidelines*, 1989 (Washington, D.C., Public Health Service, MMWR series 38, No.S-8, October 1989).

52. Masters, Johnson, and Kolodny in *Crisis* argue that the data is inadequate on this point due to the fact that kissing as a form of sexual behavior is not behaviorally or statistically isolated from other forms occurring simultaneously, and therefore it is not possible to conclude that transmission of virus did not occur from kissing. The problem they raise bedevils the entire area of AIDS research and the recommendations that flow from it. The inevitable ambiguities are exploited by those who advocate a use of mandatory testing, contact tracing, and quarantine in the AIDS epidemic. See for example the upscale, "yuppie" approach to promoting a homophobic, fundamentalist epidemic control agenda in *New Dimensions* 4, no. 3 (March 1990).

53. Compare Otis R. Bowen, M.D., Secretary of the Department of Health and Human Services, "What You Should Know About AIDS," (U.S. Public Health Service, Centers for Disease Control, 1987) with C. Everett Koop, M.D., Surgeon-General of the United States, "Understanding AIDS," (Washington, D.C.: U.S. Government Printing Office, Public Health Service, Centers for Disease Control, 1988.)

54. P. C. Fox, A. Wolff, C. K. Yeh et al., "Saliva Inhibits HIV-1 Infectivity," *Journal of the American Dental Association* 116 (1988), 635–37; P. N. Fultz, "Components of Saliva Inactivate HIV," *Lancet* 2 (1986), 1215.

55. Lawrence A. Kingsley, Richard Kaslow et al., "Risk Factors for Seroconversion to Human Immunodeficiency Virus among Male Homosexuals," *Lancet* (February 14, 1987), 348. The *Lancet* study confirmed an earlier one reported in the *Journal of The American Medical Association* by Warren Winkelstein et

al., "Sexual Practices and Risk of Infection by the Human Immunodeficiency Virus: The San Francisco Men's Health Study," *JAMA* (January 16, 1987), 321. Also see D. Lyman et al., "Minimal Risk of Transmission of AIDS-Associated Retrovirus Infection by Oral-Genital Contact," *JAMA* 255 (1986), 1703. A. R. Lifson, "Do Alternate Modes for Transmission of Human Immunodeficiency Virus Exist?" *JAMA* 259 (1988), 1353–1356. Alan Lifson, M.D., M.P.H., is an epidemiologist at the Federal Centers for Disease Control working at the San Francisco Department of Health.

56. One researcher contends that the data used by Masters et al. does not support their arguments. See E. H. Kaplan, "Crisis? A Brief Critique of Masters, Johnson and Kolodny," *Journal of Sex Research* 25, no. 3 (August 1988), 317–22. And see *AIDS Alert, The Monthly Update for Health Professionals* 3, no. 2 (April 1988), an issue in which the authors of some of the research studies cited by Masters deny that their work is being properly used by the authors.

57. Masters, Johnson, and Kolodny, *Crisis*. And see "Transmission of HIV Infection from a Woman to a Man by Oral Sex," *New England Journal of Medicine* (January 26, 1989), 251. Two clinicians associated with the Lahey Clinic Medical Center of Burlington, Massachusetts, report what they believe to be the first documented case of seroconversion due to oral sex.

58. Associated Press dispatch dated October 12, 1989, *Science/Medicine AIDS Newsgroup* (distributed electronically through the InterUniversity BITNET system).

59. See the Associated Press release of October 7, 1990, "AIDS by Oral Sex Higher than Expected," *San Antonio Express-News*, October 7, 1990, A1. There have been other clinical or anecdotal indications of some risk, but none of sufficient persuasiveness to dislodge the earlier consensus that oral sex has presented a risk so low as to be negligible.

60. See M. C. Samuel et al., " Factors Associated with Human Immunodeficiency Virus Seroconversion in Homosexual Men in Three San Francisco Cohort Studies," *Journal of AIDS* (March 1993), 303–12, and A. R. Lifson et al., "HIV Seroconversion in Two Homosexual Men after Receptive Oral Intercourse with Ejaculation: Implications for Counseling Concerning Safe Sexual Practice," *American Journal of Public Health* (December 1990), 1509–1511.

61. See "Epidemiology of Reported Cases of AIDS in Lesbians," *American Journal of Medicine* 80 (1990); "Update: Epidemiology of Reported Cases of AIDS in Women Who Report Sex Only with Women," *Journal of AIDS* 6 (1992).

62. A British social scientist states flatly that "studies of the *reliability* of self-reports of sexual behavior show that, in general, the retrospective recall of information tends to be selective, ordinally distorted and unreliable" (my emphasis). See Tony Coxon, "The Numbers Game–Gay Lifestyles, Epidemiology of AIDS and Social Science," in Peter Aggleton and Hilary Homans (eds.), *Social Aspects of AIDS* (London: The Falmer Press, 1988), 126–38.

63. Rebecca Voelker, "STDs Near Epidemic Levels, Experts Agree," *American Medical News*, June 2, 1989, 3. According to the testimony, the United States has experienced a 67 percent increase in hepatitis B since 1978, and now has about 30 million cases of genital herpes. Both of these venereal diseases are clearly implicated in the spread of HIV.

64. Apart from the risk of disease transmission, it might be noted that sodomy can be legally risky. In about one half of the states it is illegal. A Maryland trial judge in 1988 imposed a five-year prison sentence upon Steven Schochet for having

oral sex with a woman to whom he was not married. The sentence was upheld by the state court of appeals, citing as authority the United States Supreme Court's decision in *Bowers v. Hardwick*, 487 U.S. 186 (1986), a case that upheld Georgia's sodomy laws as it applied to homosexuals.

65. "The Transmission of AIDS: The Case of the Infected Cell" (Commentary), *JAMA* (May 27, 1988), 3037.

66. Peter Fryer, *Private Case–Public Scandal* (London: Secker and Warburg, 1966).

67. June M. Reinisch with Ruth Beasley, *The Kinsey Institute New Report on Sex: What You Must Know to be Sexually Literate* (New York: St. Martin's Press, 1990).

68. See the discussion "Sex Experts and Medical Scientists Join Forces against a Common Foe: AIDS," *JAMA* (February 5, 1988), 641–43.

69. Nancy J. Alexander et al., *Heterosexual Transmission of AIDS*, Proceedings of the Second Contraceptive Research and Development Program International Workshop, Norfolk, Virginia, February 1–3, 1989 (New York: Wiley-Liss, 1989), chaps. 2 and 3.

70. This was rationalized in terms of the man's honor but, in fact, had more to do with maintaining the lines of descent that established, in a feudal society, claims of control over property and power. The church elaborated rules of legitimacy to clarify lines of descent and thereby stabilize property relations and control from the king on down. The alternative was civil strife. Premarital pregnancy as well as adultery were intolerable because they both confused and endangered orderly succession to property and power. Prospective queens had to be virginal and were examined to make sure they were. Adultery with a queen was high treason. The king could sire illegitimate children without endangering the legitimate succession to the throne, but the queen could not, because only she could, as it were, palm off her child as the child of the king and legitimate heir to the throne. In illegitimacy lay the beginnings of civil war in a feudal monarchy.

71. Lawrence Kingsley et al., "Risk Factors for Seroconversion," *Lancet* (February 14, 1987), 347.

72. Warren Winkelstein et al., "Sexual Practices and Risk of Infection," *JAMA* (January 16, 1987), 24. See also "The Transmission of AIDS" (Commentary), *JAMA* (May 27, 1988), 3037.

73. Article in *News from NIAID*, June 9, 1993, entitled "Summary of San Francisco Young Men's Health Study, 1993." National Institute of Allergy and Infectious Diseases.

74. The only study I have seen that attempts to establish rough quantitative relationships between active or "insertive" anal intercourse and probability of seroconversion is found in Aggleton and Thomas, *Social Aspects of AIDS*, 136–37.

75. The data, especially from Africa, indicate that the insertive partner is at high risk of acquiring infection from in infected partner if he has genital sores (as from herpes infection) which can act as a portal for the virus. Apparently uncircumcised men are also at higher risk.

76. Thomas Peterman et al., "Risk of Human Immunodeficiency Virus Transmission from Heterosexual Adults with Transfusion-Associated Infections," *JAMA* (January 1, 1988), 55–58. "The Transmission of AIDS, The Case of the Infected Cell," 3037. Editorial, *JAMA* (October 7, 1988), 1943.

77. Norman Hearst and Stephen Bailey, "Heterosexual AIDS," *JAMA* (April 22, 1988).

78. On the point "How do you know?" see the very interesting discussion in *JAMA*

(October 7, 1988), 1879–1891.

79. Reinisch and Beasley, *Kinsey Institute New Report on Sex*.

80. Quoted in *San Antonio Express-News*, October 16, 1990, 3A.

81. "Lack of AIDS Teaching Rapped," *San Antonio Express-News*, October 6, 1990, 8B.

82. This problem is not unique to America by any means. See Rachel Sternberg, "Fighting Taboos, Fighting AIDS—Mexican Health Officials Focus on Prevention," *American Medical News*, February 3, 1989. The Muslim Middle East is another area where religious and cultural taboos get in the way of accurate reporting and counseling.

83. Warren Winkelstein et al., "Sexual Practices and Risk of Infection," *JAMA* 57, no. 3 (1987), 321. But it is not a simple matter. Multiple exposures and multiple partners are different matters and frequently difficult to disentangle. Nonetheless, the conclusion stated by one group, contains a strong implied warning and recommendation, "As infectivity estimates are revised upward or as variable infectivity levels become significant, the risk associated with multiple sexual partners increases." D. P. Francis and J. Chin, "The Prevention of AIDS in the United States," *JAMA* 257 (1987), 1357, and *JAMA* (October 7, 1988), 1879.

84. Leads from the "Morbidity and Mortality Weekly Report," Centers for Disease Control, *JAMA* (October 14, 1988), 2020.

85. James R. Thompson, "Taking Sides, AIDS: Old Disease, New Society," *This Side of Rice* (April–May 1988), 12. This publication circulates mainly at Rice University. For accessible statements on the AIDS epidemic by Professor Thompson, see "AIDS: The Mismanagement of an Epidemic," *Computers and Mathematics with Applications* 18 (1989), 965–72, and "A Simple Model of AIDS," in *Empirical Model Building* (New York: John Wiley, 1989).

86. See United Press International Release, November 17, 1993, "Warning Issued to Gay Sex Clubs," on the threat by San Francisco health authorities to close some clubs that were failing to enforce safer sex guidelines. CDC, "AIDS Daily Summary," November 19, 1993.

87. It is important to specify "proper" in this context. First, the condom must be put on correctly to minimize the possibility of breakage with no captured air bubbles except at the tip. Second, it must be of the latex variety and not be lubricated with petroleum based products which cause the latex to break down quickly. Water-based lubricants with nonoxynol-9 are preferred. Third, condoms must be used consistently to have any significant statistical safety advantage— just "once-in-a-while" will not do.

88. "Can You Rely on Condoms?" *Consumers Reports* (March 1989), 135–41.

89. See Johnston and Hopkins, *The Catastrophe Ahead*, 70-72 on condoms, and the references cited there.

90. S. C. Waller, "A Meta-analysis of Condom Effectiveness in Reducing Sexually Transmitted HIV," *Social Science Medicine* 36 no. 12 (1993), 1635–1644.

91. Gina Kolata, "AIDS in San Francisco Hit Peak in '92, Officials Say," *New York Times*, February 16, 1994, A6. Centers for Disease Control Reports, "Current Trends: Heterosexual Behaviors and Factors that Influence Condom Use among Patients Attending a Sexually Transmitted Disease Clinic—San Francisco," *Morbidity and Mortality Weekly Report*, October 4, 1990.

92. CDC, "Update: Barrier Protection against HIV Infection and other Sexually Transmitted Diseases," *Morbidity and Mortality Weekly Report*, August 6, 1993.

93. The Mariposa Foundation, Topanga, California, has studied condom effectiveness

for years. Together with UCLA and USC it tested and published condom-leakage and effectiveness ratings for over 30 brands. The scores ran from 91.3 percent impermeable to HIV to 21.3 percent. The top ten were Ramses nonlube (91.3 percent), Ramses Sensitol (91.3 percent), Gold Circle Coin (85.2 percent), Gold Circle (83.7 percent), Sheik Elite (83.7 percent), Durex Nuform (81.7 percent), Pleaser (80.2 percent), Ramses Estra (78.7 percent), Embrace Her (77.3 percent), and Hot Rubber (77.2 percent).

94. Eve K. Nichols, *Mobilizing against AIDS* rev. ed. (Washington, D.C.: NAS, 1989), 150.

95. G. J. Van Greinfven, R. A. P. Tielman, and J. Goldsmit have plotted curves comparing the probability of seroconversion as functions of type of sex and number of partners. Anal intercourse stands out dramatically as the most dangerous practice. See Aggleton and Thomas, *Social Aspects of AIDS*, 136–37, which discusses and reproduces the curves presented in the original Van Greinfven report (Van Greinfven, "Prevalence of LAV/HTLV III Antibodies in Relation to Lifestyle Characteristics in Homosexual Men in the Netherlands." Paper presented to the International Conference on AIDS, Paris, June 1986).

6

The Infected Body Politic

All natural disasters, be they earthquakes or epidemics, place the individual and the commonwealth under a multitude of strains. Some, like earthquakes or a firestorm of flu, are mercifully fast. After the event the nation pulls itself together, swings into action to clean up damage, bury the dead, and hopefully to install controls to ameliorate the cost in lives and treasure of the next episode—for there is always a next episode. Other peoples around the globe rally with assistance; all understand that "There, but for the Grace of God. . . ." The recent earthquakes that devastated Mexico City, Soviet Armenia, and California come to mind.

However, AIDS is a catastrophe of a compellingly different kind. It did not strike like a snake, rather it burrowed (and continues to burrow) insidiously like a giant mole under the walls of the republic, undermining lives and challenging the genuineness and solidity of our social, economic, and political commitments. It had already done enormous damage before the nation became aware of its existence. Between 1980 And 1983 a few courageous and prescient individuals, such as Dr. Michael Gottlieb at UCLA, playwright Larry Kramer in New York, and journalist Randy Shilts in San Francisco, warned of the danger, but their calls of alarm were lost in a wilderness of disbelief, denial, and inertia.[1]

This was the time, the early 1980s, when AIDS and its costs might have been contained, but effectively raising the alarm entailed serious political risks in all the affected communities—the political, the religious, and the homosexual. Political and religious leaders took their cue from President Reagan's deafening silence, and most national, state, and local public and private institutions dithered through the critical years (see AIDS dispersion map for 1984, Figure 7.1).

The lack of leadership can be attributed to many perfectly ordinary and understandable human reactions. There is a natural tendency to ignore bad news and hope that "it" will go away, or "it" will turn out to be nothing more than a recapitulation of the embarrassingly baseless swine flu scare of President Ford's administration. Until his friend Rock Hudson died in 1985, President Reagan apparently thought of AIDS as something like a passing epidemic of measles.[2] Clearly also, within the highest ranks of the establishment, there was a general lack of sympathy for, and sense of community with, those who were perceived to be the main victims in the early years.

However, in fairness, it must be admitted that the establishment's policy of not-so-benign neglect was matched by the myopia of gay leadership, as well as a singular lack of comment from people in contact with IDUs through the administration of drug programs. Effective action from within the nation's various gay communities, the communities most affected in these early years, was severely hampered by a Gordian's Knot of self-doubt and denial. Homosexuals are not immune to the perceptions of them encountered in the heterosexual mainstream. Indeed, most of the culture's most homophobic attitudes are internalized in the homosexual; the victim is taught to believe in the essential rightness of his oppressor's position.[3] Perhaps, many wondered, the epidemic *was* a plague sent by God. I remember an eighteen-year-old client of the San Antonio AIDS Foundation saying to me one day, "I know that I have to bear this as well as I can. I got it because I was playing around, and God is punishing me." I wondered how one so young could believe that his life, barely underway, was so corrupt and sinful as to deserve such a fate; he hadn't even had the time to become a proper sinner. In addition, the gay leadership in such cities as San Francisco and New York feared that acknowledging that there was a connection between aspects of the male gay lifestyle and viral spread would invite a majority backlash, wiping out their recent gains in establishing community identity and autonomy.[4] The silence of those working within the IDU population is harder to explain. One of the more plausible explanations is that drug users are subject to death or illness from so many causes that no one really noticed the surfacing of still another.

For all of these reasons and more, the virus went relatively unchallenged during its first years in America; it took a deep and firm hold. Too many of our political, religious, and economic leaders, both gay and straight, turned their backs on the afflicted and ignored the developing epidemic. Now all of us will pay the bill for their failure of conscience and negligence. Here and abroad, the costs will now be beyond measure.

The American philosopher George Santayana once said, "Those who do not remember their past are condemned to repeat it." Now we must relearn a lesson our ancestors of the Civil War learned the hard way, that we all live in one house; what destroys some of us, threatens all of us. We cannot isolate ourselves from the spread of the virus and the multitude of effects

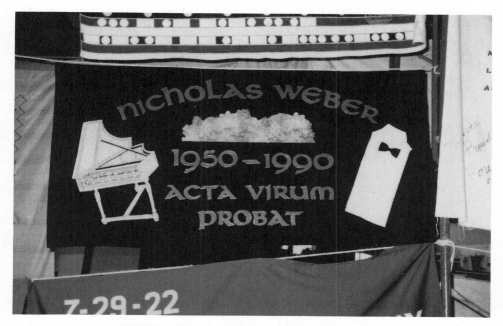

FIGURE 6.1 Panel from the AIDS Memorial Quilt:
Nicholas Weber, Harpsichordist and Composer, Panel 0155-6

that follow in its wake; we cannot run to the country as people did in the days of the bubonic plague. We are an urban civilization, and the viral carrier lives next door. As a united people we will contain this dreadful epidemic. If we divide along class, lifestyle, ethnic, or religious lines, the HIV will undermine the health of our Republic as surely as it does the lives of its individual citizens.

THE CORROSION OF GRIEF

Generations ago an action for damages could be filed for the emotional injury that resulted from being left at the altar. It was the action for breach of promise to marry. Gilbert and Sullivan, in their own inimitable way, lampooned it in *Trial by Jury*. It is no longer recognized as an independent cause of action, not because the injury is unreal or insubstantial, but because we concede that the injury is not subject to the quantitative measure that modern judges and juries insist upon before awarding compensatory damages. Everyone who has lived a little can testify that emotional injury is very real, and that grief is debilitating. But how much is the injury worth in cold cash, in hard dollars? It is all too subjective and ambiguous, too difficult to produce reasonable evidence; our legal system tends to break down when confronted with such intimate matters. It is somehow ironic that we can measure the weight of cosmic dust falling upon the earth, or the dimensions of an infinitesimally small expression of nature like the Human Immunodeficiency Virus, but we cannot measure the value or weight of the universally experienced phenomenon of human grief. But measure or not, we owe it to those who have died and will die in this epidemic to acknowledge their suffering. Properly, we must pay them homage for being the source of knowledge that may save future generations of maturing, sexual adults from the horror of AIDS.

Even if we cannot measure our sorrow, we can express it. Indeed, to stay healthy, we must express it. AIDS has stimulated the development of a whole new aesthetic of grief in plays, stories, visual arts,[5] and even displays of art in the world's galleries.[6] It has also inspired one of the most moving memorials created in our time, the AIDS Memorial Quilt. It is an enormous patchwork quilt composed of about thirty thousand coffin-sized panels bearing the names of those who have died of AIDS; portions of the quilt tour the nation.[7] It is comparable only to the Vietnam War Memorial in Washington, D.C. The War Memorial was erected by a nation grieving its dead and, perhaps even more, the death of its delusions of global invincibility. The quilt is being sewn by grieving parents, spouses, lovers, and friends in an effort to express their grief. Some representative panels of the quilt have now been added to the collection of the Smithsonian Institute. Whether on display as a public monument, or as an artifact of grief in the "nation's attic," the two are similar in that they are composed of names, and names, and more names; names of people killed in war, names of people killed in an epidemic, all of them together now in the equalitarian commonwealth of death. But there is also a melancholy difference between the two. The Vietnam Memorial with its almost sixty thousand names is finished. The quilt will not be completed in our time, for the epidemic marches on and the list gets longer. A complete quilt in a scant twenty years might well require 7 million panels in America alone![8]

It seems to me that the pain and suffering following in the wake of AIDS have some qualities with which it is especially hard to cope and that set it apart from other disasters. First, AIDS strikes hardest at the young adult; it cuts people down in the full vigor and bloom of their youth. Those who care for AIDS patients testify that this is the most demoralizing aspect of their work, with emotional burn-out a constant hazard because of it.[9] There was a seventy-year-old AIDS patient named Jake at the hospice where I volunteer. He was a wonderful, if sometimes irascible, old gentleman who put up with little nonsense from the many younger clients of the foundation. He could soundly whip all of them at any game of cards, and he would occasionally condescend to teach the skills of bridge or poker. All of the volunteers were concerned about Jake, but somehow it was not the same as their concern about the younger clients. We did not want Jake to suffer, we wanted him to be as comfortable as possible, but the greater measure of grief was reserved for the twenty-year-old to whom he was teaching poker. We knew that Jake's students would never really have the opportunity to practice and hone their new skill the way Jake had over a long lifetime. I think we all instinctively understand that it is the younger age group that holds the future of the nation in its hands; there is an enormous difference between our emotional reaction to someone dying after almost three quarters of a century of living, and one who is just beginning.

A second difficulty lies in the fact that, for the foreseeable future, there is no closure to the epidemic nor to the grief that it will cause. In war a person is killed, we conduct rites, we bury, and eventually the pain subsides to manageable proportions. There is closure. Only for those unfortunate people whose loved ones are still Missing in Action is there a special kind of continuing grief, precisely because the books cannot be closed; there is no finish, no closure. The great epidemics of the past took their toll and burned themselves out; we portrayed these deadly events as an arrival of the Grim Reaper who, with the scythe of death, mowed broad swaths through fields of people. But as reapers do, he moved on. Now with AIDS he proposes to stay a while—at least into the twenty-first century—as a major partner in our lives and loves.

Third, these problems are worsened by the fact that AIDS is a diabolically deceptive disease with a long season of dying. Those who are infected may present no outward sign of the affliction for many years. Then, when they start to show their illness, they frequently look and feel fine one month only to look and feel sick the next. The up periods generate hope, false hopes that are dashed to bits by the following down stage. The erratic character of the affliction together with the long period of general decline can find everyone, patient and survivor alike, silently praying for death, for closure at the end.

Finally, the plague-mentality endemic to our religious and cultural tradition makes it difficult for survivors to confide in and get necessary support from the circle of relatives and friends who ordinarily would be there for them. There is widespread concealment and deception on both the personal and public level. Frequently the shame of dying from AIDS affects patients so strongly that they delay notifying parents until the last minute, if at all. In my experience, the parents usually rally to the support of their afflicted children no matter what, but they often find themselves very much alone with the problem. They do not feel as though they can confide in their relatives and friends to gain the emotional support they need. The best known instance of attempted concealment was Rock Hudson's attempt to keep the information from his lover and the public. His action formed the basis of the successful damage suit against his estate. One of the striking evidences of the stigma's power can be seen in the obituary columns. In San Antonio there have been over nine hundred deaths from AIDS, but there have been very, very few obituaries that have acknowledged that fact.

None of us can live with active, corrosive, gnawing grief indefinitely. We need to put an end to it and get on with the business of living. Elizabeth Kubler-Ross's famous five stages of dying (denial, anger, bargaining, depression, and acceptance) apply not only to the patient, but also to the patient's surviving spouse, lovers, parents, and friends. I have frequently witnessed them go through the same process, especially the bargaining stage. But for survivors there must be one more stage—between depression and acceptance there must be closure for without it there is no acceptance. Twenty-five hundred years ago the Greek dramatist Sophocles had his heroine, Antigone, challenge King Creon in order to bury her fallen warrior brother. Creon's decree, denying him a soldier's burial, condemned his spirit to wander hopelessly forever, a tormented shade upon the earth. Antigone, in one of the great speeches of all drama, indicted Creon for violating the eternal laws of nature, laws that not even a king could change. Defying the king, she buried her brother to give peace to his soul and rest to her grief.[10]

But kings can be defied with more effect than disease. AIDS will give us no quick closure, no respite; it will test our capacity for compassion and grief. Many of us will try to deny it, discount it, and ignore it rather than confront and contain it. This is natural. This is understandable. It is also futile. In the end avoidance behavior will just prolong the agony, as well as enhance the guilt that all survivors feel who have failed to do what they could. The only way we can achieve closure, to close the books on grief, is to satisfy ourselves that we have cared for the afflicted with love and compassion, that we have done what we could do. Like Antigone, we must do our duty, do what is right, both for our own peace of mind as well as for the souls of our fallen kindred.

PROFIT AND LOSS

It sounds almost obscene to utter the phrase "profit and loss" in the context of such a human calamity, but if we are looking at the costs of AIDS, utter it we must. Montaigne, in one of his shortest essays, reminds us that "no profit is made save at a loss to someone else."[11] AIDS is a natural biological event just as an earthquake is a natural geological event. It is a devastating psychological event with both individual and group impact. It is a religious event with potential both for the stimulation of future good as well as the rekindling of past evil. It is also a politico/economic event of stupendous magnitude.

Anne Skitovsky, an expert in health economics, estimated that by 1991 the national economy would be absorbing a $55 billion annual loss in productivity attributable to illness and premature death due to AIDS.[12] The figure is higher than might otherwise be the case due to the fact that AIDS strikes most vigorously at those between twenty and forty years old, the age group that in gross terms is the most productive, the backbone of the workforce. However, the $55 billion figure is actually a very low estimate since a future earnings lost projection is too simple a measure to accommodate the complex character of AIDS costs.

Lost earnings projections do not, for example, factor in the extraordinary toll of major talent that this epidemic is recording. Anyone who reads the collective obituaries that occasionally appear cannot help but be impressed with the economic and creative significance of many of those afflicted.[13] Major figures in all fields have been infected; some have died; others, like Earvin "Magic" Johnson of the L.A. Lakers, are still fighting. In politics the list includes notables like Paul Gann, a leader in California Republican politics; Sheldon Andelson, regent of UCLA, whose Los Angeles home was referred to as the Western White House during the Kennedy years; Terry Dolan, master GOP fundraiser and founder of the National Conservative Political Action Committee. People in show business like Amanda Blake, the popular "Miss Kitty" of Gunsmoke, Rock Hudson, Liberace, Anthony Perkins, and the great dancer Rudolph Nuryeyev have died. Larry Kramer, playwright, author, and major AIDS activist, is still fighting for himself and others. However, in February 1994 one of the epidemic's earliest and most acute observers himself died of AIDS. Randy Shilts, national AIDS correspondent for the *San Francisco Chronicle* and author of three books, most notably, *And the Band Played On: Politics, People and the AIDS Epidemic* (1987), died at age forty-two. The fashion designers Perry Ellis and Roy Halston, as well as one of America's leading fine art photographers, Robert Mapplethorpe, have died. Actress and author Dorothy Mueller; Methodist Bishop Finis Crutchfield of Texas; Dr. Tom Waddel, Olympiad; Arthur Ashe, tennis champion; and France's Michel Foucault, one of the twentieth century's leading intellectuals, are also on the dread list.

In my home town of San Antonio, a civic leader named "Hap" Veltman succumbed in 1989. He was one of the handful of local businessmen who, years ago, had the vision and drive to inspire downtown revitalization and historic preservation; everyone in San Antonio lives in a more beautiful city partly because of him. Every major city can now record similar names and cases. The costs of losing people of this caliber are staggering, ultimately incalculable. Even more melancholy is the understanding that behind the men and women who did have the opportunity to enhance our national culture is a generation of young men and women who will not have the time to enrich us.

As we move from the intangibles of personal loss, through estimated manpower and creativity losses, to tangible matters like payouts, it is clear that the AIDS epidemic involves enormous sums. Private insurers commenced paying out over $1 billion in health and death claims in 1989. The pay-out is expected to reach $15 billion by 1995. In 1994 it was estimated by the American Council of Life Insurance and the Health Insurance Association of America that the lifetime insurance costs of treating a person with HIV infection were $119,000.[14] The estimated cost of insured care prior to a formal AIDS diagnosis was $50,000, following diagnosis the cost was $69,000. The overall costs of treatments are expected to reach $10.5 billion in 1994.[15] These amounts will have to be prorated out to all surviving private policy holders and eventually to the entire taxpaying public.

On the profit side of the ledger, HIV is rapidly generating a multibillion dollar industry. The national government's aggregate AIDS-related expenditures went over the $2 billion mark in 1989 and will continue to rise. In addition the combined states are spending over $500 million a year; this figure will also rise. These funds are funneled to scores of universities, medical research centers, and hundreds of community groups. Thousands of highly skilled researchers, laboratories, equipment companies, outreach workers, and the like are thus gainfully employed in an area that did not exist ten years ago.[16] In addition, an entirely new crop of AIDS-related companies reflecting hundreds of millions of dollars in capitalization have sprung up to produce and market everything from genetically engineered vaccines to safe-sex dolls.[17]

The market potential in all the aspects of AIDS stimulates the business oriented, including the con-man, both here and abroad.[18] One of the corporations listed in a *Wall Street Journal* review of new AIDS-related businesses, Amnion Inc., estimated a $100 million per year market in just their area of blood recycling machines. Another firm estimates a $3 billion per year market in diagnostic tests within ten years. The year 1988 experienced an international shortage (and price increase) in surgical rubber gloves and, after decades of languishing ashamedly in the pharmacist's drawer, the condom now proudly occupies its own display area in market and drugstore in addition to making an appearance on thousands of college campuses. The market for effective preventive and/or therapeutic vaccines staggers the imagination and just the suggestion that a firm may be developing an effective vaccine can boost its stock value;[19] every sexually active human being on the earth would be a potential consumer until everyone was inoculated and the virus was no longer a serious threat to our species.[20] Even televangelism is effected. AIDS has been a boon to evangelists. With the breakup of Communist Soviet Union their old fund-raising appeals, based on fighting "godless, atheistic communists," became obsolete. They now successfully appeal for money to fight against the sex and sin that God is punishing by means of an epidemic (and earthquakes). The bottom line is that the epidemic is a worldwide reality that national economies are confronting in a variety of ways. Millions will die from AIDS, billions in public and private capital will be spent to combat it, and even more billions in new income will be generated by it.

HEALTH CARE COSTS

Direct health care costs are extremely difficult to estimate at this stage of the epidemic. The Skitovsy study cited earlier estimates that by 1991 hospital costs will have reached $8.5 billion annually with PWAs occupying 1.2 percent of the available beds and accounting for 1.4 percent of the total personal health care expenditure.[21] Additional direct costs include hundreds of millions of dollars in testing, blood screening, research, and education. At the individual level it is estimated that the average total costs of care after diagnosis will be approximately $85,000.[22] Adding the indirect costs of lost productivity to this produces an estimate that approaches a $100 billion overall cost in 1991.

Although high, it does not appear that the calculable health care costs of AIDS are out-of-line with those resulting from other serious traumas. The lifetime per patient costs of persons suffering a major heart attack (myocardial infarction) is $66,837, for cancer of the digestive system $47,542, for leukemia $28,636, and for paraplegia from an auto accident $68,700. The figure of $55 billion mentioned above as the value of lost productivity may seem high, but actually it is expected to be no more than 12 percent of the total figure in 1991. AIDS is costly and getting more expensive each year, but it not so costly as to have structural impact on the American economic system. To put it another way, the American economy can absorb the impact of AIDS and, as a matter of fact, can afford and ought to allocate more funds for research, education, and treatment than it now does. This is not true for some third world economies; AIDS has the potential of breaking their backs and pushing whole nations back fifty years in developmental time.[23]

The projection of costs leads inevitably to the question, "Who picks up the bill?" In thinking about this, it is useful to apply the classic apportioning model of personal injury law. With regard to any injury (or illness), the cost can first of all be borne by the injured party. You have parked your car at the curb. Overnight an hitherto unsuspected subsurface sinkhole collapses, swallowing your car. You pay.

Or the one whose action led to the injury can be held liable for costs.

You have parked your car. Your neighbor comes home late, suffers a stroke while driving, and sideswipes your car. He pays.

Finally, the costs can be allocated among third parties who are strangers to the events leading to injury or ailment. One or both of you have purchased comprehensive insurance covering such unforeseen calamities. In that case, payment is assumed by all policyholders in the group to which you belong. The group can be privately defined, as with a Blue Cross policy, or publicly defined, as in Medicare or Medicaid.

There are, of course, many permutations, combinations, and nuances in the actual design and administration of these alternatives, but at bottom there are only the basic three to work with. Stating the alternatives is easy, but nothing else in the field of tort or personal injury law is straightforward. Except in the simplest of cases, the equities of apportioning cost raise philosophic, jurisprudential, and legal problems that tax our finest minds. Indeed the main thrust of modern practice has been legally to insist that everyone carry insurance so questions of individual apportionment do not rise at all—no-fault auto insurance and assigned risk pools are examples.

Applying this model to the costs of AIDS care leaves little room to doubt that the wisest course of public policy lies with the third alternative. Indeed, it is the only realistic one. It could be and has been argued that AIDS victims (except pediatric and transfusion) should bear the cost of their illness because it was incurred in voluntary activities such as sex or injecting drug use. This is basically the position of the American far right, especially the evangelical, fundamentalist portion of it. Whatever quasi-religious arguments can be made, the real world result would be that the afflicted would receive no care other than that which might come from private charity (presumably not the charity of the evangelical or fundamentalist). The suggestion that the cost be shared or borne by the "injurer" would lead to the same result. First, it would be difficult in most cases to establish the identity of the injuring party—who is the injurer in injecting-drug transmission? Second, even if identification were possible (as it is in some cases), the position generally leads to the shifting of costs to another sick and dying person who cannot pay his or her own bills. This is not to say that in some individual cases these positions might make some sense. However, as a matter of public or general policy, they both lead to the same result, that is, no treatment and no care. Assuming the American community evolves a compassionate response, then it must amortize over time and apportion over the entire population the costs of this disaster, just as it has done with the catastrophic costs associated with other aspects of being human, like aging or injury in an earthquake.

Although common sense appears to indicate a national insurance approach, this may not be a sufficient argument for the sorely tried taxpayer who is asked to foot the bill for a seemingly endless list of late-twentieth-century crises. What is the general taxpayer interest that justifies the expenditure of billions? The justification arises from the fact that we are all, like it or not, bound together in a hazardous urban lifestyle. The policy of the state cannot eliminate the hazards and risks of this fact. However, as President Clinton has pointed out, it can alter and distribute the attendant costs in order to alleviate the burden, a catastrophic burden in the case of AIDS, to any single individual. For example, it permits, and in some cases mandates, the shifting of accident costs, incidental to industrial process, to the large group that consumes the product. It does not demand that the individual worker or employer shoulder the entire risk of producing the article that the public wants, which cannot be produced with total safety. When you purchase a car, part of the price reflects the cost of the inevitable worker injuries that will occur in its manufacture. When you drive it on the expressway, you will, unknowingly, already have paid for the worker injuries and deaths incurred in its construction. You and the workers are bound together in an invisible community of interest. For different reasons, each of you have a vital interest not only in the production process but in the safety of that process. In addition, the state can pay costs directly out of general funds, which is another kind of apportionment by which the cost is spread through the entire taxpaying community. Examples of this approach would be the approximately $500 million in non-Medicaid disbursements from the state governments for AIDS. Federal matching Medicaid funds add another several billion.

What is the community of interest that binds together the sick and the well? Why should the well be willing to assume, as third-party payers, the costs of those caught up in this epidemic or, indeed, any epidemic? First, we are and should feel bound together by the reality of our own frailty and vulnerability as unaided individuals. Any other posture is self-destructively arrogant. We need to remind ourselves of the unpleasant truth that such very expensive programs as are now funded, for example, to defray the high but lifegiving costs of kidney dialysis—the annual cost of which is almost twice ($5 billion) that of the entire 1994 AIDS budget—might well be paralleled in a program that any of us could need in the future. To support and help the afflicted is to invest in our own future well-being. This is especially and poignantly true in the case of AIDS for the simple reason that, as pointed out in chapter 2, HIV is *our* virus. We have no really good animal models on which to test vaccines and drugs. Consequently, the only authoritative source of information that we all need for our protection is that developed in testing and treatment protocols using fellow humans as volunteers. The quality of health care available to each and every one of us is built squarely on the experience gained in caring for those who got sick before us.

In our search for treatments it is not possible to distinguish in principle between "nice" supportable afflictions and "unapproved" afflictions; the viral, bacterial, and fungal agents of our various ailments make no such distinctions. Only forty years ago having cancer was unmentionable—cancer was a sin as well as a sickness. John Wayne and his studio feared, with good cause, that if the public knew of his bout with lung cancer it would end his acting career; cancer, the "Big C," was the 1940s equivalent of leprosy. Similarly, former Congressman Coelho's childhood epilepsy was believed by his parents to be a divine punishment, and his church refused to accept him a student for the priesthood.[24] One can only hope that at least a voting majority, if not all of us, have graduated from this level of stupidity.

Second, on another level each of us clearly shares a community interest in the quality of public health. Commencing with the Pure Food and Drug Act and Meat Inspection Act of 1906, we have manifested our concern through a host of statutory regulations and programs ranging from food handling inspections to wide-ranging grants of power to track, control, or abate various infectious diseases. The federal and state Public Health Services, which have played such a prominent role in educating us, owe their very existence to this social interest. The CDC and all our national and state regulations reflect the truth that, in a crowded urban civilization, the well-being of each of us is tied to the health of all of us. HIV is not the first, nor will it be the last dangerous virus to spread rapidly in our urban culture. Virologists are constantly tracking and trying to contain pestilential agents that breakout of their home base, and more than one health care worker has died in the containment attempts. Indeed, epidemiologists are now recommending the establishment of international tracking stations, outposts that could give us fair warning that a breakout has occurred—the viral equivalent of our hurricane tracking facilities.

There is no sensible, realistic option but to express our group interests with group techniques. The application of group insurance programs to cover AIDS is the only approach that makes sense. The group can be defined as a large cohort of employees in a single firm, or the entire population of the nation, whichever works best, but it is an exercise in futility to attempt to resolve a general problem with case-by-case individual decisions. The national $500 billion bail-out of insolvent savings and loans associations is an example from outside the public health area; this failure of government to effectively regulate savings and loan management is costing each and every one of us at least $5,000 in taxes. What is the community of interest between the sick and the well in this epidemic? It is simple: the sick want to get well, and the well do not want to get sick, and in the end both are dependent upon coordinated group action to plan and fund the epidemic's containment as well as to subsidize the development of effective treatments and/or vaccine safeguards.

The epidemic has sharply underscored the fact that the United States, alone among major nations, has neither a unified, coherent health care insurance system, nor a method of rapid, effective drug testing and delivery. This is in spite of the fact that Americans spend more on illness than any other people. Medicare is a program limited to the elderly, who are largely unaffected by the epidemic, or those who have been "disabled" for two years. Medicaid for the poor is actually fifty different state programs, many of which lack benefits or access rules appropriate to a disease like AIDS. In Texas, as in other states, for example, those who become eligible for Social Security Disability automatically lose their national Medicaid entitlement. However, unlike other states, Texas does not substitute a state program for the lapsed national one. This means that there is a two-year hiatus of medical insurance coverage for the patient between the time of Medicaid's end and the triggering of Medicare. Most AIDS patients do not last that long, they die before satisfying state and national eligibility rules; as taxpayers who have helped fund these programs, they are defrauded by the rules.

Finally, about 35 to 50 million Americans have no health insurance at all. Our nation accepted a basic responsibility for the health of its citizens only in the administration of President Lyndon Johnson, although there had been agitation for action as far back as the first term of President Franklin Roosevelt in 1932. We have moved slowly, hesitantly, and with a lack of efficiency, cost, and quality control that only a very rich nation could tolerate. Gradually, and partly as a result of the AIDS epidemic, major business and political leaders are recognizing this fact of our history and speaking out for reform. In April 1989 Chrysler's Lee Iacocca suggested that "maybe we should go to school on the national health care systems in Europe and Japan and design one for ourselves."[25] More significantly, the American Medical Association is now proposing what is, in effect, a national health plan to restructure the U.S. system so that it would cover all Americans. The AMA's program is called "Health Access America," and it represents a striking departure from the AMA's older stance opposing anything smacking of "socialized medicine."[26] Finally, in the presidential campaign of 1992, President Clinton made the provision of a national health care plan one of the major proposals of his bid for the White House (see "Clinton and AIDS," in chapter 6). AIDS may be the proverbial straw that breaks the back of America's complacency and short-sightedness.

THE EMERGENCE OF NATIONAL POLICY

As has been said in this book many times, the epidemic of the HIV is a natural phenomenon obeying biologic laws of mutation, transmission, and survival. So also is politics a natural phenomenon, a natural expression of our species. Politics is basically about the continuing struggle of all us for a piece of the pie (which we now call the Gross National Product); it is about who gets what, where, and when. At its best, it is a governed and orderly competition that is geared to respond to tangible power as measured by aggregated capital and voting blocs. At its worst, it is war. But neither in peace nor in war does the political system respond to claims of compassion and humanity as readily as it does to claims of power. Like the virus, politics operates in accordance with many set rules—Machiavelli cataloged many of them in *The Prince*—and it would be foolish to expect these rules to be displaced because an epidemic entered the land.

The business of the politician, the art of governing, is that of compromising, conciliating, and finding accommodation for the various claims emerging from people's lives and dreams. The politician builds bridges among peoples and interests, does so within finite budgets and resources, and works in a twilight zone where the line between ethical and unethical conduct is sometimes hard to see. Queen Elizabeth I, a consummate royal politician, called her policy on church matters (the policy that served as the foundation for the Anglican/Episcopal Church) the path of "The Golden Mediocritie." Somehow, that says it all. When the politicians fail, we resort to force. Epidemics are hard for politicians to cope with. Epidemics are about death and dying, about pain and suffering, and they are bad for business. They confound the political system. The politician cannot run "for" an epidemic, or "against" it; both postures would be silly. Effectively coping with catastrophes such as global AIDS do call for truly great and courageous political leadership, something that is in short supply everywhere. The lack of it in America during the past few decades is one among many factors that have allowed both an epidemic and a drug culture to take firm root in the land.

Of course some issues are more amenable to political resolution than others. It is one thing to construct a coalition over the design of the new city hall, quite another to do so when emotionally charged issues like slavery, abortion, drug use, death, or sex are involved. In these areas our treasured cultural mythologies and religious codes often conflict with real world facts, making a reasonable decision difficult. Politicians quite rightly think of such issues as "no win" issues, and they shy away if possible. For example, most heterosexuals firmly believe that homosexuality is unnatural and sinful. They have been taught this by the ministers of the Western church (who enjoyed a monopoly on education until almost the twentieth century) since the days of St. Paul. Paul denounced all pleasurable, nonprocreative sex whether heterosexual or homosexual, regarded women largely as creatures who lure God-fearing men into lust and sin, and taught that, on the whole, it would be best if the species gave up all sex in order to prepare for the Day of Judgment—which he believed was just around the corner. St. Augustine and St. Thomas Aquinas seconded and elaborated on his views later. Given such a heritage, it is no wonder that today it is difficult to discuss any sexual issue rationally in the political area.

An illustration of the impact of our sex-negative origins appears in the debate on whether or not to distribute condoms in prison. AIDS has become a leading cause of inmate death in all areas (like New York) with high sero-prevalence levels. The major sexual mode of transmission is anal inter-course, which most prisoners do not regard as homosexual behavior in the closed all-male prison environment. With few exceptions, those in charge of such matters have avoided the obvious policy.[27] To distribute condoms in an all-male prison community would be to admit openly and officially that illegal sex acts are taking place. It is certain that political opponents would make it appear that the decision-makers condoned such acts. Moreover, distribution of condoms would be tantamount to admitting that the police cannot enforce the law even in prison, and if not there, where? The upshot is that lives have been and will continue to be sacrificed to the needs of myth maintenance and the political necessities of winning within America's sex-negative political arena.

Moreover, it is hard to make political capital out of an epidemic. This is not to say no one tries. In 1918 some charged that the Spanish flu, which killed over five hundred thousand Americans, had been deliberately intro-duced by German U-Boats spraying the Port of Boston with active virus. In the 1980s African political leaders denounced the West for the anti-Black, neocolonial suggestion that the virus originated there, while some American political figures were looking for evidence that it was the product of Soviet genetic engineering. The Russians, for their part, spread the rumor through-out Africa that the virus was another instrument of American biological warfare. The French, meanwhile, blamed American tourists, and we blamed Haitians and homosexuals. Oblivious to this nonsense, the virus continued to spread.

REAGAN AND AIDS

The first five years of American political reaction to the surfacing of AIDS was a compound of deprecation, derision, disbelief, and denial. Clearly the most important single variable determining political reaction was the early identification of AIDS with homosexual sex. Neither Walter Mondale nor Ronald Reagan, the presidential candidates, nor any official or party docu-ment made reference to AIDS in the campaigns of 1984 even though, by that time, public health experts and agencies were issuing alarms. It was largely Rock Hudson's highly publicized death in 1985 that forced national politics out of the AIDS closet to admit the danger and begin forming policy.

Fiscal Year	Public Health Establishment Request	Presidential Request	Congressional Request
1983	—	—	5.5
1984	—	—	28.7
1985	59.9	39.8	61.4
1986	91.0	60.5	108.6
1987	196.0	126.4	244.3
1988	351.0	213.2	355.4
1989	(Consolidated)	766.4	951.0
1990	1600.0	1300.0	1200.0

Source: *National Journal*, August 30, 1986, p. 2046.

Table 6.1 Request for AIDS Funding, 1983–1990 (in millions of dollars)

After 1990 AIDS-related appropriations are found in many different portions of the national budget. From 1991 the budgets for the National Institutes of Medicine, Centers for Disease Control, Defense Department, Social Security, Health and Human Services, Medicaid/Medicare, and the Agency for International Development contain AIDS-related appropriations. For this reason, it becomes very difficult to determine the total AIDS-related appropriation, and almost impossible to determine how much is actually being spent.

President Reagan acknowledged the existence of AIDS only when his friend died a celebrity's death while a stunned world watched. By the time he did acknowledge the epidemic, over ten thousand Americans had died.

The administration's response was slow and reluctant; public statements and administration policy indicated that a calculation had been made to the effect that those most affected were of little political consequence to the fortunes of the Republican Party and, consequently, there was no need for vigorous action.[28] No agency of the Reagan administration made an official budget request relating to AIDS until the fiscal 1985 proposals were sent to Congress. These came three years after the first alarms were sounded. In 1982 and 1983 Congress, acting on its own initiative, appropriated a total of about $34 million, and established the pattern of congressional, rather than presidential, leadership that persisted until President Clinton took office. Reagan's reluctance to address the issue ran counter to the strongly worded advice of the National Academy of Sciences and a virtually unanimous public health establishment.[29] The president's basic attitudes can best be inferred, perhaps, from the budgets he presented over the years of his administration (Table 6.1).

Only in his last going-out-of-office set of proposals for fiscal 1990 did his recommendations approximate the amounts called for within his own administration and, even then, the sum was no more than the cost of one nuclear submarine.[30] Responding to growing criticism of his inaction, Reagan established a Presidential Commission on AIDS in 1987. The opening months of the commission's life were most unpromising as the body became paralyzed by internal bickering; it was generally characterized as long on conservative politicians and short on AIDS experts. The first co-chairpersons resigned in disgust,[31] leading to the appointment of Admiral James D. Watkins (Ret.) as chairperson. Admiral Watkins turned the commission around dramatically. He proved to be another Surgeon General Koop. A conservative officer who was expected to remain quietly within Reagan policy guidelines, Watkins became an ardent and articulate spokesperson for vigorous presidential leadership and national action. Faced with the realities of the epidemic, the Presidential Commission produced a report in June 1988 with 579 recommendations—many of which called for policies strongly opposed by representatives of the ideological right in the White House.[32] The commission recommended the authorization of almost $2 billion more than the 1989 appropriation for AIDS and the related problem of drug abuse.[33] The outcome was that President Reagan declined to support his own commission's recommendations. Dr. Donald Ian MacDonald, the president's spokesperson, explained that the "White House" felt that some of the commission's central recommendations (for example, those calling for federal laws to guarantee confidentiality of HIV test results or prohibit various forms of discrimination) would amount to rewarding "disapproved" behaviors.[34] Presumably, if someone faced social, employment, or legal problems due to disclosure of positive test results, it was only just deserts. The fact that lack of confidentiality would effectively undermine any national testing program was considered irrelevant to the main moral and political issue. Instead of supporting his own commission, President Reagan issued a policy paper in August 1988 that Washington quickly dubbed the "Reagan 10-Point Inaction Plan."[35] In his term of office, President Bush implemented it.[36]

PLAGUE OR EPIDEMIC?

During the 1985–88 period AIDS-related political coalitions began to take shape, and they tended to polarize around the basic postures outlined in chapter 1, that is, the nonjudgmental, epidemic position on the one hand, and the religiously judgmental, plague position on the other. Powerful spokespersons for both positions appeared in the national and state governments. Agency officials concerned with biomedical research, public health, and epidemic control were compelled to walk a political tightrope between them. Complicating matters at the national level was the fact that the Reagan administration was publicly and firmly committed to a tight-money policy with regard to all nondefense domestic spending. The additional research and public health expenditures needed to fight the epidemic promised to "unbalance" the budget.

The leading national actors who emerged during this period representing the "epidemic" position were Surgeon General C. Everett Koop in the administration, and in the Congress by Senators Edward Kennedy (D-Mass), and Lowell P. Weicker, Jr. (R-Conn) and Representative Henry A. Waxman (D-Cal). The "plague" position was articulated in the administration by Secretary of Education William Bennett, and in the Congress by Senator Jesse Helms (R-NC) and Representative William E. Dannemeyer (R-Cal). It would be inaccurate to see the two blocks as matching a liberal-conservative or Democratic-Republican split. For example, Senator Orrin Hatch (R-Utah), a leading conservative, was and remains a strong backer of the public health approach, supporting initiatives of his Democratic colleagues in the Senate. Likewise, the leading Reagan administration "epidemic" spokesman, Surgeon General Koop, considered himself a social and political conservative. On the other hand, it is true that those coming from the "plague" perspective have tended to be mostly, but not entirely, conservative Republicans.[37] Back of each of these two groups of officials were loosely defined coalitions of social, religious, and economic interests that, for one reason or another, had and continue to have a stake in AIDS related government policy.

The fundamental difference between the two positions originates in and continues to stem from their reaction to the large number of homosexuals among the afflicted.[38] The plague position is essentially negative from the standpoint of government intervention. Federal money ought not be used for people whom Senator Helms, resurrecting Victorian terminology, refers to as "sodomites." Their sex practices are rejected by the American public and their affliction is a well-deserved punishment of God. His judgment on injecting drug users is not noticeably more benign. Consistent with this approach, Senator Helms fought the authorization of funds to help AIDS patients purchase AZT, and Representative Dannemeyer called for "routine" mandatory testing without guarantees that the results would be legally confidential. Proponents of this stance in the administration and Congress have successfully resisted efforts to modify Medicaid access rules for the benefit of PWAs who were dying before they qualified.

On the other hand, significant expenditures for research on vaccines is accepted as a long-term investment in the health of the heterosexual community, although why the nonsinful should need such protection is not clear. Money for infected children is justified as appropriately Christian. Federally financed public education is admitted to be necessary, but campaigns must be decorous in language so as, to quote a leading Victorian, "not to bring a blush to fair maiden's cheek" nor, more to the point in the 1990s, not to offend America's politically potent church conservatives.[39] Secretary Bennett successfully insisted that public educational material emphasize sexual abstinence and undefined "family values" rather than condom use.[40] Nancy Reagan's now famous motto "Just say NO!" became the battle cry for both the "war on drugs" and the "war on AIDS."

These attitudes were frequently mirrored at the state level. For example, the 1989 Texas public health budget tried to insure that not a penny fell into the hands of community groups that may be "gay operated" even though such groups have been the agencies that pioneered effective hospice programs and provided a large part of needed care to everyone regardless of the mode of infection. Following Secretary Bennett's lead, the state also severely curtailed state distribution of condoms, a stupidity that is very apt to surface later in the form of an increased incidence of teenage AIDS.[41] The Texas legislation required all educational materials to stress the illegality of homosexuality and drug usage and the virtues of abstinence. It also required the State Department of Health to trace sexual partners of infected individuals. However, few of these provisions were supported by the funding necessary to make them administrative realities. The legislative debate was more a public protestation of virtue ("We are all straight, Christian, nondrug users.") for the purpose of electioneering, than an attempt to formulate sensible policy for the state that has the distinction of ranking fourth in number of cases, eighth in population seroprevalence level, and thirty-seventh in per capita AIDS expenditures.[42]

As noted in chapter 1, this generally negative stance has deep roots in the American heritage. Senator Helms and Representative Dannemeyer forced many of their colleagues to risk political futures in order to vote for sensible federal programs to contain the epidemic. Every vote in favor of positive programs lent itself to being represented as a vote that was "soft on queers, junkies, and/or criminals." As Governor Dukakis can testify from his 1988 presidential campaign experience, being so labeled confers no advantage in American politics. It is testimony to more legislative courage than we are apt to give credit, that the "plague" position from 1987 has become increasingly a minority, rearguard action unable to stop the emergence of a coherent national policy on AIDS.

The adherents of the "epidemic" position, on the other hand, argue that the citizenry's varied sexual dispositions and habits of substance abuse[43] are irrelevant to the battle, except as factors to be considered in designing specific and targeted public health strategies. The epidemic of HIV is and should be regarded as a menace to the entire nation, and national public health policy should not be affected by any individual's moral judgment regarding the behavior of those who have been or may become infected.

It is pointed out that even where there is a very low probability of an individual's seroconverting that person is nonetheless endangered by the AIDS-assisted resurgence of other diseases such as tuberculosis. After a decade of decline, TB began a comeback in 1986.[44] The epidemic position has been clearly articulated by conservatives like Surgeon General Koop and liberals like Senator Kennedy. It is the position wthat, from 1988, set the tone (with a few exceptions) for national policy; its major legislative statements are the HOPE Act, the Health Omnibus Programs Extension Act of 1988, the national government's initial attempt at a coherent policy on AIDS,[45] and the Ryan White Act of 1990.

THE HOPE ACT AND NATIONAL POLICY

The first thing one senses in the Act is an undercurrent of urgency that was notably lacking in previous official statements. The second is that its broad divisions do recognize the various areas of policy relevant to a coherent approach to the epidemic. In summary terms and commencing October 1, 1988, Congress authorized $400 million for three years of testing, $200 million for two years' support of home health care programs, $285–$300 million for three years of research (there are other portions of the federal budget that support much additional research), $250–$300 million for three years of AIDS education, and $2 million to fund a new, permanent National AIDS Commission. The provisions of the Act can be conveniently grouped under eight policy headings:

Scientific/Medical Research. The single largest commitment of national policy up to 1988 had been to funding basic scientific research into the nature of the virus and medical research seeking effective vaccines, drugs, and treatments. The statute confirms previous priorities in the allocation of AIDS funds. However, there is a new emphasis on expediting grants and evaluations—a response to the frequent complaint that such matters were unduly delayed in the national bureaucracy. A very important change is the statutory mandate to broaden the concept of "testing and evaluation" beyond the traditional laboratory-experimental model. Scientists are mandated to devise new protocols of evaluation that are quicker, even if less certain, than the classical ones. In this vein the statute authorizes the establishment of AIDS specialized research centers, Clinical Research Review Committees, NIH Clinical Evaluation units, and methods of evaluating treatments not approved by the government. These provisions constitute a partial victory for those involved in the clinical treatment of PWAs over laboratory scientists who generally have not recognized the legitimacy of research findings unless supported by strict protocols. Provision is also made for the continuation of basic genetic research into the structure and operation of the virus as well as social science research programs connected to the impact or control of the epidemic. At the global level Congress authorized support of vaccine research elsewhere and the programs of international agencies such as the World Health Organization and the Pan American Health Organization.

Professional Information and Education. A major problem confronting those working professionally has been the explosion of research activities and information. There is so much now available that the problem is one of access, simply knowing that a particular study has been done and where to find it. Congress addressed this and similar problems by authorizing two national data banks, one for basic AIDS research and another for clinical trials and treatments. With such computerized facilities available it becomes possible to disseminate information rapidly, avoiding duplication of effort. It also authorized special educational programs to overcome both professional and lay ignorance of the uses and risks of transfusion as well as blood donation. To provide more adequate data with respect to the behavior and spread of HIV in various groups, Congress authorized the establishment of epidemiological and mortality rate databases as well as a national seroprevalence survey. This latter has helped launch possibly the most politically sensitive survey the national government has ever tried to conduct—the *National Household Seroprevalence Survey* that asks citizens to undergo anonymous blood tests and answer intimate questions about their sexual behavior.[46]

Direct PWA Care. A segment (about 13 percent) of the overall budget is dedicated to direct care through grants for home and community care services, subsidized AZT, the development of model care protocols and community based evaluation of experimental therapies. The allocation for direct care is so modest that it gives credence to speculation that Reagan made an unadmitted decision to withhold all but token aid to the one million already infected, a decision that appears to receive quiet but continued support from both the epidemic and the plague coalitions.[47] This position has been incorrectly referred to as a triage decision, but this is inaccurate. Triage is the morally justifiable division of battlefield casualties into three groups: (1) those who will die whether or not care is given, (2) those who will live whether or not care is given, and (3) those who require care to survive. Medicine and attention under battlefield conditions, where all resources are in short supply, are reserved for the third group. But no such conditions existed in the United States. We were at peace and had abundant resources; there was and there is no morally justifiable reason for the decision to withhold care and write off the infected. It was and remains a tragic departure from standard American policy in such matters. As a nation we have long since made the basic decision that we should strongly support programs for medically managing, prolonging, and generally improving the quality of life

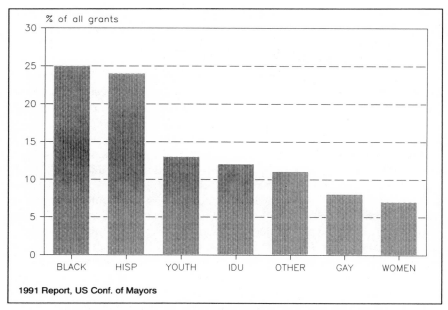

FIGURE 6.2 CDC Grants, 1985–90: Target Populations

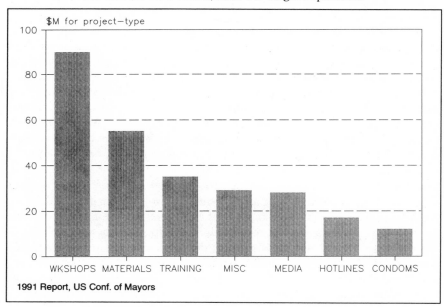

FIGURE 6.3 CDC Grants, 1985–90: Target Activities

remaining for those living with catastrophic afflictions—kidney dialysis centers and aid for various handicaps come to mind. I believe that we will, one day, classify this position as another of the sorrier moral lapses of American politics and list it with such events as the imprisonment of Japanese-Americans during World War II and the slaughter of native Americans.

Testing and Counseling. Provision is made for grants to states that operate HIV testing and counseling programs. The federal guideline calls for the testing to be anonymous and insists that there be counseling provided as an integral part of the testing program.

General Public Education. Bloc grants-in-aid to the states are provided to encourage the development of general as well as specially targeted educational programs. Special target programs might be for ethnic minorities, health care or public safety workers, or any group the unique characteristics of which call for special approaches. In addition, the Act called for the establishment of a national AIDS Information Clearinghouse and a twenty-four-hour toll-free Hotline (1-800-458-5231). The general kinds of activities for which bloc-grants were awarded during the Bush Administration can be inferred from Figures 6.2 and 6.3.

Professional Training. Funds are provided for incentive subsidies and loans to encourage students to train in the specialized subfields of AIDS treatment and research as well as continuing education coursework for those already in the profession.[48]

Felons. State grants-in-aid are provided to encourage the establishment of HIV testing of sex offenders and IV drug users.

Organizational. Congress mandated the establishment of an Office of AIDS Research directly under the director of the National Institutes of Health, emphasizing by such placement the high priority Congress placed on this activity. Further, Congress established a National AIDS Commission of fifteen members (five appointees each from the president, the Senate, and the House) to "promote the development of a national consensus on AIDS policy, and make recommendations regarding such policy."

The policy expressed in the Act of 1988 was strongly oriented toward research and preventive education but deficient in addressing the plight of those already afflicted. Further, since Congress had already appropriated its fiscal 1989 AIDS-related money prior to the passage of the HOPE Act, the funding of the Act's provisions had to await 1990 hearings and 1991 implementation.[49] Some of this deficiency was dealt with in the Americans with Disabilities Act of 1990, which extended the antidiscrimination provisions of three previous federal statutes to those who, by the act's definition, are "disabled"—a category that includes PWAs.[50] The Act makes it illegal for businesses employing more than twenty-five persons to discriminate against people with disabilities in hiring and/or firing and arms the disabled with federal remedies to fight discrimination in housing and places of public accommodation like restaurants, theaters, and hotels.[51] The language of the statute has still to receive definitive court interpretation, and there are many questions. For example, it does not prohibit discriminatory treatment of the "ill," only the "disabled," and even in that context prohibits only the application of a general rule of discrimination to all disabled. An example of a general rule in operation could be seen in the uniform exclusion of PWAs from all San Antonio nursing homes. In 1988 the president of the San Antonio AIDS Foundation tried to get a seventy-four-year-old lady with AIDS admitted to a nursing home; they refused her. The Foundation then filed a complaint with the Office of Civil Rights of the Federal Department of Human and Health Services. Two years later (long after the lady had died) that office ruled the nursing homes in violation of federal antidiscrimination regulations. If they fail to bring their admission policies into line with federal regulations, they would be denied Medicare and Medicaid funding.[52] Employers and landlords can still discriminate if they can justify their action with the facts of an individual case. The difficulty of justification will, of course, depend upon the general attitudes of the presiding arbitrator or judge.[53] President Reagan opposed the passage of the Disabilities Bill, but candidate Bush pledged to support it, and President Bush signed it into law.

Finally, in 1990, a new attitude emerged in Washington regarding the proper official position on AIDS; the "epidemic" view of AIDS became the foundation for a major piece of legislation. In early 1990 an AIDS disaster relief bill was introduced by Senators Kennedy and Hatch with nineteen others. A modified version of this passed both houses of Congress on August 4 and was sent to President Bush for signature. The Ryan White Comprehensive AIDS Resources Act (named after the Indiana teenager whose AIDS story and death captured the nation's sympathy) establishes, as a matter of public policy, that AIDS is to be conceived of and dealt with as the natural disaster which it is. The Act authorizes broad assistance to the communities that have been hardest hit by the epidemic. It applies to communities with more than two thousand cases, or a prevalence of 250 cases per 100,000 population; in 1990 this included sixteen American cities: Atlanta, Boston, Chicago, Dallas, Ft. Lauderdale, Houston, Jersey City, Los Angeles, Miami, New York, Newark, Philadelphia, San Diego, San Francisco, San Juan, and the nation's capital, Washington, D.C.

THE RYAN WHITE ACT OF 1990

The Act authorized $4.5 billion over the fiscal period 1991–96. This total included $882 million that appeared in the fiscal 1991 National Institutes of Medicine budget for emergency aid to hospitals, state programs, and special pediatric care.[54] To qualify for federal grants-in-aid, the states must provide,

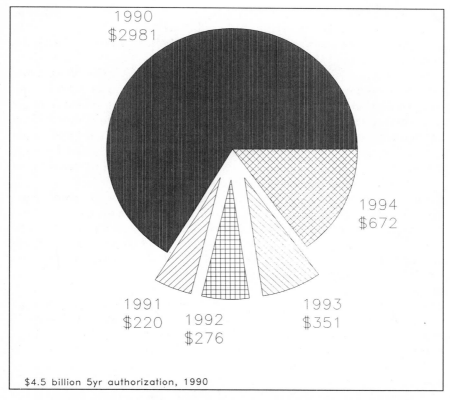

1990
$2981

1994
$672

1991
$220

1992
$276

1993
$351

$4.5 billion 5yr authorization, 1990

FIGURE 6.4 Ryan White Act of 1990: Authorization versus Appropriation.
This shows congressional appropriations for FYs 1991–93 as separate slices; the 1994 slice is President Clinton's request to the Congress. The portion labeled "1990" represents the amount of the original authorization still unappropriated.

at minimum, HIV blood testing with pre- and posttest counseling, further testing in case of positive results to determine the extent of immune system impairment, and appropriate therapeutic measures, referrals, and medical evaluations of seropositive individuals. These provisions may be the beginning of a national testing program. The Act encourages the organization of consortia of agencies, both public and private, to pool resources in order to provide a care system that, in its totality, would cover all needed services from educational outreach programs to terminal care. Other provisions authorize special studies of HIV's movement into rural areas, programs to insure the safety of the blood supply, and a partner-notification study. The Act does permit fees to be charged for various services if the individual or family is above the poverty line ($5,980 annual income per person in 1989).

However, the fees are statutorily pegged as a percentage (5 to 10 percent) of income at various levels, and, further, the Act specifically provides that, in the last analysis, services will be provided without regard to ability to pay, or current or past health condition.

The Act represented a major victory for those of the "epidemic" persuasion. As a matter of federal policy, AIDS was to be viewed as a natural and national disaster. However, it should be kept in mind that the exceedingly complex legislative-executive appropriations and spending process still offers many opportunities for those of the opposition "plague" mindset to lessen the impact of the Ryan White Act. In fact, viewing the Act from the perspective of 1994, it becomes an excellent object lesson (about which I wish citizens were more aware) on the slippage between promise and performance in politics. The Congress, first, authorizes a program with a forecast budgeted figure, then, second, it (maybe) appropriates money for the program within the authorization guideline, and, third and less immediately, oversees the actual administrative outlays under the appropriation. These are separate phases under the control of about thirteen separate committees/subcommittees and many executive agencies. So far, with 60 percent of the authorized life of the Ryan White gone, the Congress has appropriated only 19 percent of the money authorized in 1990 (not counting what it does with President Clinton's 1994 request). It is most unlikely that it will make up the "arrears"—it would require appropriations of almost $1.5 billion for each of the last two fiscal years. It is more likely that the Act will be extended with a new and equally fictional authorization. This is standard political practice.

Honest, understandable accounting is made even more difficult when administrative action is factored in. That Congress has authorized and appropriated funds for a project does not automatically mean that the executive branch will spend them. There are many examples of congressional intent being frustrated by an administration opposed to the congressional policy. For example, the Ryan White chart indicates an appropriation for 1992 of $276 million; as of the time Clinton took office, the Bush administration had spent/contracted only $152 million. It is for all these reasons that the citizen will hear loud and heated argument about who spent how much on what and when. There is so much quadruple-entry, covert bookkeeping in the national government, that only very diligent researchers or real "insiders" have access to the truth.

One of the more interesting requirements of the Act is that most of the funds to be allocated are to flow directly from Washington to "the top elected official in the metropolitan area who administers the public health agency serving the largest number of individuals with AIDS in the area."[55] There are several political implications of this directive. First, the Ryan White provisions, while not quite bypassing the central state health agencies, do diminish their significance in the expenditure of the federal money. State-level public health officers are responsible for ensuring that legitimate local consortia are formed and that a "lead agency" for the accounting of funds is designated. Beyond that, the actual allocations to various local agencies from the total money received by the metropolitan area is a matter largely for local decision. Congress hoped to produce more rapid and effective results at the municipal level where the sick reside.[56] State health agencies, reflecting state legislative attitudes, have sometimes not been overly responsive to the needs of PWAs. It is unclear whether the congressional hope is being borne out, but one indisputable result of this approach has been to set the stage for genuine dog fights among local agencies scrambling for a share of the money. Second, the budget that will be available to the municipal officer, plus the Act's emphasis on the establishment of consortia (coordinated by the municipal official), will necessarily shift the locus of control over local AIDS programs and services from private, volunteer AIDS Service Organizations to public health bureaucracies. Given the costs and complexities involved in effectively containing AIDS, a government takeover is necessary and unavoidable. But for one like myself, who has been involved in helping my local ASO, the San Antonio AIDS Foundation, there is a sadness in watching the displacement of private caring and initiative, and the development of still another government program wherein an individual, in this case a very sick person, inevitably becomes just another case number.

CLINTON AND AIDS

The 1992 campaign between President Bush and presidential hopeful Bill Clinton was unprecedented. As mentioned earlier, neither Reagan nor Mondale mentioned the burgeoning AIDS epidemic in 1984, and it played no significant role in the 1988 contest between Vice President Bush and Governor Dukakis. However, candidate Clinton made AIDS a major issue both in the nomination and the subsequent presidential contests. He delivered two speeches explicitly on the epidemic, his influence secured a spot at the National Convention for two HIV+ speakers (forcing the GOP to follow suit), his headquarters issued "AIDS policy papers," and the epidemic was among those problems given top billing in his election-night victory address. In the election of 1992, HIV politically came of age.

In his speech of October 1992 and in the AIDS Policy Papers, Bill Clinton made the following major commitments relevant to the epidemic: (1) to appoint an AIDS policy coordinator with a direct line to the Oval Office; (2) to take steps to accelerate the drug approval process; (3) to commit more resources to and organizationally streamline the research and development of vaccines and therapies; (4) to fully fund the Ryan White Act as well as increase the total AIDS budget; and (5) to promote a national AIDS education and prevention initiative in order to slow the spread of HIV. There were other commitments as well, promises of a less general nature, like ensuring that women and people-of-color were included in AIDS drug trials, but the measures mentioned are the ones that President Clinton hopes (I think sincerely) will make a difference in the national effort to contain the epidemic.

About sixteen months into his term, President Clinton had commenced implementing all of these commitments: First, in June 1993 the president appointed Kristine Gebbie, R.N., to the newly created post of White House AIDS Coordinator and made her a member of the President's Domestic Policy Council. Prior to her appointment, Nurse Gebbie was Washington state's chief public health official and had been a Reagan appointee to the National AIDS Commission. Her first act was to try to dampen expectations (aroused initially by Clinton's own campaign rhetoric and echoed by the media) that she would be a "Czar"—some kind of supreme commander, for AIDS related government action. The actual job description at the time of appointment was unclear and it remains so, but it seems to involve being a spokesperson for the president in the AIDS policy area, acting as a direct information conduit to the White House, and a facilitator for AIDS projects other than biomedical research ones. As a facilitator, for example, she was involved in the production and distribution of the primary care physicians AIDS handbook (see chapter 7) issued by the Department of Health and Human Services in 1994; she shared the spotlight in announcing its completion with the Secretary of Health and Human Services, Donna E. Shalala. In addition, she has spoken out forcefully on the issues of condoms and needle exchange programs, perhaps acting as a sensor and lightning rod for the president on these emotionally charged matters.

Second, accelerating the drug approval process was the purpose of the February 1994 creation of an eighteen-member Task Force on AIDS Drug Development. The membership includes Ph.D.s and M.D.s with major research and administrative experience, a laboratory technician, pharmaceutical research executives, as well as the heads of the National Institutes of Health, and the Food and Drug Administration. Several members are HIV+. It will be chaired by Secretary Shalala, who said that its purposes were to "identify new approaches to research and to remove any barriers to the development of effective treatments."[57] The Task Force is clearly a blue-ribbon panel, but just what it will accelerate is unclear. The big problem of the mid-1990s is turning out to be lack of new ideas from pharmaceutical houses and research centers, not bureaucratic red tape and roadblocks. After the almost frenetic search for drugs and therapies of the late 1980s and early 1990s, I think this slowing comes as a disturbing surprise to everyone working in the AIDS field. As the secretary pointed out, "the sad fact remains that not a single new drug application for an anti-retroviral" is in the pipeline. The tracks can be greased, but if there is nothing to put on them, what then?

Third, and one of the more controversial initiatives, in June 1993 the president signed the NIH Revitalization Act, a law that has the potential of dramatically altering the administration and conduct of research in the National Institutes of Medicine. In early 1994, the president appointed Dr. Harold Varmus, a Nobel laureate, to lead and invigorate the NIH. In addition to its hoped-for revamping of NIH procedures, the law greatly strengthened NIH's Office of AIDS Research (OAR) (created in 1988 but largely an advisory body) by giving its director the administrative power to design and implement trans-NIH AIDS research budgets coordinating various research operations strategically into one. Additionally, the director would have $100 million in discretionary funds to support promising research on a fast-track basis. Finally, the agency was to have a "bypass budget" for AIDS research— that is, a budget that goes straight to the president for review and transmission to Congress.[58] This bypasses the intricate NIH budget review process and guarantees that the priorities of the OAR director are represented accurately. In February 1994, Dr. Varmus and Secretary Shalala announced the appointment of Dr. William E. Paul, an internationally distinguished immunologist, to head the newly reconstituted OAR.

The NIH Act was the focal point of intense lobbying efforts by the NIH establishment opposing the bill, and an equally strong effort on its behalf by AIDS activists and others who felt that the conservative and bureaucratic NIH simply could not move fast enough for the epidemic. Clearly the pressures of the epidemic are forcing a reconsideration of our received administrative organization and behavior. The virus is demanding more coordination, more focusing, and more intensity of effort than has been called for before; the relaxed and disorganized ways of the past are fast becoming another casualty of the epidemic.[59] The exceptional stature of Drs. Varmus and Paul is a clear signal of presidential interest not only in the general performance of the NIH but specifically in its contribution to the national AIDS research effort.

Fourth, Clinton promised to "fully fund" the Ryan White Act as well as increase overall funding for AIDS. What the president should have promised is that he would request Congress to fully fund the Ryan White Act, something that it has not done yet and probably will not do in the future. In any case, what the phrase "fully fund" means is unclear to me. Probably what the president meant is that he would urge the Congress to appropriate all the money that it had authorized for the 1994 fiscal year, approximately $580 million dollars, and, in addition, to appropriate $672 million in 1994 for

1995. If Congress does follow through, the cumulative Ryan White appropriations will still fall short of the original 1990 authorization by almost $3 billion (see Figure 6.4). The president's complete budget proposal, published on February 8, 1994, calls for a total national expenditure of $2.7 billion on AIDS, $1.3 billion of which is earmarked for vaccine and therapy research.[60] President Clinton's proposal represents an overall increase of approximately 6 percent over previous budgets.

Finally, he promised to initiate a national education and prevention campaign. Part of this was started with the broadcast of TV spots promoting abstinence, safer sex, and condoms. In addition, parts of the education bill sent to Congress, and being debated as I write this in February 1994, envisage federally sponsored safer sex programs at the middle and high school levels. For the past year, "Czar" Gebbie, Surgeon General Jocelyn Elders, and Secretary Shalala have made numerous public appearances, held press conferences, and given speeches to boost AIDS awareness. Other initiatives in the campaign involved the issuance of the Red Ribbon AIDS Awareness stamp in December 1993 and the distribution of clinical AIDS guidelines to all primary care physicians. The president has backed his subordinates by participating visibly in AIDS related events. On World AIDS Day in December 1993, portions of the AIDS Quilt were hung from the balconies of the Old Executive Office Building next door to the White House. The president met with AIDS patients at Georgetown Medical Center and later delivered an emotional speech before an audience of physicians, researchers, activists, and patients. There is no question but that the president hopes, by his example and that of his highest officials, to inspire people at the local level to become more aware of AIDS, practice safer sex, and help those who are already infected.

However, our thinking as citizens about these and other measures of national policy should be circumspect. First, it is probably not the case that the failure to find an effective anti-HIV drug is a function of a bumbling administration and red tape. These are easy, traditional targets for the frustrated. The truth is that we are facing a new kind of biological competitor, and it may take a good while before we know how to deal with the viral challenge.

Second, President Clinton, or any president for that matter, has a limited number of tools at his disposal—persuasion, budgets, agencies, officials, and more persuasion. As he himself put it, "there's no way I can now keep everybody alive who already has AIDS." He can only put together an apparatus that might provide the environment within which the real gladiators, the research scientists, will hopefully prevail; the very strong appointments made in the NIH are promising in this regard.

Finally, increasing budgets alone is not a solution; there are only so many retrovirologists, virologists, molecular biologists, immunologists, bio-chemists, pharmacologists, and so on, and not all of them are working on HIV. These professional specialists require doctoral training and not even presidents can conjure them up overnight. Everyone, including me, is drawn to the analogy and image of the Manhattan Project—a great con-gregation of great scientists and technicians severely focused on one prob-lem, given full governmental resources, and solving it. Bang! The Atomic Bomb. As appealing as the image is, however, it does not really apply to biological research on HIV or coping with the social fallout. The most obvious difference is that retrovirology lacks an Albert Einstein. The people working on the atomic bomb already had the basic answers and formulae; their task was to engineer a practical application of $e=mc^2$. There is no such foundation for fighting HIV. Einstein himself once commented that the simplest social problem was infinitely more complex than the most complex problem of physical science. And whatever else AIDS is, it is not a simple biological or social problem. To repeat myself, "No one should expect a quick fix," but at least with President Clinton, the United States has a head of state willing to try.

PROBLEMS OF NATIONAL POLICY

In confronting the bubonic plague in San Francisco and New York back at the turn of the century the evolving U.S. Public Health Service (then called the Marine Health Service) employed two techniques that were to become the standard operating approach to epidemic control, namely quarantine and sanitation. Other techniques were added as the service became more com-prehensive and sophisticated, such as contact tracing of venereal or pneu-monic disease carriers, public education, data gathering, and now epidemic SWAT teams operating domestically and internationally. But one surprising oversight, in a nation that prides itself on the sophistication of its internal information system, is the lack of a uniform, national epidemic data collec-tion and surveillance system. The Federal Centers for Disease Control receives state-collected data on a number of diseases that are reported in the *Morbidity and Mortality Weekly Reports.* Many of these reportable diseases can provide the biologic basis for an epidemic, but there is no national or international surveillance system in place that can sound a warning. Had there been a tracking system in place during the 1970s our response might have been much earlier, less political, and more effective; as Joseph McCormick of the CDC put it in 1994, "Industrialized countries cannot wait for new viruses to reach their own shores. Look at AIDS. If we had spotted that disease when the cases first appeared, imagine how different the situa-tion could be today."[61] In May 1989, the Council of State and Territorial Epidemiologists urged the creation of such a system.[62] AIDS is not the first,

nor will it be the last, epidemic faced by America. There will be others produced by existing or mutant viruses. Without an early warning system, we
are like chickens in a coop, with no way of knowing the fox is coming.

A related problem has to do with the accuracy and timeliness of the data
we need to track biological killers. Currently the national reporting system
is dependent upon the efficiency of state health departments, which rely, in
turn, upon accurate reporting from physicians, coroners, hospitals, and other
local agents. Some states do a good job, some do not. But even among the
most conscientious, the methods and categories of collection vary widely so
that the data coming from different states are not necessarily comparable, a
fact that then distorts the national picture. It seems incredible, but is nonetheless true, that it is very difficult to get an accurate picture of the problems
infecting our body politic.[63] In the field of AIDS, for example, a major obsta-
cle to the collection of data has stemmed from the stigma associated with
the disease. Because AIDS is seen by so many as a sickness that results from
sin, there has been significant underreporting of the disease during treatment
and as a cause of death.[64] Patients and relatives prevail upon those responsible for reporting the data to conceal the truth.

From the standpoint of national policy, both problems place additional
strains on the federal organization of the union. Clearly the agents of viral
and/or bacterial death have no concern for the legal and political refine-
ments of national-state relations. State boundaries are our invention, not
nature's. An epidemic with national catastrophic potential, like a major
depression, is a national problem and must be confronted with a unified
national policy. The epidemic raises in an acute way the question of whether
we can continue the luxury of dealing with health problems in a piecemeal
way, state by state, and program by program. By 1989 the fifty states and
the District of Columbia had created a confusing patchwork of over one
hudnred and seventy different laws involving the many aspects of HIV
infection.[65] As surely as the Great Depression forced major changes in the
relationship of the government to the economy, AIDS will push us toward
a unified national health program including surveillance, insurance, regulation, drug development, professional certification, care, and funding.

HIV is also forcing a reappraisal of the traditional methods of coping with
disease transmission. Quarantine of those infected, as a technique, is almost
as old as epidemics themselves but seems completely inappropriate to
AIDS. The purpose of quarantine is to contain the epidemic agent within
limited physical boundaries. Entire cities (especially harbor cities) were
sealed off in an effort to contain the spread of the bubonic plague, cholera,
and yellow fever, and vessels from epidemic areas were routinely held at
anchor for forty days. Such measures made sense for diseases like the
bubonic plague, which were very easily transmitted, burned themselves

out within a limited time, and that presented readily identifiable symptoms.

But HIV infection is not such a disease. Unlike tuberculosis, for example, it is not transmissible by someone sneezing in the elevator or by a friendly social kiss. It requires participation in complex and intimate behavior, behavior we are not likely to abandon. Both sex and substance abuse of various kinds (drugs, liquor, pills) will be with us, I suspect, as long as death and taxes. And not until the final years of a long process, not until terminal AIDS sets in, does it reveal itself publicly.

Moreover, effective quarantine as a public health measure implies several nationally administered tests of the entire population within a reasonably short time.[66] It also implies rapid and accurate test protocols. However, the evidence increasingly indicates that our most widely used tests have very serious limitations, not the least of which is a possible eighteen-month lapse between the time of infection and the appearance of test reaction.[67] Quite apart from the administrative problems and astronomical costs[68] of such an endeavor, it would encounter major legal and practical difficulties. How could the legitimate objections of various religious groups, such as Christian Scientists, to such a procedure be surmounted?

Finally, the results of such a survey could rapidly be undermined by international population movement unless America were to seal its borders. Along with twenty-nine other nations,[69] the United States has instituted HIV+ travel restrictions into or through the country, but their major impacts so far have been to inspire boycotts of the Sixth International Conference on AIDS (San Francisco 1990), the 1990 meeting of the World Federation of Hemophilia in Washington, D.C., and the relocation of the Eighth International Conference from Harvard University to Amsterdam.[70] The dimensions of international population movement today make an effective self-imposed quarantine impossible. Each year there are an estimated 100 million travelers crossing borders by air transport alone, and possibly a billion if land crossings (legal and illegal) are added. Isolation from contamination either from within or without is no longer possible. Further, to quarantine a person who tests HIV+ for perhaps a decade is inhumane. To do so would transmute a blood test result into a criminal charge with an automatic life sentence. Such a process could not survive challenges under the due process, unreasonable searches and seizure, self-incrimination, and/or cruel and unusual punishment clauses of the U.S. Constitution.[71] Finally, no one in their right mind would volunteer to be tested under such circumstances. A national screening would have to be mandatory, with all the police-state implications of such an approach.

Similarly, the traditional contact tracing and sanitation techniques are much more limited in their efficacy within the AIDS context. The invasion of constitutionally protected privacy involved in tracing an infected person's sexual contacts is clearly justified in the case of, say, gonorrhea, by the fact that the infected person, once found, can be cured and the chain of transmission broken. HIV contact tracing could only serve more limited purposes. It could be important for gathering better epidemiological data, and the contact could enable social workers to warn a possibly infected person to practice safer sex lest he or she further transmit the deadly virus. However, the value society received by an individually targeted safer sex warning, or by better data, has to be weighed against not only the very high cost of contact tracing but also against the invasion of privacy entailed. Instead of a clear answer, we have cost-benefit analysis. On the other hand, there are many drugs available today that have significant prophylactic value for someone with HIV infection; episodes of *Pneumocystis carinii* pneumonia, for example, can usually be forestalled if a person knows he or she is infected and commences drug therapy. Therefore, contact tracing could be the first step in treatment, but only if the national government makes available the drugs needed for those who are found to have been infected. What would be the point otherwise?

Sanitation is, of course, an attempt to eliminate those conditions that facilitate the survival and transmission of the infectious agent. The great historical clean-ups easily come to mind: spraying or draining stagnant water areas to kill mosquito larva (yellow fever, malaria), eliminating easy access to rodent food supply and nesting areas (bubonic plague), ensuring that sewage does not drain into water supplies (cholera), and the establishment of government inspection programs for food processing, distribution, and preparation (food poisoning from botulism to salmonella). However, the breeding ground of HIV is wherever humans can have sex, inject drugs, exchange blood, or have babies, which is everywhere, and the practices that must be abated are the most hidden, intimate, and resistant to change in our entire portfolio of human behaviors. The only obvious environmental targets are the various sex emporia that cater to people looking for transient, anonymous sexual encounters. The most famous operation along these lines was the controversial closing of San Francisco's gay baths, but San Francisco's lead was not necessarily followed elsewhere, and the idea was never applied to straight sex clubs. America may be worried about the AIDS epidemic, but not so much as to seriously attack our enormous sex industry or consistently police our favorite highways and byways of assignation.

Testing and contact tracing raise the knotty problem of confidentiality which, in turn, is related to HIV+ counseling. This issue is one that separates the "plague" from the "epidemic" factions and is one poorly understood by the general public. Almost everyone admits that testing must be anonymous in a disease with so many stigma-derived implications that the mere factor of having been tested, if known, may be lead to discrimination.

No one would volunteer for testing otherwise. However, the epidemic and plague groups part company when a seropositive result is obtained. How confidential should the results be? Positive test results have been used to deny military and other employment opportunities, deny or cancel insurance, close access to the ability to practice professions from teaching to medicine, and bar or delay entrance to the United States among others.[72]

The plague position runs from the extreme of insisting that the names of infected individuals ought to be publicly known, to a position that legal duties ought to be imposed on those who know of positive test results (like physicians) to notify those who have a "need to know"—spouses, health care workers, insurance companies, employers, and the like. The epidemic position runs from the extreme that only the testee has a right to know the result and has complete control over subsequent notification to others, to a position that those who know of positive test results have a duty to make a good faith effort to insure that those who might be endangered (like sexual partners) be informed. There is no neat answer. It seems unconscionable that a physician not ensure that sexual partners of an HIV+ be notified; on the other hand, to insist upon notification violates the essential privacy of doctor-patient relationships. The situation is analogous to that faced by psychiatrists, priests, and other counselors when they come into possession of information that clearly bears upon the safety of innocent third parties. You're damned if you do, and damned if you don't.

The Ryan White Act, Title III, requires the states (as a condition of receiving federal money) to maintain confidentiality of information covering receipt of preventive or therapeutic health services, prohibits involuntary or unauthorized HIV testing, and mandates the availability of anonymous testing procedures. But the ambiguities inherent in this area, the horns of the our private and public dilemma, show up in the equivocal proviso that the Act's requirements be administered "in a manner not inconsistent with any applicable local, state or federal law," as well as provisions requiring state public health officers to trace and notify the partners of seropositive individuals.[73]

The nation, in the process of living with AIDS, is working out resolutions to many of these problems without coming to grips clearly with the principles involved. We are muddling on through.[74] Given the numbers involved, general quarantine of all seropositive men, women, and children is administratively impossible whatever might be thought of its desirability, and, at the other end of the scale, even the least compromising civil rights advocates are backing away from the protection of those who deliberately ignore the safety of others.

However, issues of testing, confidentiality, and tracing still plague our public debate and conscience. No one denies that effective counseling must be tied to testing, especially for those who receive a positive result. But there are many arguments as to how aggressive testing should be and how available the test results should be. Stephen Joseph, the Commissioner of Health, New York City, speaking to the Fifth International Conference on AIDS, predicted much more extensive, and possibly mandatory, government programs of testing, tracing, and quarantine as the epidemic picks up speed in America.[75] Aggressive, even mandatory, testing and tracing do make some sense *but only if they are securely tied to a national entitlement to treatment and antidiscrimination protection.* Otherwise these public health techniques could easily degenerate into an insidious form of trial and punishment.[76] Finally, the issue of confidentiality is gradually becoming mooted by the simple fact that so many public and private agencies are now requiring an HIV test that the facts are becoming available, although not completely in the public domain.[77] In my experience at the San Antonio AIDS Foundation, it has frequently been the seropositive individual himself or herself who has been the source of information. It is hard not to talk about something so traumatic with one's friends, and, once announced, the information circulates like all bad news, widely and quickly. As the nation moves toward the twenty-first century, the issue will not be how to protect against breaches of confidentiality, but how to protect against the employment, insurance, housing, education, health care, and other forms of discrimination that may follow.

However, to admit of all these limitations and reservations does not dispose of the genuine social, legal, and public health problems associated with "AIDS assault," that is, knowingly transmitting or attempting to transmit the virus.[78] There are many cases on record. In December 1990, San Antonio's police started searching for a thirty-one-year-old parolee who was suspected of having deliberately infected a number of women. According to the testimony of his former companions, he wooed his targets with a story that he was dying of leukemia and wanted to father a child to carry on the family name. Later he told the women that he had AIDS and had vowed to take as many people with him as possible before he died.[79] Can the law of homicide be altered to incorporate a virus as the lethal weapon, or conversely could one's infection by another in a voluntary sexual encounter become a possible defense in a retributory homicide? Every major police department and AIDS counseling agencies now knows of infected male and female prostitutes who are aware of their infection but regard it as an unavoidable risk of the profession. Can an infected person who continues sexual activity be placed in custody (quarantined) to protect the rest of us from being harmed both by our own folly and his/her unwillingness to desist? Are we prepared to give a cooperative prostitute or hustler something like unemployment benefits if he/she ceases operation? If not, can we really expect or believe that the individual will stop? Our current public policy and legal codes have no good answers for the new crop of AIDS problems. The Ryan White Act, Title III, requires the states to assure the federal government that their criminal laws are adequate to prosecute an HIV+ individual who, knowing his or her status, donates blood, semen, or breast milk with the specific intention of infecting others, or who engages in sex or shares hypodermic needles with that intention.[80] As can be seen from this provision, the response of the Congress to the need for imaginative and innovative lawmaking was to pass the buck to the states.

AIDS is clearly the kind of illness which, at the epidemic level, affects every aspect of our existence—our arts, our economy, our religious faith, our politics and law, and above all, our very lives. What is the source of this extraordinarily pervasive influence? After all, there are many other catastrophic and incurable illnesses. Why is it that AIDS almost immediately distinguished itself as something apart, something much darker, more threatening than Alzheimer's disease, lung cancer, lupus, the vicious Ebola fever, and many terminal illnesses? Some commentators have pointed to its impact on the younger, more productive age group, but, in truth, this is the same age group that is most affected by death by industrial accident, by falling, and by auto accident. How about the numbers involved? Actually AIDS has a long way to go to catch up with just one worldwide bout with the flu back in 1918. Is it due to the fact that sex is a transmission route? I think not. Syphilis was epidemic in Europe for two centuries and is reaching epidemic levels in contemporary America without causing the consternation of AIDS. But, this is the first *fatal* disease that, among other ways, can be transmitted sexually. In a sense this is true, but sex has always been a deadly game, and we have not been deterred. As part of a campaign to promote condom use, people working in AIDS education came up with a wonderful poster with the caption "I love you dear, but not enough to die for." It is a great slogan, and should be persuasive. But the truth is that, if we are genuinely caught in the throes of passion, we do not think of death. Caution is the first casualty of love. Every AIDS counselor talking to a recent seroconverter, and inquiring about whether the person practiced safer sex, has seen the sad shake of the head, the puzzled expression, and the statement, "I couldn't insist, I was in love."

There are many more explanations that have been offered to justify the special status AIDS has so rapidly achieved among the diseases rampant on this globe, but none really satisfy. I believe the explanation must be that we all realize on some gut, intuitive level that AIDS is the first, and possibly not the last, of a new series of diseases that will challenge the very existence of our species, something no other life form has been able to do until now. The afflictions may not necessarily be new in the biologic sense, although some may be. Rather they are new in the sense that, given the nature of twenty-first-century life, we are newly vulnerable to them. One does not need to be a virologist to understand that a virus that attacks the very walls that nature, over millions of years, has erected to protect us, is a challenge like none other. The Human Immunodeficiency Virus, in enlisting our very immune system to destroy us, represents the most formidable natural challenge ever mounted to the existence of our species. This is what puts AIDS in a class by itself. We are not fighting for a few more years, or a buoyant feeling of energy and good health, we are fighting for our very lives. And for all we know, the viral strategy may be a winning one.

Notes

1. Michael Gottlieb, M.D., was a research physician at UCLA, Rock Hudson's physician, and a co-founder of the American Foundation for AIDS Research, the nation's foremost private foundation for sponsoring AIDS research. He is currently a physician in Los Angeles with a large AIDS practice. Randy Shilts was the AIDS reporter for the *San Francisco Chronicle*. He wrote *And the Band Played On*, the most important single work on the beginning years of the epidemic, and more recently he wrote *Conduct Unbecoming* (1994), a scathing examination of military policy toward gay and lesbian members of the armed services. Larry Kramer is a playwright (*The Normal Heart*) and author (*Views from the Holocaust, the Making of an AIDS Activist*). He is also, arguably, the most important single AIDS activist in the United States, having been an original founder of both the Gay Men's Health Crisis in New York City and ACT UP, a confrontational group.
2. President Reagan's physician, Brig. General John Hutton (later commander of Madigan Army Medical Center, Ft. Lewis, Washington, D.C.) stated that the former president thought of AIDS as something like measles. Not until his friend Rock Hudson died of AIDS in 1985 did the president ask for an expert briefing on the epidemic. In other words, none of the warnings from university and government public health experts penetrated the phalanx of aides and advisers who controlled access to the Oval Office. See Interview and article, *San Antonio Express-News,* September 1, 1989, 1.
3. Paul Monette expresses this reaction at the personal level in his moving *Borrowed Time: An AIDS Memoir* (New York: Avon Books, 1988).
4. An example would be the defense of the gay bathhouses in San Francisco. See Randy Shilts, *And the Band Played On.*
5. The Sydney Dance Company's electrifying production of *After Venice* based on Thomas Mann's *Death in Venice*. It toured the United States in 1989. Larry Kramer's hit broadway show *The Normal Heart* (New York, New American Library, 1985); his memoirs, *Reports from the Holocaust: The Making of an AIDS Activist* (New York: St. Martin's Press, 1989); and the play by William Hoffman, *As Is* (New York: Putnam and Sons, 1988). Christopher Davis's novel *The Valley of the Shadow* (New York: St. Martin's Press, 1988); David Feinberg's

Eighty-Sixed (New York: Viking/Penguin, 1989); and Paul Monette's *Borrowed Time: An AIDS Memoir* (San Diego, Calif.: Harcourt, Brace & Jovanovich, 1988), as well as his volume of poetry *Love Alone: Eighteen Elegies for Rog* (New York: St. Martin's Press, 1988); and George Whitmore's *Someone Was Here: Profiles in the AIDS Epidemic* (New York: New American Library, 1987); Alice Hoofman's *At Risk* (New York: Putnam, 1988); and Adam Mars-Jones and Edmund White, *The Darker Proof: Stories from a Crisis* (New York: New American Library, 1988); and John Preston, *Personal Dispatches: Writers Confront AIDS* (New York: St. Martin's Press, 1989). Also Michael Klein (ed), *Poets for Life: Seventy-Six Poets Respond to AIDS* (Glendale, Calif.: Crown, 1989); Billy Howard, *Epitaphs for the Living: Words and Images in the Times of AIDS* (Dallas, Texas: Southern Methodist University Press, 1989); Andrew Holleran, *Ground Zero: Collected Essays* (New York: Morrow, 1988), and the poignant *The Screaming Room* (New York: Avon Books, 1986) by Barbara Peabody, a mother. Across the nation there have been many art shows and photography exhibits focusing on AIDS both as fundraisers and as an expression of the grief of those in the arts community.

6. The consciousness-raising memorial, "Day without Art," now involves over five thousand artists organizations, cultural institutions, museums, and galleries. For example, the rotunda of the Cultural Center of Chicago was draped in black and purple bunting and paintings were shrouded at the Metropolitan.

7. The quilt was the brain child of Cleve Jones, a gay San Francisco political activist. Motivated partly by grief over the loss of a friend, he sought a means to lighten the burden of grief, as well as to (in his words) "touch people who never really thought about the epidemic before." The quilt was first displayed in its entirety in Washington, D.C., in 1987. It now is too large to be shown completely; in 1992 it required twelve acres to lay out. Representative panels now hang in the Smithsonian, and the National Endowment for the Arts helps to defray the now considerable costs of its storage and maintenance. See: Stephen Donaldson (ed.), *Concise Encyclopedia of Homosexuality* (New York: Colliers-MacMillan, 1994).

8. For information about the ongoing AIDS Memorial write: NAMES PROJECT FOUNDATION, P.O. Box 14573, San Francisco, California, 94114 (415-863-5511). See the excellent photo essay on this memorial, Cindy Rushkin, *The Quilt: Stories from the NAMES Project* (New York: Pocket Books, Simon & Schuster, New York, 1988).

9. See the lengthy and excellent article: Donald I. Abrams, Jeannee Parker Martin, and Kenneth W. Unger, "Psychosocial Aspects of Terminal AIDS," *Patient Care* (November 30, 1989), 41.

10. A modern parallel is found in the story of a family unable to "bury" their kidnapped and murdered daughter because of the interminable legal processing of the killer, "For the Survivors, the Mourning that Never Ends," *New York Times*, National, March 2, 1989, 43.

11. Michel de Montaigne, *The Essays*, trans. George Ives (New York: Heritage Press, 1946), chap. 12.

12. Anne Skitovsky, "Estimates of the Direct and Indirect Costs of AIDS in the United States," in Alan F. Fleming et al., *The Global Impact of AIDS* (New York: Alan R. Liss, 1988), chap. 17. This overall cost includes two variables: (1) morbidity-cost = wages lost due to illness or disability, and (2) mortality-cost = present value of future earnings lost from premature death. The mortality-cost

component accounts for 94 percent of the total. In 1991 AIDS will account for 12 percent of the total indirect costs stemming from illness and premature death.

13. See "The Faces of AIDS: One Year in the Epidemic," *Newsweek* (August 1987), 22–39.

14. F. J. Hellinger, "The Lifetime Cost of Treating a Person with HIV," *Journal of the American Medical Association* (July 28, 1993), 474–78.

15. *Infectious Disease News*, January 1992, p. 15.

16. See Ron Winslow, "US Spending on AIDS Research and Prevention Reaches Level of Outlays on Other Major Diseases," *Wall Street Journal*, June 15, 1989, B4.

17. See "The New Crop of AIDS-Related Companies," *Wall Street Journal*, September 1987. The *Journal* lists Amnion Inc.; Applied Biotechnology, Inc.; Athena Neurosciences, Inc.; Biopure Corp.; British Biotechnology, Ltd.; Candace Pert Foundation; DSW Laboratories; Gensia; IDEC, Inc.; Immune Response Corp. (this is headed by Dr. Jonas Salk); MicroGeneSys, Inc.; Mikromed Screening, Inc.; Murex Corp.; Quidel Corp.; Tanox Corp.; United Biomedical, Inc.; Viro Research Laboratories, Inc. All these had been formed between 1985 and 1988. There are, of course, many more now.

18. See Kathryn Graven, "Japanese Join World Push to Cure AIDS," *Wall Street Journal*, November 10, 1988, B4. On illegitimate operations see *Info-AIDS Mailer* (University BITNET Computer Information Network), August 23, 1989. One recent con game based in Houston, Texas, even advertised its operation in the "Business Opportunities" classified section of the *San Francisco Chronicle* claiming, without authorization, that its venture had the sponsorship of singer Pat Boone (who is the Honorary National Chairman of AIDS Foundation for Children). This "business opportunity" involved the use of the Spiral Wells coin collection devices which have appeared in various shopping malls. See *San Francisco Chronicle*, Herb Caen's column, August 12, 1989.

19. For example, see *Business Week*, "An AIDS Treatment from Canada," November 29, 1993.

20. There is a parallel in the global campaign to eradicate poliomyelitis. See "Progress Toward Eradicating Poliomyelitis from the Americas," *Health InfoCom Network News*, August 30, 1989, 14.

21. Skitovsky, "Estimates," chap. 17. The burden will be spread very unevenly due to the concentration of cases in the major metropolitan areas. Although America has a surplus of hospital beds, the facilities in places like New York will be severely strained. The estimate is that PWAs will occupy 25 percent of the city's beds. It may be that we will have to distribute the burden of care over the nation's hospital system by moving some patients to where the beds are, even though that takes them away from relatives, friends, and other needed support. Another possibility is the subsidized development of a hospice network that can provide adequate care short of the hospital standard.

22. *American Medical News*, November 11, 1991, 1.

23. See the fine series of four articles by Eric Ekholm with John Tierney, "AIDS in Africa," which commenced in the *New York Times*, September 16, 1990.

24. *Congressional Quarterly*, August 8, 1989.

25. "Biting the Insurance Bullet, as Health Care Costs Rise, CEO's Warm to National Plan," *Newsweek* (August 28, 1989), 46.

26. For summaries of the AMA's plan as well as some others, see the official bul-

letin of the AMA, *American Medical News*, March 16, 1990.

27. Theodore M. Hammett, National Institute of Justice, *1988 Update: AIDS in Correctional Facilities* (U.S. Dept. of Justice, Office of Justice Programs, June 1989). For the exceptions see p. 41 of the report. Compare the 1988 report with the *1989 Update* issued in May 1990. See also "Inescapable Problem: AIDS in Prison," *JAMA* (December 11, 1987), 3215.

28. Still the most arresting account of this period is Randy Shilts's *And the Band Played On.*

29. The National Academy issued a 390-page report criticizing the president for lack of leadership. See *National Journal* (August 30, 1986), 2044; (November 8, 1986), 2733.

30. The total amount appropriated for the period commencing on October 1, 1988 for the 1989 fiscal year totaled $1.5 billion.

31. "MD Relates Reasons He Left AIDS Panel," *American Medical News*, December 25, 1987, 2.

32. *Report of the Presidential Commission on the Human Immunodeficiency Virus*, submitted to the President of the United States, June 24, 1988.

33. Ibid., Appendix B.

34. *National Journal* (August 6, 1988), 2189.

35. For a summary analysis of the Presidential Commission report, see *National Journal* (June 11, 1988). Also *Congressional Quarterly*, August 6, 1988, 2189.

36. The Presidential Commission, later renamed the National Commission on AIDS, released its final report in June 1993 after four years of work. Its final report said that it hoped that the new Clinton administration would do a better job of confronting the epidemic than previous ones, and commended its recommendations—largely ignored by Reagan and Bush—to the new president.

37. As an example, Representative Dannemeyers's attempts to add restrictive amendments to the House bill appropriating funds to fight AIDS were supported by 36 Republicans and 1 Democrat (Rep. Hall of Texas). The amendments were defeated 369–37. *Congressional Quarterly*, June 18, 1989, 1695 and 1698.

38. The ambiguity of the CDC categories make it difficult to determine the real number of what type of sexual preference is involved in each classification.

39. The Bowdler brothers, from whose name we get the term *bowdlerize*, were early Victorians who published a series of "cleansed" versions of the Bible, Shakespeare, and other great works. These editions eliminated all direct and indirect references to anything remotely resembling sex or passion so that the "fairest maiden" could read these otherwise uplifting works without embarrassment.

40. This attitude continues into the Bush administration. In October 1989, Assistant Secretary for Public Health Kay James blocked the publication of a PHS AIDS-education pamphlet on the use of condoms because it did not make clear that condoms can fail and that abstinence was the only answer. Anthony Lewis, "Bush and the Zealots," *New York Times*, October 19, 1989, 31.

41. See Rebecca Voelker, "Teens Seen as Next Group of New AIDS Cases," *American Medical News*, June 16, 1989, 11; Gina Kolata, "AIDS Is Spreading in Teen-Agers, A New Trend Alarming to Experts," *New York Times*, October 8, 1989, 1.

42. For summaries of the session on AIDS see the May 24, 1989 coverage in the following: *San Antonio Light, Houston Chronicle, The Austin American-Statesman, Dallas Morning News.* The Texas caseload and seroprevalence rank-

ings are from the September 1989 *AIDS Surveillance Report* of the Federal
Centers for Disease Control. The cumulative total for Texas is 7,289 reported
cases, 13.7 cases/100,000 population, and a per capita expenditure of 14 cents.

43. The focus of substance abuse is, of course, IV drug use. However, it should be
kept in mind that both alcohol and marijuana use are definitely implicated in
the spread of AIDS in that both lower or eliminate the cautions and/or inhibi-
tions that might otherwise encourage safer sex.

44. Gary Slutkin et al., "The Effect of AIDS on the TB Problem and TB Programs,"
in Fleming, *The Global Impact of AIDS*, chap. 4.

45. For a summary of provisions, see *Congressional Quarterly*, October 22, 1988,
3068–3071. The formal designation of the AIDS provisions is Title II of the Labor
and Health and Human Services of Act of 1989.

46. A trial survey was commenced in the fall of 1989 in Dallas County, Texas. The
Department of Health and Human Services mailed letters to thirty four hundred
household soliciting their participation. This first attempt was really the culmi-
nation of administrative initiatives going back to the Reagan years rather than
a direct outgrowth of the statute. However, both initiatives were and are on the
same track—the effort to get better data with respect to the sexual behavior of
the American population as it relates to the spread of HIV. The results of the
Dallas County survey produced an estimate of 0.4 percent seroprevalence for
adults ages 18–54. The estimated number of HIV+s is 4,000 (95 percent confidence that the population is between 2,200 and 7,500). This figure is lower than
previous estimates based on epidemic models.

47. At current case levels the direct care allocation amounts to approximately $1,000
per patient annually. Triage thinking may have been behind the decision by
Congress, in effect, to "fake" an allocation of money for support of AZT.
Congress authorized, but did not appropriate $30 million for a continuation of
the Public Health Emergency Fund that subsidizes AZT purchase. In testimony
before the House oversight subcommittee with jurisdiction over the Public
Health Service, the assistant secretary of health, Dr. James O. Mason, told the
committee that, barring new money from Congress, the only place that he
could get money for AZT programs was from biomedical research, prevention
programs, infant mortality, cancer, or some other portion of the health budget.
Health InfoCom Network News, August 19, 1989, 9.

48. The National Institutes of Health is currently offering a program under which
a health care professional can have up to $20,000 annually repaid on his/her
student loan if work on NIH sponsored AIDS research is undertaken. Program
Director: Marc Horowitz (301-496-0357).

49. The formula for the allocation of national money to the states is as follows: each
state/territory would receive for education and prevention programs the greater
of: (1) A minimum of $200,000, or (2) the amount determined equally from: (a)
a percentage equal to the state's population divided by the total US population;
and (b) a percentage equal to the number of new AIDS cases reported by the
state to the CDC divided by the total new cases nationally. (3) In addition, states
that register 1 percent or more of the total national AIDS cases, must pass on
at least one half of the national money they receive to migrant, community
health, or private nonprofit ASOs.

50. The Americans with Disabilities Act extended the antidiscrimination provisions
of the Civil Rights Act of 1964, the Rehabilitation Act of 1973, and the Fair
Housing Act of 1988 (*Congressional Quarterly*, May 13, 1989, 1121). Its exten-

sion of the concept of "disability" to PWAs followed the line of reasoning suggested by U.S. Supreme Court Justice Brennan, who stated in *School Board of Nassau County, Florida v. Arline*, 480 U.S. 273 (1987), "The fact that *some* persons who have contagious diseases may pose a serious health threat to others under certain circumstances does not justify excluding from the coverage of the Act [Rehabilitation Act of 1973] all persons with actual or perceived contagious diseases." J. Brennan explicitly excludes AIDS from his argument, stating that it was not before the court in this case, but his line of argument could be and was applied later to AIDS by the Congress in drafting the Americans with Disabilities Act.

51. The U.S. Supreme Court in *School Board of Nassau County, Florida vs. Arline*, 107 S. Ct. 1123 (1987), ruled that Section 504 of the Rehabilitation Act applied to a case of tuberculosis with reasoning that clearly would apply to AIDS as well. The Department of Justice, which initially held that AIDS was not a "handicap" under the Act, changed its position in October 1988. The Americans with Disabilities Act of 1989 picks up this development and embodies it in statutory terms.

52. The ruling was an application of Section 504 of the Rehabilitation Act of 1973. "SA Nursing Homes Discriminating," *San Antonio Express-News*, October 13, 1990, A1.

53. Wendy E. Parmet, "Legal Rights and Communicable Disease: AIDS, The Police Power and Individual Liberty," 14. Paper delivered at the 1988 Annual Meeting of the American Political Science Association, September 1–4, 1988. The author is an associate professor of law at Northeastern University Law School.

54. For a summary of the bill, see *Congressional Quarterly*, August 18, 1990, 2683–2686; for a review, see *New York Times*, August 6, 1990, A12.

55. *Congressional Quarterly*, August 18, 1990, 2683.

56. On the other hand, the formula-grant provisions of the 1988 HOPE Act provide that funds be awarded through a single formula at the state level, instead of directly to state and municipal health departments. Federal policy is thus ambiguous, not an unusual situation.

57. Philip J. Hilts, "Panel Is Created to Speed Effort on AIDS Drugs," *New York Times*, December 1, 1993, A1; "Clinton Administration Names AIDS Panel to Speed Drug Search," *New York Times*, February 7, 1994, A1.

58. The FY 1994 NIH budget for AIDS research is $1.3 billion. Derek Hodel, "Washington Watch," *Gay Men's Health Crisis Treatment Issues*, (February 1993).

59. It is interesting to note that the United Nations is also reorganizing its programs and for the same reasons. By 1996 all AIDS programs will be coordinated and administered by one lead agency. This will merge operations previously found, and separately administered, in the World Health Organization, the UN Development Fund, the UN Population Fund, UNICEF, and UNESCO. "AIDS Work to Be Unified," *New York Times*, January 23, 1994, A4.

60. For a comparison and perspective, the FY 1993 budget contained $1.9 billion for cancer research.

61. Cynthia Johnson, "Health Officials Fear Man Losing His Advantage over Microbes," *Reuters*, February 2, 1994, as reprinted in CDC, *AIDS Daily Summary*, February 4, 1994.

62. See "Surveillance for Epidemics—United States," *Health InfoCom Network News* 2, no. 38 (1989), 14. A parallel proposal from the World Health Organization suggests the establishment of global tracking stations.

63. For example, local Texas health departments, at the request of the Texas Department of Health, began collecting data on the epidemic in accordance with the 1993 Revised Definition of AIDS a year prior to its official adoption by the national Centers for Disease Control in January 1993. Therefore, all Texas figures will be out of phase for several years until the reported AIDS cases are factored back into the year of diagnosis.

64. The Federal Centers for Disease Control estimates a rate of underreporting from 10 percent to 30 percent. However, a report from South Carolina health authorities in 1989 indicated a 40 percent rate of nonreporting in that state with a much higher likelihood of nonreporting for Blacks and women than for Whites. "Many AIDS Cases Go Unreported," *New York Times*, November 28, 1989, 20. It is not a problem unique to the United States. Medical experts meeting under the auspices of the World Health Organization agreed that the same problem occurs in the Muslim countries of the Middle East. They have a significant AIDS problem but refuse publicly to acknowledge it for religious and social reasons. See *New York Times*, International, February 19, 1990, A5.

65. For a brief review of state legislation, see Larry O. Gostin, "Public Health Strategies for Confronting AIDS," *JAMA* (March 17, 1989), 1621.

66. The six-month interval is necessary to eliminate the so-called window of negativity during which a recently infected person would not test positive. Only Cuba has effectively imposed a total quarantine policy. However, it should be noted that apart from this extreme measure some forms of partial quarantine are not only possible but have been tried in the United States. For example, HIV+ school children have been denied admission to school or when admitted have been physically segregated from other children. Some states have tried to isolate individuals who refused to follow a court order to refrain from sexual activity. Insurance companies have "red flagged" entire metropolitan areas that were known to house a large gay population.

67. Stephen M. Wolinsky et al., "Human Immunodeficiency Virus Type I (HIV-1) Infection, a Median of 18 Months before a Diagnostic Western Blot," *Annals of Internal Medicine* 2, no. 12 (1989), 961 et seq. The disturbing conclusion of this study is "There is a long and variable interval between virus acquisition and a diagnostic serum antibody response." See Elaine Sloand et al., "HIV Testing: State of the Art," *JAMA* (November 27, 1991), 2861.

68. The United States military spent $43 million between 1986–88 to test 3.2 million people. It identified 5,890 HIV+ individuals at an average cost of $7,300.00 each. No one asserts that its procedure identified all the positives. To project this experience to the national population involves, at minimum, a multiplication by 75, and the acknowledgment that a civilian population would be much more difficult to test completely and reliably.

69. The following nations have instituted some AIDS-control travel and/or immigrations measures. In many cases, the measures seem more attuned to meet domestic politics than practical public health problems: Belize, Bulgaria, China, Costa Rica, Cuba, Cyprus, Ecuador, Egypt, East Germany, Bavaria (W. Germany), Greece, India, Iraq, South Korea, Kuwait, Liberia, Libya, Marshall Islands, Mongolia, Pakistan, Papua New Guinea, Philippines, Qatar, Saudi Arabia, South Africa, Soviet Union, Syria, Thailand, United Arab Emirates, United States of America. Anyone considering travel to these nations should check with the consulates to obtain the current restrictions. For a summary of the requirements as of August 1989, see *New York Times*, August 13, 1989, Travel, 3.

70. "Hemophilia Groups May Boycott or Move," *AIDS Treatment News*, October 20, 1989. Ultimately Harvard declined to host the conference to protest Bush administration policy. See also *Visiting the USA: A Legal Guide for Persons with HIV* (San Francisco, Calif.: National Gay Rights Advocates, 540 Castro St., CA 94110).

71. There have been sporadic quasi-quarantine methods employed such as the refusal to allow attendance of infected children or their physical segregation in the school environment, segregation of workers in the work space or prisoners in jails, and insurance "red flagging" of whole city districts known to be the living space of homosexual populations. Most of these efforts have fallen before legal challenge.

72. See the instructive debate in the New England Journal of Medicine May 11, 1989 and November 2, 1989 issues inspired by the publication of "The Case for Wider Testing for HIV infection," in volume 320, pp. 1248–1254, by F. S. Rhames and D. G. Maki.

73. *Congressional Quarterly*, August 18, 1990, 2685.

74. For an excellent general review of the myriad concrete problems that arise, see the biweekly newsletter covering legislation, regulations, and litigation, *AIDS Policy and Law* (Washington, D.C.: Buraff Publications).

75. "Steven Joseph Envisions the Future of AIDS," *The New York Native*, June 19, 1989—the text of the Commissioner's speech to the 5th International Conference on AIDS.

76. Currently less than one half of states' Medicaid programs support prescriptions for drugs commonly used in AIDS treatment. "Medicaid's Hodgepodge on AID," *New York Times*, May 25, 1989, B18.

77. For example, all federal employees with overseas assignments (foreign service, peace corps, etc.), the FBI and CIA, all military, an increasing number of general admissions to hospital care, patients seeking surgical intervention (especially orthopaedic), those receiving trauma or emergency care, most life and health insurance, inmates of federal and state penitentiaries, entering aliens and those applying for amnesty, health care workers, blood or organ donors, sperm bank donors, and the newborn and their mothers. The AMA advocated an even broader requirement, "those whose history or clinical status warrant this measure [involuntary testing]."

78. For example, an HIV+ sailor who had consensual intercourse without warning his partner was held to have been properly convicted of aggravated assault under the Uniform Code of Military Justice in September 1993.

79. "Police Seeking Man Accused of Spreading AIDS," *San Antonio Express-News*, December 9, 1990, A1.

80. *Congressional Quarterly*, August 18, 1990, 2685.

7

Into the Twenty-First Century with AIDS

The Human Immunodeficiency Virus has been in the human community for at least 75–100 years. Its earliest appearance was restricted to remote villages of sub-Saharan Africa, and it was just one more killer in a land that gave birth to many. Then it reached out to the greater world. A young man in St. Louis died of "unknown causes" in 1969, having been infected years earlier. Attending physicians were puzzled by his array of symptoms so they stored frozen samples of his tissue and blood for later analysis; that was the end of it. Now we know that he did have HIV antibodies in his blood, that he did die of opportunistic diseases associated with AIDS, and that there were other cases here and abroad. Usually the dead were not public figures, people whose death would be a matter of public comment. When a prominent person was involved, physicians attributed death to standard causes.[1] The signals sent forth by the virus were lost within and indistinguishable from the background noise generated by a galaxy of incurable afflictions and unaccountable deaths. Finally, by the 1980s HIV confronted physicians in sophisticated metropolitan centers with enough inexplicable cases to inspire scientific curiosity and then to raise alarms. The rest is history—unfortunately it is a continuing history.

In the United States, we have knowingly lived with AIDS for about fourteen years, and certain facts are becoming abundantly clear. First, the epidemic involves living entities in competition, and its profile changes with the dynamics of that competition. *Biological examples* of the process emerge from the changing incidence and impact of opportunistic infections suffered by PWAs. For unknown reasons, the incidence of Kaposi's sarcoma is dropping in America while mycobacterium tuberculosis is rising in some cities like New York—an epidemic on its own. In the early days of the epidemic, Kaposi's sarcoma and *Pneumocystis carinii* pneumonia were the two most common expressions of AIDS. Now there is a rising incidence of other opportunistic infections, such as Mycobacterium Avium Complex and tox-oplasmosis of the brain. People are still dying, but of different causes.[2] Another, and important, example of biologic change is signaled by the detection of HIV-2 infections in America. So far the numbers have been small, but sufficient nonetheless for the FDA to require blood banks to commence screening for both types of the virus.

Geographic examples of the dynamic can be found in Asia. Through the 1980s, this part of the globe seemed relatively unaffected. Epidemiologists talked of a different "pattern" of spread, and Indian and Chinese politicians preened themselves on the cultural virtues which were, seemingly, holding the virus at bay. Now the virus is spreading very rapidly; the "virtue" barrier turned out to be nothing more than a time lag.[3]

Within the continental United States, those parts of the nation previously untouched are losing their immunity. Peter Gould, Pennsylvania State University's Evan Pugh Professor of Geography, has created a series of maps that dramatically display HIV/AIDS dispersion in the United States; Figures 7.1, 7.2, and 7.3 show his maps for 1984, 1986, and 1990. Until 1984 five U.S. cities accounted for 63 percent of the cases; by 1990 their share has dropped to 38 percent, and the virus was found to be moving into other cities as well as rural America with sufficient speed to inspire a specially funded congressional study.[4] *Demographic examples* can be drawn from the data which indicate that the rate of new cases in the American homosexual population is decreasing and dramatically increasing within the drug culture, among women, and among teens.[5] In the next fifteen years it is likely that the American epidemic will come to parallel the African/Caribbean and become a dominantly heterosexual phenomenon. The twists and turns the epidemic may take in the future surely no one can know. For example, in Asia the epidemic has spawned a child prostitution industry, and the infection is spreading into younger and younger age groups. Children are being bought and sold as sex objects for the pleasure of men; the men hope to avoid HIV by employing only children too young, presumably, to have been infected. One more unexpected AIDS nightmare. However, one thing is dismally certain: HIV, like so many other microparasites, is now irreversibly part of the global human culture. It has joined the human race, and will never just "go away."

Second, AIDS is far more than a new or recently named illness caused by a heretofore secreted virus; it is an event of global and historic proportions that touches every aspect of human existence. It is forcing us to rethink many of our basic attitudes and approaches. For example, twentieth-century Americans have embraced a model of "health" that equates it with youth and beauty. The healthy person is the person bursting with youthful grace and vigor; aging is something to be fought back at the gym, on the

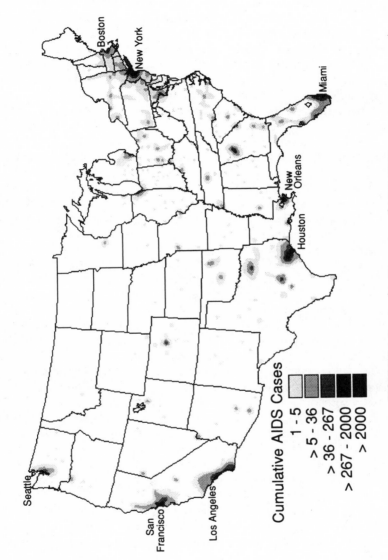

FIGURE 7.1 Geographic Dispersion of AIDS: 1984

Source: Peter Gould, *The Slow Plague* (London, New York: Blackwell, 1988).

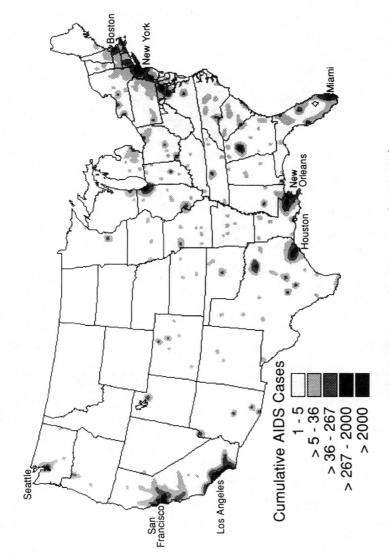

Cumulative AIDS Cases

1 - 5
> 5 - 36
> 36 - 267
> 267 - 2000
> 2000

FIGURE 7.2 Geographic Dispersion of AIDS: 1986

Source: Peter Gould, *The Slow Plague* (London, New York: Blackwell, 1988).

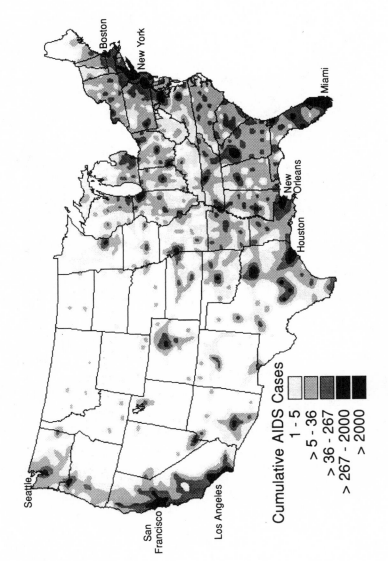

FIGURE 7.3 Geographic Dispersion of AIDS: 1990

Source: Peter Gould, *The Slow Plague* (London, New York: Blackwell, 1988).

jogging trail, and in the consumption of "natural" foods and cosmetics. Age, together with its gradual accumulation of disabilities and wrinkles, is almost an embarrassment—even seventy (plus)-year-old President Reagan declined to appear in public with his grey hair. However, in this time of AIDS, a young person can be afflicted with a deadly disease and still function for many years as a strong and vigorous person. When he or she does reach the terminal stage, then the aging process accelerates past anything we have experienced before. AIDS confuses our usual expectations and images—the healthy young person can be afflicted and infectious and a very aged person can be young. We have idealized the qualities of the younger age groups and used them as a litmus of health, but, ironically, this is a group within which AIDS has become a major cause of death. The impact of AIDS on youth is reminding many of the merit in aging.

PWAs have insisted that their infection alone not be taken as evidence of poor health or of disability. Rather, they insist that the measure should be functional—whether a person "can do a job," should be the test of health. This has been roughly the approach taken by Congress in the Americans with Disabilities Act. Increasingly, it appears that this would be a sensible approach for all of us—to define "health" functionally and circumstantially; a person is "healthy" if he or she can achieve realistically stated and selected goals. Such an approach allows those who are afflicted by a wide range of tribulations, from mental retardation to HIV, to be considered as healthy and active partners in American life.

Finally, we are at the beginning, not the end of this event. Dr. Jonathan Mann, director of the International AIDS Center at Harvard, put the situation bluntly in 1990, "The worst is yet to come."[6] At the beginning of the decade, 163 nations reported 418,403 cases; 89 percent of the nations reporting to the World Health Organization recorded some AIDS. WHO projects about 14 million HIV+ worldwide, a number that will triple by the year 2000.[7] Harvard's Global Programme on AIDS calculates a maximum figure of 110 million seropositives. In no nation can anyone do more than statistically estimate how many people will be infected with HIV, will progress to AIDS, and will die as we move into the early years of the twenty-first century. Different assumptions about behavior change, developing medical technologies, and the size of the existing pool of infected individuals affect everyone's forecasts. One of the more convincing studies I have seen for the United States postulates three scenarios by the year 2002: a "worst case" figure of 14,553,000 HIV infected, a "best case" figure of 1,583,000 (approximately the present number of HIV+s), and a "middle" estimate of 5,861,000 which the authors, in an "optimistic" frame, hope will be the correct figure.[8] Another mathematical model projects a cumulative total of 7 million Americans infected over the next twenty years.[9] Health care costs will be roughly $50 billion annually in the United States by mid-decade. Whatever set of figures proves ultimately to be right, clearly the closing decade of the twentieth century and the opening decade of the twenty-first century will be the Time of AIDS. It will be a time during which the Human Immunodeficiency Virus will come to play a part in the life of every person reading these words. Some of its effects are clearly foreseeable, others are not.

HIV, AIDS, AND HEALTH CARE

The more easily foreseeable effects are in biomedical research and medical care. Research talent and facilities have been mobilized for a forced march on AIDS; viral research, which would normally have taken decades, is being compressed into years. It took forty years of poliovirus research to accumulate the amount of detailed information scientists have developed in the past ten years on HIV. Just ten years ago the virus was a retroviral mystery and seemed invulnerable to attack. Its complex interactions within the human system gave it so many attack routes that it seemed impossible to cover them all. Now major points of possible vulnerability in its life-cycle are being isolated and defined by researchers. Still, however, too much remains too hidden; retroviral research, including HIV research, has a long way to go before unlocking the secrets and the threats posed by viruses and retroviruses. If anyone ever questioned the importance of basic research, the absolute need to unravel the viral life-cycle should put doubts to rest, for it is only with this knowledge that we will be able to devise effective counterattacks.[10] And counterattack is a "must priority" for society, not just for HIV, but for its many cousins as well. As Nobel laureate Joshua Lederberg warned, "Our only real competition for dominion of the planet remain the viruses."[11]

New Perspectives on Containment

The failure of classical approaches over the past decade to develop an effective remedy for the virus itself has led some to consider whether the assault might better proceed from other directions—that HIV may be largely impregnable to our usual vaccine and/or drug approach.[12] The standard model of biomedical research is what I call the "shooting gallery model"; that is, one identifies a pathogen, then invents guns and ammunition that will shoot it down (with as little damage to the surrounding environment as possible). The gun, or instrument of delivery, can be as simple as a pill or as complex as a computer controlled laser beam. The ammunition can range from a household antibacterial, like plain iodine, to complex manufactured compounds that insinuate themselves into living cells and subtly alter their functions.

The shooting gallery model is most successful when the target is clearly defined and stands still. This was the case with the poliovirus. Its rate of mutation was glacial, its internal viral structure simple and well defined, and it was, therefore, vulnerable to the vaccines developed by Drs. Sabin and Salk. However, when the target moves, scores become more problematic, as in the case of the influenza virus. The strains of this virus can produce from two to four mutations per year, a sufficient number to keep our virologists and drug manufacturers busy devising variants to stave off national epidemics. Unfortunately, HIV makes the influenza virus look slow. It not only has many more variable sites on its genome, it can respond to the host environment with changes at an extraordinary rate, many times that of influenza. It is like comparing a jogging duffer, with an olympic sprinter. Something of its ability in this regard can be gathered from comparing it to its cousin, the human T cell leukemia/lymphoma virus type 1. HTLV-1 and HIV infects many of the same cells, but HTLV-1 has nothing like HIVs pathogenicity or mutation rate. Constantly in a running search for transmission and survival strategies that work, HIV can effect changes in its genome within a few years that would require literally centuries for HTLV to bring about.

If you keep in mind that full dress drug development from concept to distribution can easily consume ten years, and that HIV can change *all* of its hypervariable genome sites, and some of its variable sites, in thirty years, then the problem of confronting it resolves into focus with stark clarity. In ten years HIV can change often enough to exhaust the capacity of our immune system to challenge it. It can also change its genomic character sufficiently to at least partially nullify the drug that moved into the development pipeline a decade earlier.Nobel laureate Manfred Eigen, thinking about this, suggests that perhaps the only approach that will really work is one opposite the classical model. Instead of trying to slow and hit this fast-moving target, speed it up. Devise drugs that will accelerate the error rates (or mutation rates) in viral replication until such time as "they cross the critical error threshold that defines their quasispecies, [and] experience a catastrophic loss of [genetic] information."[13] That is, speed-up HIV until it crashes. Now you are no longer shooting at stationary or moving ducks in a gallery, you are sabotaging the machinery itself.

Professor Paul W. Ewald, the Smithsonian's Burch Fellow of Theoretical Medicine, suggested another approach to viral control —one that has strong implications for human behavior.[14] Approaching HIV from the standpoint of evolutionary epidemiology, he suggests that we might be able to promote a more benign co-existence with the virus by adopting behaviors that induce it to select mutations that are less harmful to us:

In the absence of an evolutionary view, the future will repeat the past.

When we impede versatile pathogens with a drug, they will evolve resistance. A pathogen's potential for change will undoubtedly lie beyond our ability to anticipate its mutability. It is for such more formidable pathogens that we desperately need a new perspective. Virulent pathogens may be transformed into mild ones not because benign coexistence is the inevitable end point of evolution, but because we will have made it the most favorable outcome.[15]

To roughly paraphrase Ewald's argument, assume that HIV evolved in a highly stable sexually monogamous environment, a culture where partner exchanges were few and far between—an African tribal culture. In such an environment, a sexually transmitted pathogen would naturally select for viral mutations that favored low virulence combined with a long incubation period. It would make no sense for the virus to kill its host before, on average, it had an opportunity to transmit its genome to another host; like us, HIV is programmed for species-survival. Low-level, long-lasting virulence is exactly what HIV displays; only after a decade does the host immune system collapse and allow other fatal pathogens to operate. Because we focus on the youthful targets and the end result of HIV infection, we tend to think of HIV as exceptionally virulent, but it is not. The virus that produces Ebola hemorrhagic fever qualifies as highly virulent—an 88 percent mortality rate in 5–8 days.

However, HIV was a virus that evolved in one type of society and was transplanted by war, commerce, and population movement to less stable urban areas with high rates of interpersonal interchange of every kind, including sexual. In such communities it could produce much greater havoc than ever it could in close-bound tribes. Because of frequent sex-partner exchanges, it was able to rapidly infect the most sexually active age groups, and, from them, percolate via other transmission routes to infants and older people. Further, there was no further evolutionary incentive for it to continue selecting mutant genes expressing less virulence.

If something like this was and is the case, then by behavioral changes we could restrict HIV to its original role, and perhaps even offer it incentives to select for less destructive genes. Speaking for myself, and focusing on sexual transmission, the logic of the case points to a few major choices: (1) We can abstain from intercourse until we mate, and then mate monogamously for life. An infection carried into a sexual union, by any means, would end there. (2) We can abstain, then mate monogamously, but with the possibility of infrequent exchanges such as occur with divorce and remarriage. This would slow the infection rate. (3) We can employ barrier protection like condoms consistently in sexual relations until such time as we mate monogamously. This would tie the incidence of new infections to the rate of condom failure and encourage the production of condoms better than those now in use. (4) We can employ condoms consistently without regard to marital status, partner, or partner exchange. This also would reduce the incidence of new infections while leaving sexual expression virtually unrestricted. From the viral standpoint, any of these options would present HIV with the problem of surviving in a stable society with infrequent partner exchanges and few opportunities for transmission.

In the first option HIV would probably collapse as a viable species; in the second, it would survive, but not thrive; in the third and fourth, it would transmit more than in (1) and (2) depending upon our consistency of use and the quality of barrier protection. However, in none of these cases would we be contending with an epidemic; there would be individual infections, as there are of measles, but no epidemic. It may be that options (1) and (2) embody values generally associated in Western society with the best of all possible worlds, but options (3) and (4) are more realizable in the entire world and in the short run. In any case, transmission of its genetic materials is what is critical to HIV; whatever stops that transmission presents the virus with an evolutionary choice: death or change.

In 1983 Luc Montagnier and his colleagues of the Pasteur Institute isolated the Human Immunodeficiency Virus; in 1993 Montagnier appealed to the leader of his faith, Pope John Paul II, to reconsider his church's uncompromising opposition to condoms. In that intervening decade, research gradually revealed how evasive, how insidious, and how dangerous HIV is in contemporary societies. Pandora's Box is open wide. However, as Montagnier's plea underscores, there is a cheap, over-the-counter, and effective defensive weapon available, the simple condom. No billion-dollar scientific effort is called for, no genius is required, just the use of a simple condom shuts the box. I cannot help but support his plea. It seems to me that in those areas of human behavior where the parameters of moral conduct are arguable (both within and between denominations), the right course of action is to do what we can do to save living, uninfected people. Then I will trust in a compassionate God to sort out whether the lives saved were saved morally.

OPPORTUNISTIC INFECTIONS AND THE PWA

Most of the foregoing arguments and considerations relate to a broad concern for public health, not the narrow one of individual health and survival. Those who are already HIV+ are understandably most concerned with the impact of research and medicine on their health now, not the course of an international epidemic twenty years from now. As mentioned, no really effective drug has been developed that confronts HIV directly. AZT and other drugs like it, called nucleoside analogs, have demonstrated a modest ability to slow the replication of the virus, but in the end HIV prevails.[16] With regard to other compounds that attempt to disrupt various viral functions—the production of its envelope, its docking, its budding from the host cell, and so on—many have been effective *in vitro* and with laboratory developed HIV cell-lines but not in actual individuals infected with natural HIV cells. There are, for example, an increasing number of possible therapies emerging from the intersection of molecular biology, virology, and genetics.[17] These engineered gene therapies may be the therapeutic wave of the future but are still in primarily experimental stages today.[18] And that is where we are in 1994.

However, there is an increasing arsenal of weapons with demonstrated effectiveness against the opportunistic infections that arise in late-stage HIV infection, in AIDS. In January 1994, the American Pharmaceutical Association reported that there were seventy-four pharmaceutical manufacturers researching 103 possible treatments. Eleven of these are awaiting FDA approval, while twenty-three have entered final testing stages.[19] The treatments that survive all stages will join the twenty-one FDA-approved drugs now available. To illustrate, there are now four FDA-approved drugs effective, either prophylactically or therapeutically, against *Pneumocystis carinii* pneumonia, the deadliest infection during the first years of the U.S. epidemic; no person should now drown in his or her own lung fluids. Blinding by *Cytomegalovirus retinitis* is preventable with Cytovene and Foscavir. As an aside, CMV-related afflictions offer a good example of the impact of HIV; it is estimated that by age fifty about one half the population unknowingly has CMV infection, but with a normal immune system nothing happens. Without one, CMV can inflame and cripple many organs including the eyes. For *Mycobacterium avium complex*, now the most common bacterial opportunistic infection, the drugs rifabutin, azithromycin, and clarithromycin are effective. Some of the lesser manifestations of AIDS like thrush respond to Fluconazole, while Acyclovir is effective for herpes simplex or zoster blisters. TB screening and therapy is becoming a routine part of HIV examination. Similarly, the new sensitivity to female-specific manifestations represented in the 1993 Revised Definition surfaces in a routine use of pap smears and pelvic examinations in cases where HIV infection is known or suspected. "Wasting syndrome" is being met with better nutritional and antidiarrhea regimens. Some infections, like progressive multifocal leukoencephalopathy (PML), remain very difficult to treat.

The key to the effective use of available therapies is a combination of *self* and professional monitoring. In 1994 the Department of Health and Human Services released a free 196-page guide for physicians who might care for HIV infected people. The guide especially targets family-practice physicians, pediatricians, nurse practitioners, and other primary care, non-AIDS specialists who need help in diagnosing and treating the complex presentations of the syndrome. Simply stated, there are not enough infectious-disease specialists in America to care for the volume of patients developing, so other health care providers must be encouraged and helped to upgrade their knowledge. The new professional guide, together with others targeting PWAs and parents of HIV+ children, represents one manifestation of President Clinton's pledge of more national involvement in the care and treatment of PWAs.[20] An HIV+ can upgrade his or her self-knowledge by reading the excellent bulletins and newsletters published by *Project Inform* of San Francisco and/or the *Gay Men's Health Crisis* of New York.[21]

It is important, I think, to keep some matters in central focus. Without effective anti-HIV drugs, there is little we can do about the length of HIV's residence in the body—that is a function of the virus's genetic program. So what is really important to an HIV+ is the survival time he or she can expect *after* an AIDS diagnosis. In the fall of 1987, when I commenced research for this book, the average survival time was seven months. When it was finished and published in fall 1991, the time following diagnosis had stretched to two years on average. Now, with the 1994 second edition, physicians are advising patients that the prospects are 36–50 months, again on average. This lengthening is ample evidence of the improvement in care and available therapies. Even in the absence of effective anti-HIV drugs, I expect this time to gradually stretch until AIDS takes its place alongside other lengthy and eventually destructive diseases for which we have no cure (for example, many cancers, acute renal failure, schizophrenia, bacterial heart infection, North American blastomycosis).

However, I do not want to be misunderstood. No matter how effective our therapies for opportunistic infections become we must never diminish efforts to find an agent effective against the virus itself. It is clear that America is beginning to accept the continued presence of HIV. Compared to the late 1980s, there has been a major shift of public attitude—congressional debates no longer exhibit a sense of urgency, the nation now accepts a large HIV-related bureaucracy as normal, and media attention has shifted elsewhere. From one standpoint this is normal and perhaps good; formerly very troubled waters are calmer. However, it could lead to socially damaging results if it promotes the belief that AIDS is "just another" incurable disease. Putting HIV infection in company with other intractable ailments should never cloud our understanding that HIV has a social impact far beyond any other contemporary pathogen. As a social problem it is in the league with history's greatest killers—epidemic cholera, the bubonic plague, and smallpox. Both AIDS and acute renal failure kill, but renal failure cannot displace entire generations and disrupt whole societies. AIDS can and does.

However, these are broad considerations. For the individual, the truth is simpler. Until science produces HIV-controlling drugs, infected individuals, like others similarly situated, should give thought to their mortality and plan their remaining life accordingly. I think Mickey Hays, who died a few years ago at age twenty from Progeria-induced old age, said it best, "Live your life fully one day at a time. None of us are promised tomorrow."

New Relations and Policies

Pushed by the HIV epidemic, scientists are making significant advances in our understanding of and ability to cope with other viral ailments and immune system malfunctions.[22] There has been more progress in our understanding of the immunology, viral cell functions, and advanced medical possibilities such as gene therapy in the past ten years than in the preceding fifty. In addition, important changes are being forged in medical training, research networking, care of the terminally ill, and drug testing protocols.[23] In all these areas, but especially in drug testing, AIDS is driving the scientific community to adopt techniques and possibilities that it would have rejected out-of-hand ten years ago. The future care of everyone will benefit from these advances.[24]

Not least among new developments is the emergence of the "informed patient." The standard model of doctor-patient relationship in the pre-AIDS era was one in which the patient deferentially accepted the *ex cathedra* diagnoses of his benign and all-knowing physician. All that changed with AIDS. Because of the newness of the disease, the physician had little genuine expertise; there was precious little to have. Furthermore, in America the epidemic struck first at the urban homosexual community, which has a highly educated, professional upper class. Patients drawn from such origins, and under a death sentence, were not easily put off with Latinized "medispeak" concealing the reality that no one knew much about AIDS. A new, refreshing, and sometimes painful candor, as well as a new style of patient-doctor collaboration in fighting disease is rapidly emerging as the model for the future. As one physician put it after attending an International AIDS Conference in Montreal, "When I went to [the meeting], I was flanked on either side by a half a dozen of my own patients reading the same posters I read. I don't see an end to that. I see patients becoming more and more empowered to be involved in the process, and that's a good thing."[25]

The restructuring involves more than the private patient-doctor connection, reaching to a public or civil relationship as well. PWAs, and following their lead other sick people, are gaining access to channels of medical information and decision-making that have always been closed to the nonprofessional. The afflicted are now becoming part of the process by which testing protocols are developed, and drugs are tested and distributed. The national government has responded to the demand for authoritative information by inaugurating a public health "first"—open access data banks both for the professional health care worker and for the concerned citizen. Clearly, the national government has accepted a major responsibility for the level and quality of public knowledge on the epidemic. Any person wishing information about the disease, or current clinical drug trials, should phone 1-800-874-2572 or 1-800-243-7012 (TTD/TDY) or write the National AIDS Information Clearinghouse, P.O. Box 6003, Rockville, Maryland 20850.[26]

By the turn of the millennium these many developments may eventually start to contain AIDS with a variety of medical and public health strategies. Gradually it will be reduced to the status of the most serious disease that lurks in the shadow of human sexual behavior but not an as inevitably fatal one in the short term.[27] Perhaps by then we will have learned to live with HIV rather than die from it. Eventually all of us will look back, as did Dr. Russell V. Lee, reflecting upon his involvement as a young intern in the great Flu Epidemic of 1918: "We were humbled by our incapacities, but challenged by the responsibilities. [It was] . . . a great teacher, but a dear one."[28]

AIDS may be a great teacher in another sense. It is obliging us, as citizens, to consider some hard and uncomfortable questions about the connection between medico/scientific intervention, private ethics, and public policy. It shares this role with the debate over abortion and the use of extraordinary life maintenance equipment. As we move into the twenty-first century, medical tests and genetic engineering will become available, making it possible to control eugenically for hereditary disease, as well as for other less clearly disadvantageous traits (like left-handedness, for example). We will need to consider how far we care, or dare, to go in playing God with the evolution of our species. Clearly we will have the technological skill.

We will need convincing answers to questions as to whether we should make use of the entire array of applicable medical interventions, regardless of cost, for people who present terminal, incurable illnesses. Should we discriminate in the allocation of services based on the patient's age, sex, wealth, occupation, mode of getting the disease, or previous or possible future social contribution? Should we treat the business person but not the street person, the infant but not the adult, the heterosexual but not the homosexual? As taxpayers should we pay the bill for the education of a child born with a disease that makes it unlikely that he/she will live to the age of twenty? Should such a birth be aborted or, if not, who pays for the extraordinary costs of life maintenance—the public or the parents? Given the short supply of transplant organs, should alcoholics get new livers or heavy smokers get new hearts? These difficult questions are the raw material of personal, medical, and social debates; AIDS is helping to propel them into the public forum where, ultimately, they must be resolved by the people whose lives will be enhanced or diminished by the answers.

Furthermore, AIDS will require us to search our hearts to decide how much we are willing to pay for some of our ancient beliefs; in effect, it is asking us to calculate the human mortality costs of preserving traditional dogmas. From time immemorial political and ecclesiastical officials have been willing to sacrifice live people to protect the purity of abstract doctrine, ignoring the fact that there is no necessary relationship between logic and real life. Perhaps the devastation of AIDS, when its full impact is felt, will help convince us that it is time to stop all forms of human sacrifice, the subtle as well as the blatant. We do need logic to form a scaffolding for thought, but it ought never to be confused with the substance of it. Life or death, nature's binary, are the only absolute mundane values; all else is negotiable.

Furthermore, the epidemic is putting our health care delivery nonsystem under such an increasingly heavy strain that eventually we will be compelled to rationalize it, nationalize it, and guarantee Americans access to care.[29] All major unions of health care workers, led by the American Medical Association and the American College of Physicians, are calling for a reexamination and overhaul of our health care delivery system.[30] Canada, Australia, and other nations have provided necessary drugs like AZT from the beginning, accepting a responsibility about which we still vacillate. AIDS will force hard decisions upon us. For example, it will compel us to decide whether we wish to continue spending 40 percent of all Medicare funds on patients with no hope of recovery during the last six months of their lives or whether it is socially just to continue spending 55 percent of the nation's health care dollars on 5 percent of the population. Can we continue to leave tens of millions of Americans with no effective health coverage?[31]

AIDS may well be one of the stimuli that will prod our reluctant nation to provide an effective level of health care as a statutory entitlement, as President Clinton's plan envisages, and it may be the force that will demote the profit motive from its present commanding position as the system's driver. Expanding the reach of health insurance will not be as radical a change as many Americans think because we are almost there now. At taxpayer expense, the national government already covers all members of the military, all veterans, all members of Congress and their staffs, the president and vice president and their staffs, the executive and independent regulatory bureaucracies, the judges and magistrates of the court system and supporting staff, the elderly and the disabled or handicapped. In addition most political and administrative state employees, employees of larger businesses, and teachers at all levels in public and private systems are covered by some form of insurance. Essentially, national health insurance means extending benefits already enjoyed by the bulk of the workforce to everyone.

The biggest problem will not be extension, but cost-containment because that is tied to the profit motive. All existing actors in the system—physicians, hospitals, and drug companies—stand to gain from keeping things as they are; there are no incentives for anyone in health care to control and contain costs. Consequently, unless we are willing to pay a major share of our tax dollars to the health care industry, the currently dominant influence of the profit motive will have to be severely diminished by statutory regulation of medical service and drug pricing.

AIDS AND CULTURAL VALUES

More problematic, more difficult to discern are the broad-gauge social impacts. One that may emerge is an America where the homosexual no longer need hide—the elimination of the last great outcast group. Truly this would be a radical change since homosexuals have had to conceal their sexual identity since the intolerant, sex-negative Judeo-Christian culture displaced the tolerant Graeco-Roman one.

IN GROUPS/OUT-GROUPS

Every nation has its outcasts, people who suffer severe legal and social discriminations imposed because of their sex, race, religion, ethnicity, or class. It is one of the more destructive tendencies of our species to classify people into "them" and "us," "Greek" and "Barbarian" categories. Mainstream Americans built social and legal discriminations around many groups—Irish, Mormons, Catholics, Orientals, Slavs, Turks and Middle Easterners, Central and Eastern Europeans, American Indians, and Mexican Americans.[32] Jews, Blacks, women, and homosexuals were the largest groups subject to pervasive discrimination. In each case, the White Anglo-Saxon male majority rationalized its action on egregious biblical interpretations—Jews were responsible for the execution of Christ, Blacks bore the Mark of Cain, women were derivative of and intended to be servants of men, and homosexuals acted contrary to the "Order of Nature." Jews, Blacks, and women have been beating down the barriers by using every technique from outright physical assault to the choreographed violence of litigation. They made little real progress until they mobilized in their own interests.

In the next decade, a major social significance of AIDS may be the mobilization of America's millions of gays and lesbians and the creation of the sense of community that is the base for effective politics. AIDS has made political action, and its consequent visibility, a condition of survival. It has dragged many gays out of their protective closets and diminished the significance of the straight world's homophobic sanctions. Before the AIDS epidemic there was little more than the loose network of the Metropolitan Community Churches that could be called a gay community infrastructure.

Today an elaborate collection of political action groups, businesses, social clubs, community service and health care organizations, churches, and publications have emerged to respond to an increasingly visible and vocal gay population.[33]

In this epidemic, gays have become an important influence in compelling a conservative government and biomedical establishment to reevaluate its traditional approaches and techniques of drug evaluation and delivery. For example, one of the most important documents delivered at Montreal's Fifth International Conference on AIDS was "A National AIDS Treatment and Research Agenda" prepared by the AIDS Coalition to Unleash Power (ACT UP). This study inspired a major reevaluation of procedures in the National Institutes of Health. Only a few years ago, it would have been inconceivable that government agencies (especially large bureaucracies like the National Institutes of Health and the Federal Drug Administration) would respond directly to an openly gay pressure group, especially one that had stormed New York's St. Patrick's Cathedral to protest Cardinal O'Connor's orthodox homophobia.[34] ACT UP is an activist, confrontational gay pressure group focusing on AIDS issues. It has adapted Carry Nation's advice to the American farmer back in the 1890s, "Raise less corn, and more hell."[35]

In the 1990s gays, prodded by AIDS, will likely be more insistent and more organizationally effective in their petition for reconsideration by the culture.[36] They will demand status acceptance, if not approval, with all that such acceptance implies in terms of benefits and protection under the Constitution and laws of the United States. In politics, mainstream churches, and the military, the one-time absolute barrier stemming from being a known homosexual is under siege and giving way.[37] Indeed, the 1992 Democratic Convention represented a milestone in American political history in that not only were gay Americans recognized as a constituency by presidential candidate Bill Clinton, but they were allowed openly to express their concerns in various panels concerned with drafting the platform. Gay and lesbian Americans have long been a significant part of the political process as well as the administrative, legislative, judicial, and military apparatus regardless of which party was in power; the main difference is that after Bill Clinton, the truth is being acknowledged. In the twenty-first century it is likely that America's secular and religious intelligentsia will finally and utterly abandon the defense of our ancient, destructive mythologies. We then will be able to welcome in our last major outcast group.[38] Supreme Court Justice Harlan's famous 1896 dissenting comment will finally become the law of the land: "The Constitution . . . neither knows nor tolerates classes among its citizens."[39]

Yet, it is not beyond the realm of possibility that, as the epidemic spreads, Americans led by home-grown demagogues, of whom we have always had a plentiful supply, could violently react against the groups they identify as the source of the epidemic. By 2005, projecting from the current HIV+ pool, the epidemic will have a very different focus than it had in the early years. The original hetero-homosexual ratio of the early years will have reversed. In addition, there will be a large component of female PWAs. If current projections are correct, it will become predominantly an epidemic of the "marginal classes" (as seen by White middle-class America), that is, Blacks, Hispanics, gays, ghetto teens, the homeless, Eskimos, and American Indians. The potential in this situation for the surfacing and exacerbation of class, racial, and religious hatreds is obvious. Stephen Joseph, former New York City commissioner of Health, thinks it very probable that public attitudes will revert back to the "us against them" stance of the early and mid 1980s. This, in turn, will make politicians reluctant to fund epidemic control and AIDS treatment and care at the levels needed.[40] The scapegoating that led to the herding and burning of Jews during the Black Death could recur. To go beyond this would require a level of panic sufficient to threaten our basic institutions, but it could happen. It is painful, but wise, to remember that Adolph Hitler and his Nazis were not a perversion of the Western cultural tradition. On the contrary, they were the apocalyptic administrators of some of its most consistent hatreds.

The Nazi extermination of Jews, homosexuals, and Gypsies was the tragic apotheosis of the Old Testament, Greek, and early Christian doctrine which taught that people should be separated into "Chosen" or "Natural" categories of moral superiority and inferiority and that those who were inferior could be dispensed with. Our surest protection against such a movement in America will be the selection of national leaders capable of exerting a strong but compassionate leadership, the kind we associate with Lincoln.

SEXUAL RELATIONS

On another direction of thought, it is more than conceivable that AIDS will bring about major changes in our sexual practices and mores. There can be no doubt that the transmission characteristics of AIDS enhances the value of cautious, limited, and eventually exclusive sexual pairing; the fact that 20 percent of all Americans have now been infected by some STD other than HIV simply underscores the point. The Judaic, Christian, and Muslim traditions have always taught that limitation and exclusivity was the morally correct path. So it might be thought that AIDS is, in effect, recommending a "return to" conservative sex practices of the past. This would be true were it not for the fact that there is no evidence indicating that earlier generations pursued sex with less enthusiasm or more restraint than contemporary ones. It is just that in previous times those in positions of authority were more emphatic in their ritualistic condemnations of "loose living." I think that the truth is not that AIDS recommends a return to the past, but rather that it recommends that we need to consider, for the first time, taking traditional teachings a bit more seriously.

This line of thought cannot be taken too far. The epidemic of HIV (and other STDs) does not legitimate the "family" as defined in any traditional religion or period of time (such as the Victorian); what it does do is emphasize the importance of restricting the exchange of possibly infected body fluids by whatever behavioral strategies that work. Definitions of "family" from earlier times incorporate the values of those times (heterosexuals are "good," homosexuals are "bad"; males are "superior," women are "inferior," Whites are the "served," Blacks are the "servitors," for example) which people either accept or deny, usually in accordance with what they have taught. However, an epidemic is an empiric set of facts (people dying), and logically facts cannot validate values. What HIV says is, "Whatever patterns of pairing and sex you employ, and however you define them in law and custom, take account of me!"

AIDS is raising questions at this most basic and profound level. It is not a judgment of God, but it most definitely is a trial. It will be a great test to determine whether the ruling White, heterosexual community can move beyond the myopia of self, which so easily flows from power, and throw off the prejudices that have been cancerous within our culture for over two thousand years.[41] As Karl Mannheim pointed out in *Ideology and Utopia*, when people are immersed in a certain ideology or religion, they lose their ability to see certain facts; they are blinded not by optic degeneration but by internalized templates that allow only parts of the real world to pass, just as polarized lenses filter some of the light.[42] It is not easy to shatter these lenses once installed; it is not easy to alter the mindset of an entire culture, no matter how wrong-headed the ideas may be. But it can be done. Between 1300 and 1800 Western church-state officials (mostly male) burned alive hundreds of thousands of witches (mostly female); now most of us no longer even believe in witches. AIDS sets the stage for one of the great challenges of the twenty-first century, one that will require all our good will and intellectual resources—the challenge of exorcising homophobia from the mind of America.

AIDS AND THE SOCIAL CONTRACT

Many factors contribute to the changes of history, frequently in unexpected and unforeseeable ways. For example, epidemics crippled the French military presence in the Caribbean, so Napoleon wisely sold Jefferson the Louisiana Territory he could no longer defend. America, until then an insignificant shoestring republic tied to the East Coast of a vast continent, was launched upon one of history's most extensive and successful territorial conquests. It was like winning an unbelievably rich lottery at the beginning of one's career. Similarly, the great fourteenth- and fifteenth-century visitations of the bubonic plague helped kill feudalism, especially in England. So many people died, especially in the urban areas, that a manpower shortage developed which, in turn, raised the value of urban labor. In spite of legal measures designed to "keep them down on the farm," the serf left the feudal estates to seek a better life in the city. Looking from our time forward, AIDS might well accelerate very basic changes that are taking place in the organization of the global community.

We are told that the Great Wall of China is the only human artifact observable from space. It is appropriate that this be so. The construction of walls dividing people from people has been one of the most enduring traits of the human species. We have built them of everything from the concrete blocks of the Berlin Wall, through electronic walls in space, to elaborate codes of prejudice like America's Jim Crow and South Africa's apartheid laws. The walls are even present within the community of those dying from AIDS; they can be encountered within any AIDS Service Organization trying to meet the interests of all kinds of clients. There is a gulf, unbridgeable even by common affliction and destiny, between various groups of PWAs—for example, those from the gay middle and upper class, and those from poor circumstances or from the streets. There is little understanding or sympathy between the IV and non-IV group. And those who acquired the virus through blood or blood product transfusion tend to keep strictly to themselves, mounting separate "innocent victim" campaigns for assistance from the government. I suppose that, from Troy to the present, the building of garrison, city, national, class, religious, and ethnic walls have had some survival value for the world's cultures. All of our great moral leaders from Christ to Schopenhauer, Ghandi, and Martin Luther King tried to teach us otherwise, but we nonetheless built walls, walls, and more walls.

Tampering with our walls is a traumatic and dangerous business for we have entire cultures invested in them. Still, the fact remains that they no longer serve to protect us from anything more than the necessary next phase of cultural evolution—the development of a global human community neither confined nor deformed by national or psychological boundaries. Everywhere there are signs that old walls are tumbling down. The disintegration of both the American and Soviet empires opens rich new possibilities of East-West exchange. The gradual realization of the European Economic Community, and the proposal of many others, will intertwine our various interests such that violent conflict will be suicidal.

Signs of the coming times are the emergence of the World Trade Centers network to promote direct international contact between small businesses, and, of course, the gradual domination of all economies by the new leviathans, multinational corporations and banks. Profound structural

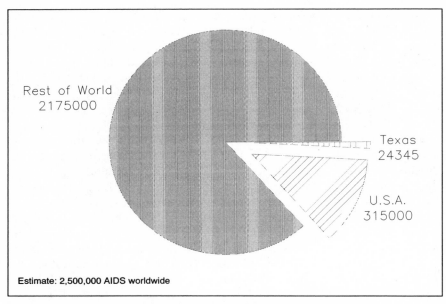

Rest of World
2175000

Texas
24345

U.S.A.
315000

Estimate: 2,500,000 AIDS worldwide

FIGURE 7.4 AIDS Cases, 1994: Global, U.S., Texas

changes at the top, like the cartelization of global commerce, are matched in importance at the "people" level by population movement in a volume unprecedented in history. On every continent millions of migrant laborers wash across boundaries like tidal waves. Today's workers flee poverty in their homelands, just as England's serfs fled the feudal estates six centuries ago. America's experience with migration from Mexico and Central America shows that quotas and boundary checks are no more effective a dam to the flow than were the statutes of Edward III in 1351.[43] Besides, the immigrants are wanted! Flying over their heads are the very businesspeople who will hire them.

The increasing interconnectedness of economies and peoples means that we can no longer fence out problems. The weakness of Latin American economies and the global decline of petroleum values spread so much sickness in American lending institutions that now only the entire taxpaying public can generate enough revenue to defray the recovery costs. Likewise America cannot contain its share of a global AIDS epidemic without attending to patients abroad. In 1987 Professor Thomas H. Weller, Nobel laureate, in an article that should be read by everyone concerned with AIDS, predicted that the epidemic will not be contained unless and until we accept two facts: (1) that AIDS threatens and affects everyone on the planet, not just politically impotent minorities like New York junkies, Bangkok prostitutes, or Mexico City's homeless street urchins;[44] and (2) that it cannot be conceptualized as just a public health problem to be dealt with by health measures alone.[45] He points out that while AIDS is, on its surface, a problem of public health, it is actually far more. Weller contends that a successful strategy of containment must attack a broad front of late twentieth-century dilemmas, problems that are reflections of the gross maldistribution of wealth both within and among nations.

For example, AIDS has killed Haitians and Haiti's critical tourist industry; it threatens to do the same in Thailand. It will probably lead to major ecological collapse in Central Africa as villages lose the manpower to keep land under cultivation. AIDS will probably undermine all the advancements made in third world economies since the 1950s and nullify the effect of billions in foreign aid over the last twenty-five years. Instead of a brighter, more viable economic future, the view from AIDS is famine. No third world nation can afford the multimillion dollar cost of a thoroughly screened blood supply; without help they will necessarily remain a continuing source of HIV infection. Typical treatment for AIDS in Tanzania, which has one physician per thirty-two thousand people, is bedrest and a few aspirin. The total budget of Zaire's largest hospital is comparable to the cost of treating ten patients in America. The United States spent $43 million to identify 5,890 infected military, a sum greater than Central Africa's total health budget.[46]

These kinds of discrepancies are commonplace between rich and poor nations, but with AIDS it is no longer just a matter of the number of phones, indoor toilets, or even caloric intake per capita. Clearly it is now a case where the "haves" must help the "have nots" if they are concerned with the state of their own health. Self-interest dictates that the great nations launch an integrated global strategy, or AIDS will return again and again, as did the bubonic plague, to infect them.[47] Modern China, using the controls of a police state, tried to build a wall of protection against the spread of AIDS just as, long ago, it tried to shut out the Mongol armies. Both attempts failed.[48] We cannot fence out the world's politico-economic woes or its diseases. Both are endemic to the body of Mother Earth.[49] Nor can AIDS be fenced in! Every nation has what the politicians like to call "Pockets of Poverty," suggesting by the imagery of the phrase that almost everyone is fat and happy. Nationally and globally, it is a lie. What we really have are "Pockets of Wealth" sewed with threads of pain and deprivation on an otherwise poor fabric. Politically and economically, America is owned and operated by a very small percentage of its population, and America has an equitable distribution of wealth and power compared to nations like Mexico or Saudi Arabia.[50]

So what? What is the connection to an epidemic? The connection is that the conditions and services that make for a healthy population, as well as the literacy and education that makes that population susceptible to health warnings, are closely tied to significant private discretionary resources. The middle and lower classes, the majority of all nations, have few, if any. Without a broad-based attack on the epidemic, the American and global underclass will bear a disproportionate share of the epidemic's burden in a manifestly unjust way, and class injustice has a way of coming back to haunt the societies that perpetrate it—as every White American ought to know. It is an exercise in self-deception and futility to frame policy that addresses AIDS without also targeting poverty, illiteracy, drug addiction, and, ultimately, the barren, empty lives that result. Those fortunate enough to live in the Upper Manhattans of this world cannot wall in the huge areas of hopelessness—the urban ghettoes will function as encapsulated foci of endemicity, they will be the reservoirs from which AIDS will draw ever renewed vitality.

The problems resulting from growing interconnectedness will be more acute in just a few years. It is possible that by the year 2000, 75 percent of the world's five billion people will live in urban areas; in 1900 it was over 75 percent rural. As noted in chapter 3, epidemics are metropolitan events. Cities are and always have been the playgrounds of epidemics. If we continue to develop sprawling and pestilential barrios, favellas, ghettoes, and slums like Calcutta's ironically named City of Joy,[51] we will guarantee the continued vitality of not only the Human Immunodeficiency Virus but other, perhaps deadlier, agents now waiting in the wings. One answer to the problems that arise in living next door to poverty—one that will be tried—will be to create physical and electronic barriers, a new form of *cordon sanitaire*, around the comfortable classes. Walled islands of wealth will be scattered in the troubled ocean of poverty. We try, rather ineffectively, to use these now to frustrate the car thief and house burglar—but how does one fence a virus in or out?

The AIDS epidemic in the next two or three decades should provide us with the stimulus to depreciate the things that divide us and search for ways as a global family to stop the destroyer within our collective body. Today Americans read about four hundred thousand American cases; all too soon the figure will be 1 million, and there will be millions more abroad. Our leaders will need to work the subtle alchemy needed to transmute our interconnectedness into a global community.[52] Perhaps only the threat posed by the Human Immunodeficiency Virus, with its weighty sanction of mass death, can provide the incentive to abandon our walls, to set aside our ancient investment in hatred, prejudice, and separateness. We can then jointly attack our common nonnational, nonreligious, nonracial, nonhuman adversary. We can realize our most noble aspirations and build a new global and humane union. Changes of this magnitude in human organization are so basic and profound that they find an analog only in movement of the very earth we walk upon, the shift of major continental plates. Whether this be our path or not, whether we succeed or not, we will at least come to understand the truth of Bishop Cyprian's final thought on the epidemic of his time and its application to ours: "[How] suitable, how necessary it is that this plague and pestilence which seems horrible and deadly, searches out the justice of each and every one, and examines the minds of the human race."

Notes

1. Very technically speaking there were no "AIDS" or "HIV" deaths prior to 1987. Before that, deaths were routinely described by such recognized medical categories as "cell-mediated immunity deficiencies" or "*Pneumocystis carinii*." The international standard for ascribing the cause of death is the *World Health Organization's Manual of the International Statistical Certification of Diseases, Injuries, and Causes of Death* (Geneva, 1977). The *Manual* was updated to include HIV infection in 1987. See Federal Centers for Disease Control, *Mortality and Morbidity Weekly Report (MMWR)*, Human Immunodeficiency Virus (HIV) infection codes: official authorized addendum ICD-9-CM, 1987:36 (no.S-7). This classification time lag was the basis for some conflicts of ascription among private attending physicians, public coroners, and the media in "celebrity" deaths. For the 1987 revision of the syndrome see MMWR 1987:36 (no. 1S).
2. See the report of Dr. Marcus Conant on the 6th International Conference on AIDS, San Francisco, June 1990, in *AIDS Treatment News*, July 6, 1990.
3. Lecture of Dr. Anthony Fauci, Director of NIAID, December 6, 1989, National Institute of Health Clinical Center, as summarized in *Washington HIV News*, January 1990.
4. *The 57th Annual Meeting of the United States Conference of Mayors, Task Force on AIDS, 1989 Report*. And see "AIDS Enters Rural Areas; 150 [Texas] Counties Report Cases," *San Antonio Express-News*, May 7, 1990, 7C. The rate of increase in new cases in rural America is 37 percent, while the urban rate is 5 percent. Congress funded a special study in Title IV of the Ryan White AIDS Act of 1990.
5. See Ronald Smothers, "Spread of AIDS in Rural Areas Testing Georgia," *New York Times*, April 18, 1990, A8. And see also U.S. Department of Health and Human Services, *HIV/AIDS Surveillance: US AIDS cases reported through January 1990* (Washington, D.C.). The World Health Organization predicts that by 2000 A.D. three fourths of HIV infections will be from heterosexual contact, or 80 percent of the worldwide total. *HIC Medical News*, December 9, 1990.
6. Dr. Mann's address to an international AIDS symposium in Atlanta, Georgia, in September 1990 (Associated Press). *San Antonio Express-News*, September 28, 1990, A13.
7. *AIDS Surveillance Report* (Update), July 1, 1990, World Health Organization. And see Dr. James Chin, Chief, Surveillance, Forecasting and Impact Assessment, WHO Global Programme on AIDS, "Understanding the Figures," >*World Health, The Magazine of the World Health Organization*, October 1989. In the same issue Dr. Jonathan Mann, "Global AIDS in the 1990s."

8. William B. Johnston and Kevin R. Hopkins, *The Catastrophe Ahead* (New York: Praeger, 1990), 7, Table 1.1. The authors also break the total projections down into White, Black, and Hispanic subgroups.

9. Rebecca Voelker, "Model Predicts Huge Jump in AIDS in Coming Years," *American Medical News*, December 22/29, 1989, 4. Mathematician Yakov Fuxman developed his models in response to insurance industry needs for long-term projections. The methods used by the Federal Centers for Disease Control cannot accurately forecast on the long term. The Center's projection anticipates 365,000 cases by the end of 1992.

10. See Broder, "The Life-Cycle of the Human Immunodeficiency Virus as a Guide to New Therapies," in Vincent de Vita et al. (eds.), *AIDS: Etiology, Diagnosis, Treatment and Prevention*, 79–87. Gina Kolata, "AIDS Research Finds 13 Vulnerable Spots in Virus Life Cycle," *New York Times*, October 2, 1990, B6. Kolata summarizes Dr. Broder's most recent article on the same subject which appeared in *Science* (October 1990).

11. Quoted in Stephen S. Morse and Robert D. Brown, "The Enemy Within," *Modern Maturity* (June-July 1993). Dr. Morse is a virologist at the Rockefeller University and editor of two relevant works: *Emerging Viruses* (New York: Oxford University Press, 1993), and *Evolutionary Biology of Viruses* (New York: Raven Press, 1994). Also on the topic of human-microbe competition, see Avrion Mitchison, "Will We Survive?" and Warner C. Greene, "AIDS and the Immune System," both in *Scientific American. Special Issue: Life, Death and the Immune System* (September 1993).

12. What follows is a summary and, in some cases, personal speculative extension of the innovative and provocative suggestions made by Paul W. Ewald, Ph.D., associate professor and chair, Biology Department, Amherst College, and Manfred Eigen, Nobel laureate in Chemistry, director of biochemical kinetics research at the Max Planck Institute, Gottingen. See Paul W. Ewald, "The Evolution of Virulence," *Scientific American* (April 1993); Manfred Eigen, "Viral Quasispecies," *Scientific American* (July 1993).

13. Eigen, "Viral Quasispecies," 49.

14. In 1991 the Smithsonian Institution appointed Professor Ewald as the first George E. Burch Fellow of Theoretical Medicine and Affiliated Science.

15. Ewald, "The Evolution of Virulence," 93.

16. The original research upon which low-dose AZT protocols were based: Paul Volberding et al., "Zidovudine in Asymptomatic Human Immunodeficiency Infection," *New England Journal of Medicine* (April 5, 1990), 941. See also "Early Treatment for HIV: The Time has Come!" (Editorial), same issue; Gay Men's Health Crisis, "AZT Update: News from San Francisco," *Treatment Issues* (August 30, 1990). However, it should be noted that early, low-dose protocols may not affect the AIDS death rate. See also "Federal Studies Questions Ability of the Drug AZT to Delay AIDS," *New York Times*, February 15, 1991, A1. Remarks of Dr. Basil Vereldzis, *Washington HIV News*, January 1990. And see "Long Term AZT Treatment," *Internal Medicine, World Report* (December 1, 1989), 22; and, "Low-Dose AZT plus Acyclovir Safe for Asymptomatic HIV Infected Patients," February 1, 1990, 1; and "The 1989 AIDS Survey" (of primary care physicians), same issue. The famous British *Concorde Study* of AZT, the results of which were issued in late 1993, indicated a very slight effect from AZT.

17. For example, Genetic Immunotherapeutics is an attempt to boost the natural capacity of the immune system to deal with viral intruders. Antisense therapy

attempts to alter the HIV genome so as to prevent replication. Dominant-negative mutant or decoy therapies hope to cripple the HIV by introducing weakened or false genes into the genome. See National Association of People with AIDS, "Gene Therapy," *Medical Alert* 2, no. 1 (January/February 1994).

18. G. I. Buchschacher et al., "Molecular Targets of Gene Transfer Therapy in HIV Infection," *Journal of the American Medical Association* (June 9, 1993).

19. "103 AIDS Medicines Now in Development," *Wholesale Drugs* (January 1994), 20.

20. Warren E. Leary, "U.S. Offers Guide for Doctors on Care of Those with HIV," *New York Times*, January 21, 1994.

21. Project Inform, 1965 Market St., Suite 220, San Francisco, CA 94103, National Hotline: 1-800-822-7422; GMHC, Medical Information, 129 West 20th St., New York, NY 10011.

22. See, for example "The Cutting Edge: Advances in Medical Technology, Polymerase Chain Reaction Diagnostics," *Internal Medicine World Report* 5, no.4 (1990), 9.

23. See William A. Check, "Growing Up Fast: A New Generation of AIDS Physicians," *Observer* (American College of Physicians) 9, no. 10 (November 1989), 1. See also the developments looking toward more expedited drug delivery resulting from the PCP/steroid treatment delay. See *New York Times*, November 14, 1990, A1.

24. Sari Staver, "AIDS Fight Focusing on Improved Access to Care, Drugs," *American Medical News* (January 7, 1991), 46. "Benefits of Treating AIDS at Home," *New York Times*, November 11, 1989, 26. Gina Kolata, "Radically Wider Testing of AIDS Drugs Is Urged," *New York Times*, March 26, 1990, A1; "Many Recommend Disputed AIDS Drug," *New York Times*, March 19, 1990, A13; "New System for Staging Clinical AIDS Proposed," *Internal Medicine News*, February 1–14, 1990, 28A. John F. James, "Toward Faster Anti-viral Development: 'Rapid Screening' Trials Proposed," *AIDS Treatment News*, September 7, 1990.

25. The comments of Dr. Marcus Conant in *Internal Medicine News*, January 15–31, 1990, 28a.

26. This service is a U.S. Public Health Service project provided collaboratively by the Centers for Disease Control, the Food and Drug Administration, the National Institute of Allergy and Infectious Diseases of the NIH, and the National Library of Medicine. It is operated by the National AIDS Information Clearinghouse and was authorized and funded by the Omnibus 1988 Act discussed in chapter 6.

27. One of the most interesting and potentially valuable developments is the establishment of specialized AIDS research laboratories capable of focusing world-class research efforts on the virus' vulnerable processes. An example is the AIDS Research Center of New York City funded by private donation and government grant. See "Big Lab for AIDS to Open in Manhattan," *New York Times*, January 31, 1990, A20.

28. Dr. Lee's remembrance of 1917 epidemic and his comparison to the present one are worth reading. See *Internal Medicine News*, January 1–14, 1988, 17.

29. See the excellent summary of national health care problems and possible governmental interventions. "Health under the Knife," *National Journal* (March 24, 1990).

30. See "National Health Insurance, Has Its Time Come?" *Observer* (ACP) 10, no. 1 (January 1990), 1; American Medical Association, "AMA's Health Access America," *American Medical News*, March 16, 1990, 1.

31. Linda Marsa, "Phoenix Rising," *OMNI* (December 1989), 50.
32. For example, prior to the 1940s when the U.S. Supreme Court declared them unenforceable at law, most homes in the "better" areas had racially restrictive covenants upon them which effectively excluded almost everyone who was not of English/Scottish or Western European origin.
33. See the excellent summary article, Carol Matlack, "Gay Clout," *National Journal* (January 6, 1990).
34. *New York Times*, December 11, 1989, A17, and December 12, A24.
35. ACT UP was founded by the playwright Larry Kramer, among others. Kramer, who is personally fighting AIDS, was also one of the founders of the New York City's Gay Men's Health Crisis, the nation's largest single private, volunteer AIDS service organization. See his *Reports from the Holocaust: The Making of an AIDS Activist* (New York: St. Martin's Press, 1989). For a description of some ACT UP initiatives, see Gina Kolata, "Advocates' Tactics on AIDS Issues Provoking Warnings of a Backlash," *New York Times*, Week in Review, March 11, 1990, 5E.
36. Eliza Carney, "Raising the AIDS Banner," *National Journal* (June 20, 1992). Ms. Carney makes the point that the gay lobbyists are becoming more professional and more successful. Groups like the AIDS Action Council, which was important in getting the Ryan White Act passed, are forming effective alliances on health issues with old-line groups like the American Academy of Family Physicians and the American Hospital Association.
37. See *Newsweek* (September 25, 1989) for feature articles on homosexuality and politics. Mireya Navarro, "A Gay Man Is Ordained as an Episcopal Priest," *New York Times, December 17, 1989, p.24. See also New York Times*, January 29, 1990. The unusual feature is not that a homosexual was ordained but that an open and admitted homosexual was ordained. The priest in question is the Reverend J. Robert Williams, Episcopal Diocese of Newark, N.J. Elaine Sciolino, "Report Urging That Military End Ban on Homosexuals Is Rejected," *New York Times*, October 22, 1989, 1.
38. The temporary suspension of editorial commentator Andy Rooney by CBS for remarks offensive to homosexuals and Blacks is an example of withdrawal of powerful institutional support for inaccurate and offensive public statements. (Mr. Rooney, in effect, equated homosexual sex with unsafe sex in the context of the AIDS epidemic.) In the same vein, Congress enacted and President Bush signed in April 1990, legislation to gather data on "hate" crimes, those inspired by bigotry of any kind. Presumably this will be preparatory to legislation dealing directly with this phenomenon.
39. *Plessy v. Ferguson* (1896). J. Harlan's original comment, like the case, related to Blacks and racial segregation. The underlying premise applies to all.
40. Stephen C. Joseph, *Dragon Within the Gates: The Once and Future AIDS Epidemic* I New York: Carroll and Graf, 1992), 36.
41. There are hopeful signs such as congressional consideration of bills punishing "hate crimes." See "Senate, 92–4, Wants U.S. Data on Hate Crimes Spawned by Bias," *New York Times*, February 9, 1990. Universities, including mine, are gradually recognizing gay student clubs (sometimes under court order). There are a scattering of antidiscrimination housing and benefit ordinances.
42. See chap. 1.
43. Statute of Labourers, 25 Edward III, st.1, 1351. For a brief discussion of the impact of the Black Death on English law of the period, see Thomas Pitt

Taswell-Langmead, *English Constitutional History*, 10th ed. (London: Houghton, Mifflin Co. 1946), 203–5.

44. A lengthy Associated Press story appearing in the *San Antonio Express-News* on November 5, 1989 talks of as many as 2 million abandoned or runaway youths in Mexico City showing signs of harboring an AIDS infection. "AIDS Stalking the Street: Lost Children of Mexico," *San Antonio Express-News*, November 5, 1989, 2B.

45. Thomas A. Weller, Richard Pearson Strong Professor of Tropical Public Health Emeritus, Harvard School of Public Health, "Lessons for the Control of AIDS," *Hospital Practice* (November 15, 1987), 41. Dr. Weller was a co-recipient of the Nobel Prize in Physiology and Medicine in 1954.

46. See the fine series of four articles by Eric Ekholm with Jon Tierney, "AIDS in Africa," which commenced in the *New York Times*, September 16, 1990, A1.

47. There are now about 160 private agencies in addition to the usual public health government bodies dealing with various aspects of AIDS in the developing countries. There is the beginning of some action and coordination through the Global Programme on AIDS of the World Health Organization, the Pan American Health Organization, the U.S Agency of International Development, and the Fogarty International Center of the U.S. National Institute of Health. So far, it is only an underfunded beginning. See World Health Organization, Global Programme on AIDS, *Inventory of Nongovernmental Organizations Working on AIDS in Developing Countries* (preliminary version 1989).

48. Sheryl WuDunn, "Outbreak of AIDS among Drug Users Alarms China," *New York Times*, March 30, 1990, National, A12.

49. Recognizing this fact of international life, the U.S. Centers for Disease Control recommended in February 1990 that the United States drop AIDS from its list of illnesses that are used to bar people from visiting or immigrating. See *New York Times*, February 28, 1990, A15.

50. See the following analysis James W. Lamare, *What Rules America?* (St. Paul, Minn.: West Publications, 1988); Michael Parenti, *Democracy for the Few*, 5th ed. (New York: St. Martins Press, 1989).

51. Dominique Lapierre, *The City of Joy* (New York: Warner Books, 1985).

52. For example there is the 1994 proposal that Japan and the United States are negotiating to the effect that they will participate in a multibillion global AIDS and population-control effort. *San Antonio Express-News*, February 10, 1994.

Appendix 1

Bibliography
AIDS Information Resources and
Further Readings

AIDS is one of the defining events of the twentieth century, and the volume of material it generates—good, bad, and indifferent—is sufficient to dismay the most intrepid and dedicated inquirer. Moreover, it is a sensational event and gets a sensationalist press. In the mass of information, it is often difficult to sort out the wheat from the chaff, the information from the misinformation that bombards everyone. The obvious tabloid material is easy enough to spot (close to the supermarket checkout counter). Still, there remains the question, "Where does one go to get the best information, the most thoroughly examined and documented information, the data which currently is believed valid by responsible people?" There is a veritable flood of materials, a flow so vast that specialized journals and newsletters have been developed simply to summarize and disseminate information. In 1987 Stephen A. Berger, an Israeli physician at Tel-Aviv Medical Center, with tongue-in-cheek, calculated that, given the rate of increase in AIDS articles between 1982–86, that by the year 2263 the AIDS category of the *Index Medicus* (an international index of all medical articles) would require a volume to itself in order to accommodate a projected 1,036,348 reports for that year (*New England Journal of Medicine* [December 3, 1987], 1479). What Dr. Berger thought was a learned joke is turning out not be no joke at all.

NEWSLETTERS

Those who want to keep current on events, treatments, debates, and so forth, should follow *AIDS Treatment News*, published by John James in San Francisco (P.O. Box 411256, San Francisco, CA 94141 [1-415-255-0588]). It is an established newsletter that targets the nonprofessional reader. It can be had for a modest annual subscription.

Those who want more professional reviews of research literature can read *ATIN, AIDS Targeted Information Newsletter, Abstracts and Critical Comments from the Current Literature*, Williams and Wilkins, Box 23291, Baltimore, MD 21203, 1-800-638-6423. This is an expensive monthly newsletter sponsored by the American Foundation for AIDS Research and is distributed in cooperation with the World Health Organization's Special Program on AIDS. *ATIN* summarizes articles from over one hundred professional journals in molecular biology, virology, immunology, epidemiology, clinical medicine, and treatment, as well as articles germane to the public policy issues raised by the epidemic.

The contents of the May 1988 issue are illustrative and typical of the rich mine of information contained in *ATIN*. The issue opens with an article summarizing the results of the American Foundation for AIDS Research Forum that took place in Washington, D.C., on April 9, 1988. This conference brought together some of the nation's leading researchers in a major confrontation and debate on the causes and development of the AIDS syndrome. The Forum did not settle all the issues, but it did crystalize the majority and minority positions relating to the causes of AIDS. *ATIN* then goes on to digest, or give bibliographic notice to, some 318 articles or conference proceedings which had appeared since the previous month. For example, a leading article in the *British Medical Journal* examined the nature and character of heterosexual transmission of AIDS. Another from the *Journal of Infectious Diseases* examined the appearance of cryptococcal meningitis in AIDS patients. An article by a group of immunologists examines the prospects for the development of a vaccine. The examples could go on and on through the 318 references of the May issue. This one issue represents the research of thousands of scientists participating in a global effort not only to isolate causes and develop treatments, but also to confront the nonmedical dimensions of the epidemic. It is an example of the periodicals designed to render AIDS information manageable.

For up-to-date information on treatments, drug trials, and the like, see The Gay Men's Health Crisis' *Treatment Issues—The GMHC Newsletter of Experimental AIDS Therapies* (129 W. 20th St., New York, NY 10011); the San Francisco AIDS Foundation's *Bulletin of Experimental Treatment for AIDS* (1-415-863-2437); *AIDS/HIV Treatment Directory* published by the American Foundation for AIDS Research (1-212-719-0083); various bulletins from Project Inform (347 Dolores St. No. 301, San Francisco, CA 94110, 1-800-822-7422).

UNIVERSITY TEXTS

DeVita, Vincent T., Jr., Samuel Hellman, and Steven A. Rosenberg (eds.), *AIDS: Etiology, Diagnosis, Treatment, and Prevention* 3d ed. (Philadelphia: J. B.

Lippincott, 1992); Kaslov, Richard A., and Donald P. Frances (eds.), *The Epidemiology of AIDS, Expression, Occurrence and Control of Human Immunodeficiency Type-1 Infection* (New York: Oxford, 1989). These are medical school reference texts. There are other professional works, such as, Jay Levy et al. (eds.), *AIDS Pathogenesis and Treatment* (New York: Marcel Dekker, 1992) and Gary Wormser et al. (eds.) *AIDS* (Noyes, 1992). All of these target the serious professional reader and clinician. None are light reading, but a perusal of any of them is sufficient to give you a sense of the unbelievable complexity of AIDS, its manifestations, and its treatment. In these tomes you encounter the grim real world, as distinct from the phony world portrayed in the tabloids and ten-second sound-bite summaries thrown out (or up) by the evening news.

Institute of Medicine, National Academy of Sciences, *Confronting AIDS: Directions for Public Health, Health Care, and Research* (1986) and *Confronting AIDS: Update 1988* (Washington, DC: National Academy Press). These were the two early semiofficial summaries of what was understood about the virus and the epidemic.

Gould, Peter, *The Slow Plague. A Geography of the AIDS Pendemic* (Cambridge, MA: Blackwell, 1993). The book embodies a geographer's approach to the epidemic. Dr. Gould has applied classic geographical mapping techniques to HIV data and developed some maps that visually portray the past and (probable) future spread of the virus much better than words can.

Joneson, Albert R., and Jeff Stryker (eds.), *The Social Impact of AIDS in the United States*, Report of the Panel on Monitoring the Social Impact of the AIDS Epidemic, Committee on AIDS Research and the Behavioral, Social, and Statistical Sciences, Commission on Behavioral and Social Science and Education, National Research Council (Washington, DC: National Academy Press, 1993). Soporific reading (in the way of most committee reports), but it has lots of good information.

McNeill, William, *Plagues and Peoples* (New York: Doubleday, 1976). This is the classic review of historical epidemics and their social impacts. It is very useful to put the HIV epidemic into perspective. McNeill is Professor Emeritus of History, University of Chicago, and the author of many stimulating historical essays.

Nichols, Eve K., Institute of Medicine, National Academy of Sciences, *Mobilizing against AIDS* rev. ed. (Cambridge, MA: Harvard University Press, 1989).

Stine, Gerald J., *Acquired Immune Deficiency Syndrome* (Englewood Cliffs, NJ: Prentice Hall, 1993). This is an intermediate-level college text with a strong biomedical focus; an introductory course in biology or microbiology would be a helpful background for reading this book. But it is accessible enough (and good enough) to be worth extra effort for those without such a background. It has good summaries of the major biomedical arguments raging within the research community.

Walker, Robert S., *AIDS: Today, Tomorrow. An Introduction to the HIV Epidemic in America* (Atlantic Highlands, NJ: Humanities Press International, 1994).

DATA COMPILATIONS/BIBLIOGRAPHIES

Mann, Jonathan, M.D., Daniel J. M. Tarantola, M.D., and Thomas W. Netter (eds.), *AIDS in the World* (Cambridge, MA: Harvard University Press, The Global AIDS Policy Coalition, 1992). A convenient source of global demographic-epidemiologic data.

For the Unites States there is no substitute for the Centers for Disease Control *HIV/AIDS Surveillance*, issued quarterly. Department of Health and Human Services, Public Health Service, Centers for Disease Control, Atlanta, GA 30333. National Library of Medicine, *Monthly Bibliography for AIDS*. This comprehensive publication can be found in any library with a government documents section. Ask the reference librarian.

AIDS ONLINE

For those with computer modems, print sources can be supplemented with a constant flow of current information from one of the nineteen national and international computer information networks now existing. One of the largest of the electronic networks is the *HIV/AIDS Information BBS*, which is the hub of the AIDS Education and General Information System (AEGIS). For access information write to Sister Mary Elizabeth, Sisters of St. Elizabeth of Hungary, P.O. Box 184, San Juan Capistrano, CA 92693-0184. Students and faculty in universities that subscribe to either the INTERNET or BITNET systems, or individual subscribers to services like *Delphi*, usually have access to a number of AIDS related forums such as the *sci.med.aids* newsgroups that are available on INTERNET or BBITNET (aids@uscum.bitnet or aids@cs.ucla.edu). *Sci.med.aids* transmits AIDS-related information on a daily basis and has available for e-mailing documents covering basic information such as "risk of transmission," "origins of the HIV," "experimental treatments," and so on. Schools that are part of the "Gopher" system, likewise, enable their students and faculty to access AIDS databases all over the country, like that at the University of California at San Francisco. In addition, the 90,000 mostly technical references of the National Library of Medicine's three online AIDS databases are available without search charge. The necessary interfacing search software, passwords, and other information are available from: National Institutes of Health, National Library of Medicine, Bethesda, MD 20894. A very complete collection of AIDS-related materials can be accessed on Ben Gardiner's *AIDS Info BBS* in San Francisco (1-415-626-1246); this BBSalso maintains a complete up-to-date listing of all electronic bulletin boards that feature AIDS information or forums.

Other groups or agencies that maintain information resources for interested people are: (1) Mothers of AIDS Patients, P.O. Box 3132, San Diego, CA 92103 (619-293-3985); (2) National AIDS Information Clearinghouse, P.O. Box 6003, Rockville, MD 20850 (1-800-458-5231); (3) National Institutes of Health, Hotline for AIDS Clinical Trials Information (1-800-TRIALS-A) for information on federally sponsored clinical trials (Monday through Friday, 9:00 AM to 7:00 PM EST); (4) Pharmaceutical Manufacturers Association, 1100 15th St., NW, Washington, DC. For current information on AIDS medicines, drugs, and vaccines in various stages of development and testing, write: The Editor, "AIDS Medicines in Development" at the above address;

(5) PWA Coalition, Inc., 31 West 26th St., New York, NY 10010 (1-212-532-0290). The PWA Coalition publishes a monthly newsletter called *PWA Coalition Newsline* written "by and for People with AIDS"; (6) U.S. Centers for Disease Control, Aids Program, Center for Infectious Diseases, Division of HIV/AIDS, 1600 Clifton Rd., Bldg. 6, Room 285, Atlanta, GA 30333. The Centers is the source of all official statistics on AIDS. It publishes the monthly *CDC HIV/AIDS Prevention Newsletter*, a quarterly funded under the HOPE Act which saw its first edition, Vol. 1, No. 1, in October 1990. For copies write to the editors: Linda Cayton and Carol O'Connell, 1600 Clifton Road, MS/E41, Atlanta, GA 30333.

TRADEBOOKS

[So-called trade books are aimed at a mass market rather than a narrow one like undergraduate or graduate students in particular courses. They are often easier reading than textbooks (which assumes that there is an instructor lurking about somewhere), have a simpler organization, and generally present much less information for digestion. They range in quality from Kubler-Ross's thoughtful book on AIDS to Magic Johnson's instant book on AIDS. The ones listed here are, among many, worth reading.]

Altman, Dennis, *AIDS in the Mind of America* (New York: Doubleday, 1986). Good for a look back at the attitudes that were shaping and controlling American reaction to the HIV epidemic during its early years in the United States.

Bateson, Mary Catherine, and Richard Goldsby, *Thinking AIDS: The Social Response to the Biological Threat* (Redding, MA: Addison-Wesley, 1988). Thoughtful essays view the epidemic from the standpoints of biology and cultural anthropology.

Dreuilhe, Emmanuel, *Mortal Embrace, Living with AIDS* translated from the French by Linda Coverdale (New York: Hill and Wang, 1988). Here is AIDS from the inside, from a man suffering all the real physical and social effects of the syndrome. It is simultaneously sad, terrifying, revealing, and beautiful.

Johnston, William B., and Kevin R. Hopkins, *The Catastrophe Ahead, AIDS and the Case for a New Public Policy*, published in cooperation with the Hudson Institute (New York: Praeger, 1990). This is an interesting and sometimes provocative discussion of the basic policy issues that the epidemic raises. It also employs and discusses the use of statistical models projecting the course of the epidemic.

Kramer, Larry, *Reports from the Holocaust: The Making of an AIDS Activist* (New York: St. Martin's Press, 1989). A very personal book about the organization of private, community-based volunteer aids service organizations such as the Gay Men's Health Crisis and ACT UP. The author, a leading playwright and an impassioned activist, was a major figure in the creation of both those organizations. There is no person more important than Larry Kramer in setting the tone and the agenda of AIDS activism in America.

Koch-Weser, Dieter, and Hannelore Vanderschmidt (eds.), *The Heterosexual Transmission of AIDS in Africa* (Cambridge: ABT Books, 1988). A good look at a very different transmission setting than the American.

Kubler-Ross, Elisabeth, *AIDS, The Ultimate Challenge* (New York: MacMillan, 1987). The sad and revealing story of the author's attempt to establish a hospice for dying AIDS children. You can learn a lot about bedrock American attitudes toward AIDS and its victims from this book.

Miller, Heather G., and Charles F. Turner, Lincoln Moses (eds.), *AIDS, The Second Decade* (Committee on AIDS Research, National Research Council, Washington, D.C.: National Academy Press, 1990).

Miller, Norman, and Richard C. Rockwell (eds.), *AIDS in Africa, the Social and Political Impact*, Studies in African Health and Medicine, Volume 10 (Lewiston: Edwin Mellen Press, 1988).

Morse, Stephen S. (ed.), *Emerging Viruses* (New York: Oxford, 1993). The point of this book is really that HIV is the beginning, not the end of our troubles. And we still do not have an international tracking system in place.

Pierce, Christine, and Donald Van DeVeer (eds.), *AIDS, Ethics and Public Policy* (Belmont, CA: Wadsworth, 1988). Some very good readings on many aspects of AIDS—testing, privacy rights, and so on.

Rodwin, Marc A., *Medicine, Money and Morals: Physicians' Conflict of Interest* (New York: Oxford, 1993).

Rogers, David E., and Eli Ginzberg (eds.), *Public and Professional Attitudes Toward AIDS Patients, A National Dilemma* Cornell University Medical College 5th Conference on Health Policy (San Francisco: Westview Press, 1989).

Randy Shilts, *And the Band Played On, Politics, People, and the AIDS Epidemic* (New York: St. Martin's Press, 1987). No one can get into the American epidemic without reading this book (the HBO version does not cut it). It is a passionate and all too accurate indictment of our national reaction—or lack of it—in the opening years of the epidemic.

MAGAZINE SUMMARIES

Science, The AIDS Issue, vol. 239, no. 4840 (February 4, 1988). Dated now, but still a good beginning point for those interested in basic epidemiology and bio-medical research.

Scientific American:
1. vol. 259, no. 4, October 1988, "What Science Knows About AIDS";
2. vol. 263, no. 2, p.50, August 1990, "AIDS-Related Infections," by John Mills and Henry Masur;
3. vol. 269, no.3, September 1993: Warner C. Greene, "AIDS and the Immune System," and Avrion Mitchison, "Will We Survive?"

DISSIDENT VIEWS

Most of the foregoing material is in the "HIV causes AIDS" mainstream of thinking. However there are other positions with regard to what causes or caused AIDS and what to do about it. The debate is a very serious matter and has implications for all research and treatment. In addition to the serious material in this category, there is a ton of crap—conspiracy theory books and articles (The Devil Did It) blaming AIDS on the CIA, or Communists, or mad scientists, or whatever. They sell at least as well as the JFK assassination stuff, contribute to the income of their publishers and authors, and satisfy some peoples' "minds." But they are not significant contributions to the literature on AIDS. The following are.

Peter H. Duesberg, "Human Immunodeficiency Virus and Acquired Immunodeficiency Syndrome: Correlation But Not Causation," *Proceedings of the National Academy of Sciences* vol. 86 (February 1989), and "AIDS Epidemiology: Inconsistencies with Human Immunodeficiency Virus and with Infectious Diseases," *Proceedings* vol. 88 (February 1991). Professor Duesberg's works are essential reading for those interested in alternative hypotheses. His critique of the "HIV causes AIDS" hypothesis is the fountainhead of all departures from the mainline.

Robert S. Root-Bernstein, *Rethinking AIDS: The Tragic Cost of Premature Consensus* (New York: The Free Press, 1993). This is a sober, serious, and thorough critical analysis of the mainline position, together with the proposal of a rather complex alternate hypothesis on AIDS.

CANADIAN INFORMATION RESOURCES

1. AIDS Calgary Awareness Association, 1021 10th Ave. SW, Suite 300, Calgary, Alberta T2R OB7, Canada (403-228-0155)
2. Canadian AIDS Society, 170 Laurier Ave. West, Suite 1101, Ottawa, KIP 5V5, Canada (613-230-3580)
3. Emergency Drug Release Program, Ottawa (613-993-3105)
4. Federal Center for AIDS, 301 Elgin St, 2nd Floor, Ottawa, Ontario K1A OL2, Canada.
5. Laboratory Center for Disease Control, Tunney's Pasture, Ottawa K1A OL2, Canada (613-998-8784)

INTERNATIONAL

World Health Organization, Surveillance, Forecasting and Impact Assessment Unit (SFI), Global Programme on AIDS, 1211 Geneva 27, Switzerland. WHO publishes a monthly, *World Health*, which covers AIDS as well as other public health matters. The October 1989 issue was devoted to AIDS.

Appendix 2

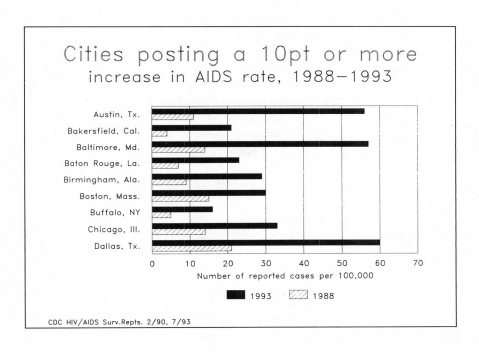

Cities posting a 10pt or more
increase in AIDS rate, 1988–1993

Austin, Tx.
Bakersfield, Cal.
Baltimore, Md.
Baton Rouge, La.
Birmingham, Ala.
Boston, Mass.
Buffalo, NY
Chicago, Ill.
Dallas, Tx.

0   10   20   30   40   50   60   70
Number of reported cases per 100,000

■ 1993   ▨ 1988

CDC HIV/AIDS Surv.Repts. 2/90, 7/93

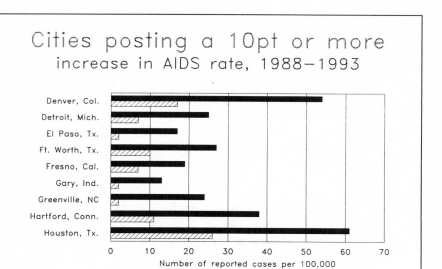

Cities posting a 10pt or more
increase in AIDS rate, 1988—1993

Denver, Col.
Detroit, Mich.
El Paso, Tx.
Ft. Worth, Tx.
Fresno, Cal.
Gary, Ind.
Greenville, NC
Hartford, Conn.
Houston, Tx.

Number of reported cases per 100,000

■ 1993   ▨ 1988

CDC HIV/AIDS Surv.Repts. 2/90, 7/93

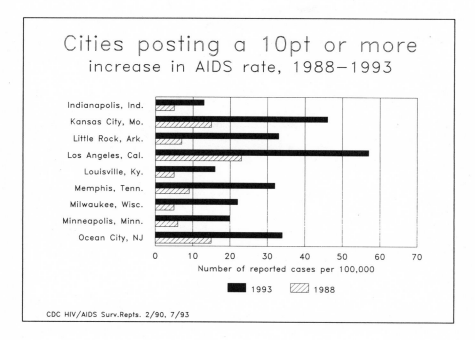

Cities posting a 10pt or more
increase in AIDS rate, 1988—1993

Indianapolis, Ind.
Kansas City, Mo.
Little Rock, Ark.
Los Angeles, Cal.
Louisville, Ky.
Memphis, Tenn.
Milwaukee, Wisc.
Minneapolis, Minn.
Ocean City, NJ

Number of reported cases per 100,000

■ 1993   ▨ 1988

CDC HIV/AIDS Surv.Repts. 2/90, 7/93

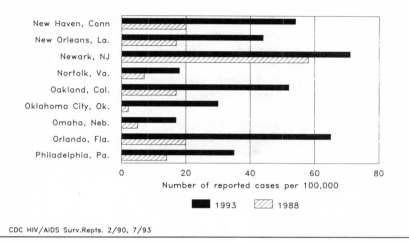

Cities posting a 10pt or more
increase in AIDS rate, 1988—1993

New Haven, Conn
New Orleans, La.
Newark, NJ
Norfolk, Va.
Oakland, Cal.
Oklahoma City, Ok.
Omaha, Neb.
Orlando, Fla.
Philadelphia, Pa.

Number of reported cases per 100,000

■ 1993   ▨ 1988

CDC HIV/AIDS Surv.Repts. 2/90, 7/93

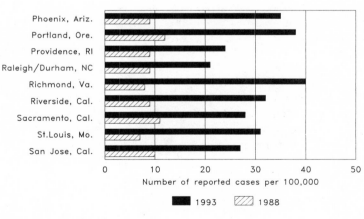

Cities posting a 10pt or more
increase in AIDS rate, 1988—1993

Phoenix, Ariz.
Portland, Ore.
Providence, RI
Raleigh/Durham, NC
Richmond, Va.
Riverside, Cal.
Sacramento, Cal.
St.Louis, Mo.
San Jose, Cal.

Number of reported cases per 100,000

■ 1993   ▨ 1988

CDC HIV/AIDS Surv.Repts. 2/90, 7/93

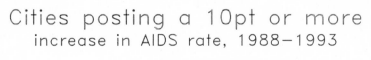

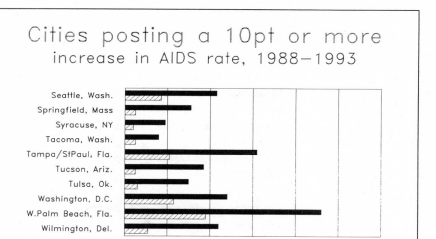

Cities posting a 10pt or more
increase in AIDS rate, 1988–1993

Number of reported cases per 100,000

■ 1993   ▨ 1988

CDC HIV/AIDS Surv.Repts. 2/90, 7/93

Index